BINOCULAR ANOMALIES
THEORY, TESTING & THERAPY
Fifth Edition

Volume 1
THEORY & TESTING

John R. Griffin, M.Opt., O.D., M.S.Ed.
Distinguished Professor Emeritus
Southern California College of Optometry
Fullerton, CA

Eric J. Borsting, O.D., M.S.
Professor
Southern California College of Optometry
Fullerton, CA

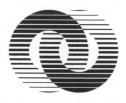

OEP FOUNDATION

Revised and updated by arrangement with Butterworth-Heinemann, a division of Elsevier Science. Originally published in 1976 by Professional Press.

Every effort has been made to ensure that the drug dosage schedules within this text are accurate and conform to standards accepted at time of publication. However, as treatment recommendations vary in the light of continuing research and clinical experience, the reader is advised to verify drug dosage schedules herein with information found on product information sheets. This is especially true in cases of new or infrequently used drugs.

Printed in the United States of America

Published by Optometric Extension Program Foundation, Inc.

1921 E. Carnegie Avenue, Suite 3L

Santa Ana, CA 92705-5510

ISBN 978-0-929780-16-0 (2 Volume Set)

Library of Congress Cataloging-in-Publication Data

Griffin, John R., 1934-
  Binocular anomalies : theory, testing & therapy / John R. Griffin, Eric J. Borsting. -- 5th ed.
    p. ; cm.
  Includes bibliographical references and index.
  ISBN 978-0-929780-16-0
  1. Binocular vision disorders. 2. Visual training. I. Borsting, Eric J. II. Optometric Extension Program Foundation. III. Title.
  [DNLM: 1. Vision Disorders--diagnosis. 2. Vision Disorders--therapy. 3. Vision, Binocular. WW 140]
  RE735.G74 2010
  617.7'62--dc22
                    2010037068

Optometry is the health care profession specifically licensed by state law to prescribe lenses, optical devices and procedures to improve human vision.

Optometry has advanced vision therapy as a unique treatment modality for the development and remediation of the visual process. Effective vision therapy requires extensive understanding of:

- the effects of lenses (including prisms, filters and occluders)
- the variety of responses to the changes produced by lenses
- the various physiological aspects of the visual process
- the pervasive nature of the visual process in human behavior

As a consequence, effective vision therapy requires the supervision, direction and active involvement of the optometrist.

Volume 1 - Theory & Testing
Table of Contents

Preface ix

1 Normal Binocular Vision
Value of Normal Binocular Vision 1
Anatomy of the Extraocular Muscles 3
Neurology and Characteristics of Eye Movements 3
Sensory Aspects of Binocular Vision 8
Physiologic Diplopia 11
Pathologic Diplopia 11
Types of Sensory Fusion 12
Theories of Sensory Fusion 14
Binocularly Driven Cells and Ocular Dominance 15

2 Visual Skills Assessment Part 1
Case History, Eye Movements, and Accommodation
Background and Rationale for Vision Skills Testing 16
Patient History 17
Maladaptive Behaviors 18
Educational History 19
Vision Skills and Reading 20
Testing For Visual Skills 21
Ranking Visual Performance 21
Saccadic Eye Movements 21
Pursuit Eye Movements 30
Fixation 32
Management of Deficits in Saccades and Pursuits 33
Accommodation 33
Testing of Accommodation 34

3 Visual Skills Assessment Part II
Vergence Testing and Heterophoria Case Analysis
Vergence Symptoms and Differential Diagnosis 46
Tonic Vergence and Accommodative-Convergence/Accommodation Ratio ... 47
Absolute Convergence 49
Relative Convergence 52
Fusional Vergence at Far 52
Fusional Vergence at Near 54
Vergence Facility 54
Summary of Vergence Testing 55
Diagnosing Vergence Disorders Using Case Analysis (Graphical Analysis) ... 56
Zone of Clear, Single Binocular Vision 57
Morgan's Normative Analysis 59
Integrative Case Analysis 60
Fixation Disparity Analysis 60
Criteria for Lens and Prism Prescription 68
Effectiveness of Prism Prescriptions 70
Recommendations for Prism Prescription 72
Vergence Anomalies 73
Normal Zone with Symptoms 77
Bioengineering Model 77

4 Strabismus Testing

History   82
Summary of Clinical Questions   85
Measurement of Strabismus   85
Comitancy   91
Signs and Symptoms   101
Subjective Testing   101
Frequency of the Deviation   105
Direction of the Deviation   107
Magnitude of the Deviation   109
Accommodative-Convergence/ Accommodation Ratio   110
Eye Laterality   111
Eye Dominancy   111
Variability of the Deviation   112
Cosmesis   112

5 Sensory Fusion and Sensory Adaptations to Strabismus

Sensory Fusion   114
Suppression   119
Amblyopia   126
Amblyopia as a Developmental Disorder   129
Case History   131
Visual Acuity Testing   132
Fixation Evaluation   140
Eye Disease Evaluation   144
Screening for Amblyopia   146
Anomalous Correspondence   146
Testing   154

6 Diagnosis and Prognosis

Establishing a Diagnosis   165
Prognosis   166
Modes of Treatment   175
Case Examples   181

7 Types of Strabismus

Accommodative Esotropia   190
Infantile Esotropia   195
Primary Comitant Esotropia   199
Primary Comitant Exotropia   201
A and V Patterns   204
Microtropia   206
Cyclovertical Deviations   209
Sensory Strabismus   210
Consecutive Strabismus   211

8 Other Oculomotor Disorder

Neurogenic Palsies   213
Myogenic Palsies   217
Mechanical Restrictions of Ocular Movement   220
Internuclear and Supranuclear Disorders   224
Nystagmus   227

Preface

The first edition of *Binocular Anomalies* was published in 1976 by Professional Press. This was written by Dr. John Griffin in response to requests of practitioners and students for a practical text on the management of patients with binocular anomalies. They asked for a book that outlines the efficient clinical steps toward diagnosis and treatment.

The second edition by Dr. Griffin was published, also by Professional Press, in 1982. This edition was in accord with the first edition; however, with expansion of testing procedures and vision training techniques.

The third edition, by Dr. Griffin and Dr. David Grisham, was published in 1995 by Butterworth-Heinemann. The clinical approach for primary health care was emphasized. Discussion of vision therapy, including all modes of treatment of binocular problems, was expanded.

The fourth edition, by Griffin and Grisham, was published in 2002 by Butterworth-Heinemann, an imprint of Elsevier Science. Elaborations on vision training techniques were given in detail and outlined for clinical practicality.

This fifth edition by Dr. Griffin and Dr. Eric Borsting updates and amplifies information of the previous editions as regards to theory, diagnosis and therapy. We have added results of research from the Convergence Insufficiency Treatment Trial and the Pediatric Eye Disease Investigator Group studies on strabismus and amblyopia. The first part of the book provides the theoretical foundation for understanding binocular vision as it relates to diagnosis and prognosis. Emphasis in the second part of the book on therapy includes all modes of treatment (e.g., lenses, prisms, surgery, pharmaceuticals and, especially, vision training techniques). Related topics of binocular anomalies, such as the effect of poor visual skills on reading fluency are discussed in detail.

The authors purposely kept the clinical tone of the book, notwithstanding their pertinent presentations of psychological-physiological foundations of visual science that are necessary for understanding normal, as well as abnormal, binocular vision.

These easily readable discussions are melded into clinical discussions on both testing and therapy.

This latest edition runs the gamut from the science of binocular vision to the therapies for its anomalies. As convenience to students and practitioners, the text is an all-inclusive book in two parts. Volume 1 covers theory, testing, and diagnosis and volume 2 covers treatment with an emphasis on vision therapy training techniques. The textbook is applicable for students taking a curricular series of courses in binocular vision at a professional academic institution, as well as for the practitioner who wants and needs the information all in one convenient source.

We would like to thank the following individuals for their help in making this new edition possible: Judy Badstuebner, Jamie Lam, Dr. James Saladin, Dr. James Bailey, Dr. Lawrence Stark, Donnajean Matthews, Pam Bickel, Sally Corngold, Kathleen Patterson, Robert Williams, and support from the administration of the Southern California College of Optometry. We would like to thank our families for their support and understanding of the many hours we devoted to this effort.

JRG
EJB
Fullerton, California

To students and practitioners of binocular vision

CHAPTER 1 / NORMAL BINOCULAR VISION

Value of Normal Binocular Vision	*1*	*Egocentric Direction*	*9*
Anatomy of the Extraocular Muscles	*3*	*Retinal Correspondence*	*9*
Neurology and Characteristics of Eye Movements	*3*	*Panum's Fusional Areas*	*9*
Accommodation	*4*	*The Horopter*	*9*
Conjugate Gaze Movements	*4*	*Physiologic Diplopia*	*11*
Saccades	*4*	*Pathologic Diplopia*	*11*
Vestibulo-Ocular Eye Movements	*5*	*Types of Sensory Fusion*	*12*
Pursuits	*5*	*Theories of Sensory Fusion*	*14*
Vergences	*6*	*Binocularly Driven Cells and*	*15*
Sensory Aspects of Binocular Vision	*8*	*Ocular Dominance*	
Monocular Considerations	*8*		

Disorders of binocular vision are among the most common disorders that the eye care professional will encounter in clinical practice. Common disorders include, strabismus and amblyopia (2 to 5%), convergence insufficiency (approximately 2 to 8%) and accommodative disorders (5 to 10%). In order to understand disorders of binocular vision, it is important to understand principles of normal binocular vision.

Binocular vision pertains to the motor coordination of the eyes and the sensory unification of their respective views of the world. This is a unitary process but, for the sake of analysis, it can be broken into sensory and motor components.

The sensory side starts with light emitted or reflected from physical objects in the external environment that are brought into focus on the retina by each eye's optics. This pattern of light energy is transformed by retinal photoreceptors into neuro-electrical impulses and is transmitted to the visual perceptual areas of the cerebral cortex and certain subcortical areas. The result of complex neural processing, which is only partially understood, is the sensation of object attributes (i.e., form, color, intensity, and position in space) that, in turn, culminates in an immediate, vivid perception of object identity and of the relations of objects in the external environment.

The motor positioning and alignment of the eyes completely subserve the primary sensory function of image unification and allow visual perception to proceed efficiently. The task of the motor system is to direct the alignment of both foveas (foveae) to the object of attention within the visual field and to maintain them in that position as long as the individual requires. The motor system holds the eyes in alignment and sustains clear focus, thereby ensuring the maintenance of binocular vision. Frequently, however, the complete remediation of binocular vision anomalies requires attention to both sensory and motor aspects.

VALUE OF NORMAL BINOCULAR VISION

One distinctive perceptual attribute of humans, among all primates, is a high degree of stereoscopic binocular vision. Our skills in hunting, food gathering, and tool making have helped to direct our evolution. In the competition for food, shelter, and safety, stereopsis is one of several attributes that evidently provided important advantages to those who possessed it. In the modern age, stereoscopic vision continues to provide individuals with important information about their environment. Stereopsis significantly aids in making judgments of depth, whether at school, the workplace, or the sports field. It also helps to stabilize sensory and motor fusion and can be considered a "barometer" of the status of binocular vision.

Besides stereopsis, there are other benefits that derive from normal binocular vision. The most obvious benefit of having two eyes is that, in case of injury to one, there is an eye in reserve. This might be called the "spare tire" concept whereas the loss of sight in one eye can cause some significant problems for an individual, the loss of sight in both eyes can be devastating.

The binocular individual also has the advantage of a large field of vision (Figure 1-1). The binocular field of vision usually is at least 30 degrees larger than the monocular field.

Binocular visual acuity normally is better by approximately one-half line of letters on a Snellen chart, as compared with either eye alone.[1,2] The difference is even greater, from our clinical expe-

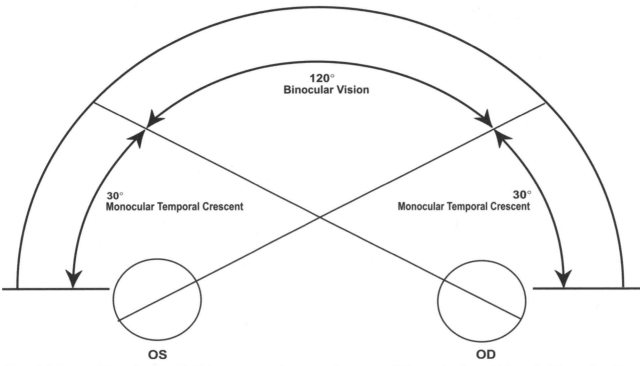

Figure 1-1. Extent of binocular visual field showing monocular temporal crescents. (OD = oculus dexter [right eye]; OS = oculus sinister [left eye].)

rience, when uncorrected ametropia is present in each eye.

Binocular vision, in contrast to monocular vision, minimizes the effects of many ocular diseases. Binocular summation of ocular images significantly heightens contrast sensitivity, by approximately 40%.[3] In practical terms, this is helpful for driving at night and working under low-illumination conditions. Individuals with certain ocular diseases (e.g., optic nerve demyelination in multiple sclerosis) may demonstrate profound differences in contrast sensitivity between binocular and monocular sight.

There are several vocational and avocational performance benefits of having good binocularity. Sheedy et al[4] described superior task performance under binocular versus monocular viewing conditions (Table 1-1). Differences favoring binocular viewing were notable in such tasks as card filing, needle threading and, surprisingly, speed of word decoding. No significant difference was noted, however, in letter counting on a video display terminal or in throwing beanbags accurately. These investigators concluded that stereopsis provides a performance advantage for many different jobs, particularly those requiring nearpoint eye-hand coordination. Persons in several occupations (e.g., machinists, microsurgeons, cartographers) are aided by stereopsis in performing their tasks safely and efficiently.

Recent research has also suggested that motor control is improved when under binocular condition for certain visually guided tasks.[5,6] For example, Jackson et al[6] found that subject's motor movements were faster and more accurate when reaching for a target amongst flanker targets under binocular as opposed to monocular viewing conditions. Although the binocular advantage is small, this has potential implications for dynamic activities such as sports where accurate visual motor responses are critical and small improvements can yield significant changes in performance.

Strabismus affects only a relatively small percentage of the population (1.3-5.4%),[7] but other deficiencies of binocular vision, such as convergence insufficiency and accommodative infacility, are much more prevalent and may result in bothersome symptoms and inefficient performance. Except for those individuals who have acquired strabismus and experience persistent double vision, most constant strabismics report few extraordinary visual symptoms. On the other hand, many nonstrabismics with binocular vision dysfunctions experience a variety of anomalies that are visual in origin, such as intermittent blur at far or near, tired eyes after reading or viewing a computer monitor,

Table 1-1. Superiority of Task Performance under Binocular Conditions as Compared with Monocular Conditions

Task	Percentage of Improvement of Scores under Binocular Conditions	Significance (Student's t-test)
Putting sticks in holes	30	0.001
Needle threading	20	0.001
Card filing	9	0.001
Placing pegs in grooves	4	0.001
Reading (word decoding)	4	0.05
Letter counting on video display terminal	2	NS
Beanbag tossing	-1	NS

NS = not significant.

Source: Adapted from JE Sheedy, IL Bailey, M Muri, E Bass. Binocular vs. monocular task performance. Am J Optom Physiol Opt 1986;63(10):839-846.

"eyestrain" at day's end, the appearance of jumping or moving print, vision-related headaches, reduced depth perception, and mild photophobia. Many of these symptomatic individuals experience "binocular efficiency dysfunction" (see Chapter 3).

ANATOMY OF THE EXTRAOCULAR MUSCLES

Three pairs of extraocular muscles control the movements of each eye: a pair of horizontal rectus muscles, a pair of vertical rectus muscles, and a pair of oblique muscles. The rectus muscles, the superior oblique muscle, and the levator muscle (controlling the upper eyelid) are attached to the bones at the back of the orbit by a tendinous ring (the annulus of Zinn) that surrounds the optic foramen and part of the superior orbital fissure. The four rectus muscles, optic nerve, ophthalmic artery, cranial nerve VI, and two branches of cranial nerve III form a muscle cone (Figure 1-2). The insertions of the rectus muscles are not equidistant from the corneal limbus but form a spiral, known as the spiral of Tillaux, with the superior rectus inserting farthest away from the limbus (7.7 mm) and the medial rectus inserting nearest to the limbus (5.5 mm) (Figure 1-3). The more advanced the insertion, the greater the mechanical advantage of the muscle (e.g., the medial rectus as compared with the superior rectus).

As with the rectus muscles, the superior oblique muscle originates from the annulus of Zinn, but it courses along the superior medial wall of the orbit to the trochlea, a U-shaped fibrocartilage, that acts as a pulley. Near the trochlea, the muscle tissue becomes a tendon as it passes through the trochlea and then reflects back normally at an angle of approximately 51 degrees to the medial wall.

The muscle then crosses the globe superiorly, passing under the superior rectus, to insert in the posterior, superior quadrant near the vortex veins. The trochlea, therefore, becomes the effective mechanical origin for the action of the superior oblique (Figure 1-4). The inferior oblique is the only extraocular muscle that does not originate in the orbital apex; it arises from a small fossa in the anterior, inferior, orbital wall (the maxilla bone). This muscle's course parallels the reflective portion of the superior oblique muscle, again forming a 51-degree angle as it courses inferiorly and laterally across the globe and over the inferior rectus to insert in the inferior, posterior quadrant.

Evidence from magnetic resonance imaging studies of the orbit indicate that all rectus muscles pass through pulleys, structures composed of connective tissue and smooth muscle, that are coupled to the orbital wall and located just behind the equator of the globe.[8-10] In effect, these pulleys ("sleeves")—rather than the attachments of these muscles at the annulus of Zinn in the back of the orbit—act as the origin for the action of the rectus muscles. In most people, the location of these pulleys is remarkably consistent and does not shift much with rotation of the globe into the various fields of gaze. Many strabismic individuals have been found to have normal pulleys, although some do not. Abnormal location of rectus pulleys has been implicated as a cause of noncomitant strabismus.

NEUROLOGY AND CHARACTERISTICS OF EYE MOVEMENTS

The neurology of the following systems are discussed briefly: accommodation, saccades, pursuits, vestibulo-ocular movements, and vergence.

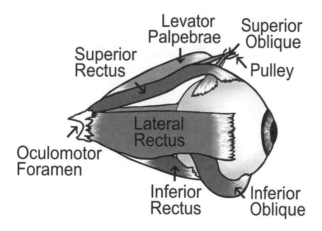

Figure 1-2. Lateral view of muscles of the right eye.

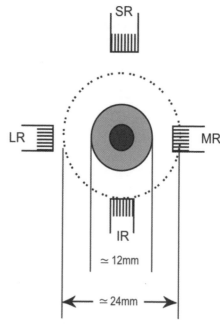

Figure 1-3. Spiral of Tillaux showing insertions of rectus muscles of the right eye. Starting clockwise with the medial rectus, the insertions become increasingly far from the limbus. (IR = inferior rectus; LR = lateral rectus; MR = medial rectus; SR = superior rectus.)

Accommodation

Accommodation is one member of the oculomotor triad that also includes pupillary constriction and accommodative convergence, all mediated by the third nerve nucleus in the midbrain. Accommodation is a reflex initiated by retinal blur; it can, however, be consciously controlled. The afferent pathway extends from the retina to the visual cortex and projects from area 19 to the pretectum and superior colliculus before entering the Edinger-Westphal nucleus of the third nerve complex. Projections from the frontal eye fields (traditionally referred to as Brodmann's area 8) also enter the third nerve complex that, in part, mediates conscious control of accommodation. The efferent component of the reflex arc from the third nerve complex synapses in the ciliary ganglion and again in the ciliary muscle which, in turn, effectuates the change of lens power (Figure 1-5).

Conjugate Gaze Movements

Conjugate eye movements are tandem movements of the two eyes, known as versions. These are saccades, vestibulo-ocular movements, or pursuits. These three eye movement systems share a common final pathway to the extraocular muscles, but they are neurologically distinct, with different central pathways and dynamic properties.

Saccades

Saccadic eye movements refer to ballistic-type eye movements that carry the eye quickly from one target in space to another (i.e., a change in fixation). Saccadic eye movements are abrupt shifts in fixation and are classified as fast, as compared with pursuit and vergence eye movements.[11] A good clinical average velocity is approximately 300 degrees per second, which is approximately 10 times greater than the velocity of pursuit and vergence movements (approximately 30 degrees per second).[12] Saccadic eye movements are mainly voluntary, the other eye movements being mainly involuntary. The duration and velocity of a saccade are proportional to the magnitude of the eye movement. For example, a 40-degree sweep would have a greater velocity and a longer duration than would a 5-degree sweep. The velocity of a saccade changes during its course, being faster at the beginning and slower toward the end of the sweep. Although this may be shown in the laboratory, its observation clinically is difficult, even with recording instruments such as the Visagraph (see Appendix J).

There are two primary types of saccades (1) reflexive (nonvolitional) saccades that occur in response to any new environmental stimulus; and (2) voluntary saccades that carry the eyes from one target to another predetermined target.[13] In recent research, saccades and fixations have been considered part of a system that generates reflexive and voluntary saccades.[14,15] The fixation system insures the direction of gaze and keeps the visual world stable. However, fixation has to be disengaged for a saccadic eye movement to occur and shift fixation to a new target either reflexively or voluntarily.

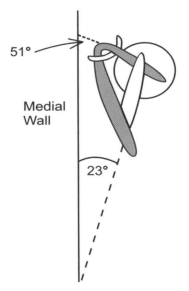

Figure 1-4. Relation between the superior oblique muscle and the superior rectus muscle. (Note: Both the inferior and superior oblique muscles form a 51-degree angle with the medial wall, and both the inferior and superior rectus form a 23-degree angle with the medial wall. The action fields for clinical purposes are approximately 50 and 25 degrees for the oblique and vertical recti, respectively.)

Javal may have been among the first to note that vision turns off as a saccadic eye movement is occurring. This makes sense; otherwise, the world would appear to be a swimming, blurry mess as we scan our environment. This perceptual inhibition, which has been called saccadic "blindness," is more aptly named saccadic suppression. According to Solomons,[16] each saccadic eye movement is preceded by a latent period of approximately 120-180 milliseconds before the eye movement actually begins, and saccadic suppression begins to occur approximately 40 milliseconds before the movement commences. The inhibition increases until visual perception is almost zero during the first part of the movement. Probably not until after the saccadic movement has ended does the saccadic suppression completely cease.

The anatomy subserving voluntary saccades has been partly established by monkey studies and clinical observation in humans. For example, if there is an intention for dextroversion (eye movement to the right), stimulation occurs in Brodmann's area 8 (frontal eye field) in the frontal lobe of the left hemisphere. Impulses then travel to the right pontine gaze center and are forwarded to the ipsilateral nucleus of cranial nerve VI. Subsequently, the lateral rectus muscle of the right eye contracts. Simultaneously, impulses travel from the ipsilateral pontine gaze center up through the medial longitudinal fasciculus that decussates to the left third nerve nucleus. That results in contraction of the medial rectus of the left eye (Figure 1-6). Because yoked muscles have equal innervation (Hering's law),[17] the two eyes move in tandem. Versions are not restricted because of the simultaneous relaxation of the antagonistic yoked muscles (Sherrington's law of reciprocal innervation)[17] (Figure 1-7).

Vestibulo-Ocular Eye Movements

The vestibulo-ocular system stabilizes the eyes on a target during head movements and can be tested with the *"doll's-head"* maneuver. The dynamics of vestibular eye movements are relatively fast, having a latency of only 16 milliseconds as compared with the 75-millisecond latency of the pursuit system.[18] As the head turns, vestibulo-ocular reflexes are initiated by the movement of fluid within the semicircular canals of the inner ear. For example, stimulation of the left vestibular nucleus causes impulses to travel to the right pontine gaze center. From there, the pathway to the extraocular muscles is the same as that described for saccadic eye movements. Stimulation from the left vestibular nucleus by a left head turn causes compensatory dextroversion.

Pursuits

According to Michaels,[19] pursuits are unlike saccades in that vision is present (without suppression, as in saccades) throughout the eyes' excursions. The speed of pursuits is limited to approxi-

AFFERENT

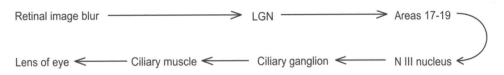

EFFERENT

Figure 1-5. Neural pathway for accommodation. (LGN = lateral geniculate nucleus; N III = cranial nerve III [oculomotor nerve].)

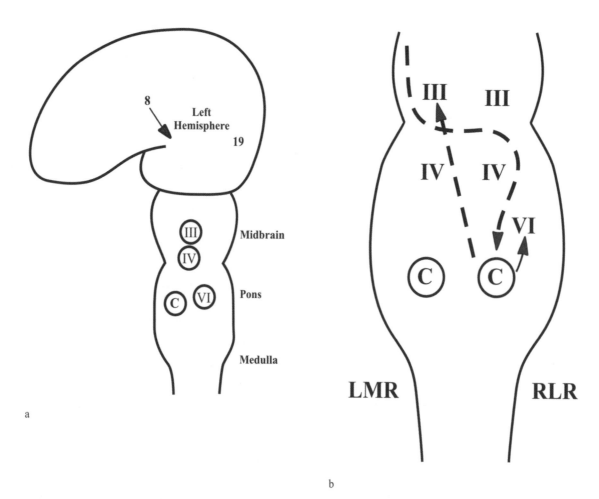

Figure 1-6. Neurologic pathways for saccades. a. Side view. Versional eye movements are initiated in area 8 (supranuclear). A signal from area 8 in the left hemisphere causes a versional movement of the eyes to the right. Axons travel down the left side of the midbrain and then decussate to the right side at the level of the pons-midbrain. These axons then innervate the right pontine conjugate gaze center, which in turn innervates the ipsilateral abducens (VI) and the contralateral oculomotor (III) nerve, b. Posterior view. (C = conjugate gaze center; IV = trochlear nerve; LMR = left medial rectus; RLR = right lateral rectus.)

mately 30 degrees per second. They may be considerably slower but not much faster. If the target velocity is too high, the pursuits break down into a jerky motion. The attempt to keep tracking requires the faster saccadic responses to come into play in order for the patient to regain fixation of the target. In infants, pursuit eye movements start to manifest at approximately 6 weeks of age and increase in tandem with the development of sustained visual attention to moving targets.[20]

The pursuit system mediates constant tracking of a moving target and is the slowest of the three eye movement systems. Pursuit eye movements are mediated via the occipitomesencephalic pathway. Impulses travel from the occipital lobes (presumably from Brodmann's area 19) to the midbrain and pontine gaze centers and on to the nuclei of the third, fourth, and sixth cranial nerves to innervate the extraocular muscles. Each occipital lobe

is involved in the pursuit of a target, in both directions, horizontally or vertically.[21] The assumption is that the right and left occipital areas are connected to each right and left pontine gaze center, so that stimulation from one occipital lobe may stimulate both the left and right pontine gaze centers for left or right pursuit movements. Because of this double coverage, pursuits may sometimes be intact despite an extensive lesion in one hemisphere of the brain that could also cause a homonymous hemianopic visual field loss (Figure 1-8).

Vergences

Vergence refers to disjunctive eye movements, or rotation of the eyes in opposite directions. The two main types of vergence movements are accommodative vergence, stimulated by blur, and fusional vergence, stimulated by retinal image disparity. Vergences are consciously controlled to some degree, but they usually are involuntary

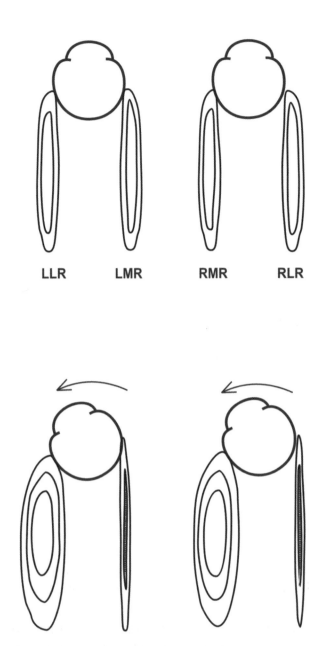

LLR   LMR   RMR   RLR

Figure 1-7. Hering's law and Sherrington's law evident during levo-version. The right medial rectus (RMR) and the left lateral rectus (LLR) (yoked muscles) contract, in accord with Hering's law. The left medial rectus (LMR) is the antagonist of the left lateral rectus, and it relaxes, as does the right lateral rectus (RLR) (antagonist of the right medial rectus), in accord with Sherrington's law.

Occipital Lobes

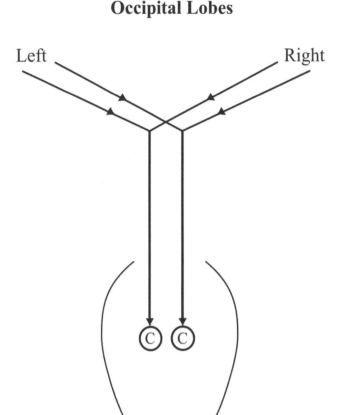

Figure 1-8. Neurology of pursuits, showing that either left or right hemisphere goes to the left or right parietal lobes and, ultimately, to the conjugate gaze centers (C), providing double coverage neurologically.

psycho-optic reflexes.[22] Vergence movements are slow and show a negative exponential waveform (velocity diminishing from fast to slow). For most visual tasks, both vergence and saccadic eye movements are used in combination to place objects on the foveas.

Little is known about the supranuclear pathways subserving vergence eye movements, although convergence in the monkey was produced as early as 1890 by electrical stimulation of sites in the cortex.[23] Vergence eye movements probably are synthesized bilaterally in the cerebral cortex[24] (Figure 1-9). Impulses travel from the cortex to the pretectum and rostral mesencephalic reticular formation. Innervation is integrated from several sites, including the cerebellum. In the midbrain, convergence is mediated by the bilateral nuclei of the oculomotor nuclear complex (cranial nerve III) that sends efferent signals to both medial rectus muscles. There is probably no single convergence center, contrary to what once was believed (the so-called "nucleus of Perlia"). Regarding vergences, it is not certain whether Hering's law of equal innervation of yoke muscles is the operative principle. In the real world, vergence stimuli often are presented asymmetrically to the eyes, and asymmetric responses have been found by close inspection.[25] Hence, each eye appears to be responding independently to that eye's view of the target. Therefore, vergence testing can be done using symmetric stimuli (e.g., Risley prism procedure)

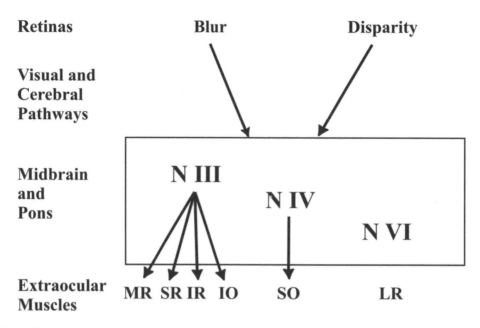

Figure 1-9. Simplified illustration of neurology of vergences showing retinal blur stimulating accommodation, which in turn results in accommodative vergence, and retinal disparity resulting in disjunctive eye movements. Indirect stimuli (e.g., proximity and volition) are not depicted, nor is cerebellar integration. (IO = inferior oblique; IR = inferior rectus; LR = lateral rectus; MR = medial rectus; N III = oculomotor nerve [cranial nerve III]; N IV = trochlear nerve [cranial nerve IV]; N VI = abducens nerve [cranial nerve VI]; SO = superior oblique; SR = superior rectus.)

or an asymmetric stimulus (e.g., step prism procedure).

Divergence once was accepted as merely the relaxation of convergence innervation. However, divergence usually is an active neurophysiologic process, as indicated by electromyographic recordings from the lateral rectus muscles.[26] The pathways that subserve divergence remain essentially unknown.

SENSORY ASPECTS OF BINOCULAR VISION

The ability to integrate information from the two eyes into one fused image and to extract depth information depends on the primary visual cortex (mainly in the calcarine fissure) located bilaterally on the medial aspect of each occipital lobe. Other functions of the primary visual cortex (V1, formerly Brodmann's area 17) include detecting spatial organization of the visual scene, brightness, shading, and rudimentary form organization. Specific points of the retina connect with specific points of the visual cortex (e.g., the homonymous right halves of the two respective retinas connect with the right visual cortex). In other words, the primary visual cortex is organized like a map of the retina. Because the eyes are separated by a distance of approximately 60 mm in humans, each eye's view of the environment is from a slightly

different perspective. The sole basis for stereopsis is the horizontal disparity between the two retinal images. A little understood neural mechanism presumably located within the visual cortex compares the retinal images from each eye for disparity information. Further neural processing in this visual pathway (also not fully understood) gives almost all people with normal binocular vision a vivid sense of three-dimensionality (e.g., volume) in their visual perception of the external world.

Binocular vision seems so natural to most people that they are hardly aware that their perception of the world arises from the unification of two separate and slightly different images. Most people are surprised if diplopia occurs. What is truly remarkable, however, is that we usually do see single images—a fact that requires an explanation. Fusion of two ocular images requires adequate functioning of each eye and sufficient stimulation of corresponding retinal points in the two eyes to produce single binocular vision.

Monocular Considerations

Our perception of space with one eye depends on oculocentric localization where the position of objects in space is based on retinotopic mapping and local sign.[27] The coordinate system is centered on the fixation point which is typically the foveal area. The fovea or area of highest acuity is the principle visual direction and all other points are considered secondary visual directions. The fovea or principle visual direction is perceived as straight ahead and the secondary visual directions are relative to the fovea. When the eye moves both the straight ahead position and secondary visual direction change according to how objects are imaged on retinal points. The practitioner needs to understand oculocentric localization when assessing monocular fixation in a patient with amblyopia. In some cases of ambylopia the principle visual direction can shift away from the fovea to an eccentric retinal position. (See Chapter 5.)

For normal binocular vision, the best possible visual acuity of each eye should be attained, whether by means of spectacle lenses, contact lenses, surgical intervention (e.g., to correct for cataract), or other possible treatments (e.g., vision therapy for amblyopia). Poor acuity of either or both eyes is a deterrent to sensory fusion. This is particularly true when the vision of one eye is much poorer than that of the other eye. The discrepancy may be due to such functional reasons as anisometropic amblyopia and strabismic amblyopia, or it may be due to organic causes, such as macular degeneration, cataract, and optic nerve atrophy. Any organic disease must be ruled out or managed correctly before functional testing is continued and vision training techniques are begun.

Egocentric Localization

When looking with both eyes the two oculocentric visual directions need to be reconciled to avoid diplopia and visual confusion. Under binocular viewing conditions the visual system uses an egocentric point located between the two eyes which serves as the body's spatial localization reference point.[27,28] That is, we judge the position of objects in space relative to our sense of a stable egocentric localization that is located in the head midway between the eyes. This solution allows us to localize objects relative to a stable head centered point that can be independent of eye movements. One critical feature of this solution is that the visual system has to process corresponding points in each eye in order to match the two visual inputs.

Retinal Correspondence

Retinal correspondence refers to the subjective visual direction and the spatial location of objects in the binocular visual field. An individual is said to have normal retinal correspondence when the stimulation of both foveas (and other geometrically paired retinal points) give rise to a unitary percept. (The correspondence actually occurs in the cortex, but clinically it is easier to conceptualize retinal points.) The existence of corresponding retinal elements with their common subjective visual direction is fundamental to binocular vision. Stimulation of corresponding retinal points results in haplopia (singleness of vision), whether correspondence is normal or anomalous. (Anomalous retinal correspondence is discussed in Chapter 5.) Conversely, double vision results when noncorresponding retinal points are sufficiently stimulated.

Panum's Fusional Areas

Rather than a point-to-point correspondence between the two eyes, there exists a point-to-area relationship subserving binocular fusion. This relationship was first described by Panum, a Danish physiologist, in the middle of the nineteenth century.[29] Panum's area is "an area in the retina of one eye, any point of which, when stimulated simultaneously with a single specific point in the retina of the other eye, will give rise to a single fused percept."[17] Panum's areas are oval and larger horizontally than vertically. Foveal Panum's areas are very small, only a few minutes of arc, as compared with peripheral Panum's areas, which may be several prism diopters in extent. The increasing size of these areas in the periphery may be related to anatomic and physiologic differences known to exist between central and peripheral retina, receptors being densely packed at the fovea but widely separated in the peripheral retina. Panum's areas parallel the increase in size of the retinal receptive fields, but they are functionally part of the visual cortex, where binocular information comes together.

The Horopter

Corresponding points in the two eyes can be mapped out both theoretically and experimentally and is referred to as the horopter.[27,28] The horopter is defined as the locus of all object points that are imaged on corresponding retinal elements at a given fixation distance and can be generating using a variety of criteria.[30] The theoretical or geometrical horopter is an idealized map of all points that when imaged on each eye subtend equal visual

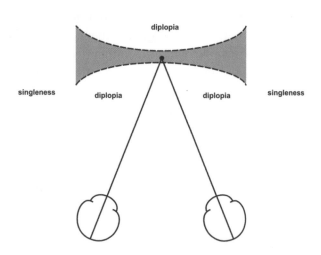

Figure 1-10. Singleness (haplopia) horopter. Diplopia can occur for an object that is not within the horopter.

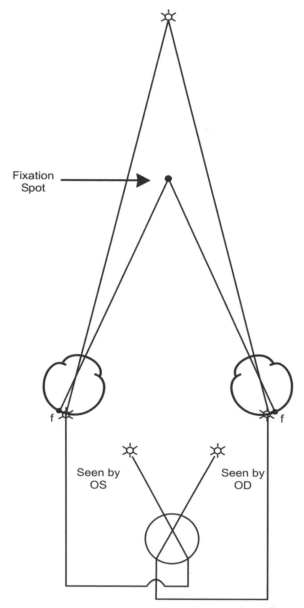

Figure 1-11. Homonymous ("uncrossed") physiologic diplopia, (f = fovea.)

angles and is called the Vieth-Müller circle.[27,28] The geometric horopter predicts the shape of the horopter based on the angular arrangement of corresponding points in each eye and assumes perfect optics exist in each eye. The measured horopter discussed below typically differs from the Vieth-Müller circle, and Ogle developed an elegant analysis of the deviation which is beyond the scope of this chapter.[28]

Because we cannot stimulate corresponding points in each eye directly in human subjects a variety of criteria have been used to measure the horopter in human subjects.[27,28] Classically, there are five criteria that have been used when measuring the horopter.[27,28] The identical visual direction (IVD) horopter is a locus of object points in which images on the two retinas give rise to a common visual direction and is considered the most accurate horopter. The IVD horopter usually is represented as a single horizontal line passing through the fixation point and having no thickness. The apparent frontal parallel plane horopter (AFPP) is the easiest horopter criteria for a subject to appreciate and is defined as the location of points that are perceived as lying in the same distance from the observer as the fixation point. The minimum stereoacuity threshold horopter finds the location where stereoacuity sensitivity for an individual is optimal. This criterion is very time consuming to measure and is rarely performed in practice. The zero vergence horopter assumes that points seen as equidistant will not stimulate a motor fusional vergence response.

Finally, the singleness horopter uses the concept of Panum's fusional areas and is easily visualized by using the horopter criteria of singleness (haplopia). The singleness horopter criteria is represented as having thickness corresponding to Panum's areas expressed by the anteroposterior limits through which a nonfixated test object may be displaced and still be seen as single (Figure 1-10).[17] The actual horopter is the midpoint between the areas where diplopia noticed. Note that the horopter is thicker in the periphery, corresponding to the increasing size of Panum's fusional areas. The significance of the singleness horopter, is that any object seen outside the horopter necessarily falls on diplopia-producing, noncorresponding points. In other words, the visual world outside the single-

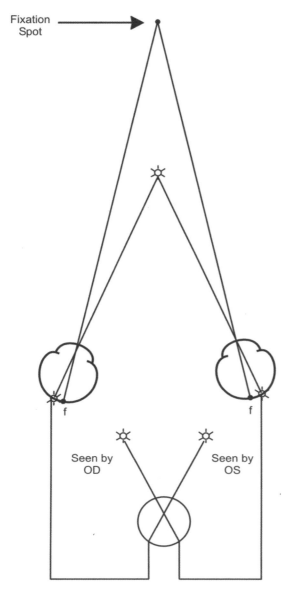

Fixation Spot →

Seen by OD

Seen by OS

f   f

Figure 1-12. Heteronymous ("crossed") physiologic diplopia, (f = fovea.)

ness horopter should theoretically appear as double when retinal stimulation is sufficient. Fortunately, our neurological system is highly adaptable and *physiologic suppression* usually eliminates physiologic diplopia so that most people can go about living normal lives, at least visually without noticing diplopia. Similarly, the neurological system provides sensory antidiplopic mechanisms for the strabismic individual in the forms of anomalous retinal correspondence and pathologic suppression (as discussed in Chapter 5).

PHYSIOLOGIC DIPLOPIA

The doubling of a nonfixated object is known as physiologic diplopia, because there is nothing abnormal about this phenomenon. With normal binocular vision, all objects falling outside

the singleness horopter can be seen as double if sufficient attention is paid to the stimulus object. Homonymous physiologic diplopia (also called "uncrossed" diplopia) occurs when objects are beyond the point of bifixation. Conversely, heteronymous ("crossed") diplopia occurs when a farther object is bifixated with a nearer object in view (Figures 1-11 and 1-12). Because of physiologic suppression, these physiologic diplopic images usually are unnoticed under ordinary viewing conditions.

Most patients consider seeing double to be abnormal and seek help from an eye doctor. If the examination does not reveal a paretic muscle or a motor fusion problem and physiologic diplopia seems the most likely explanation, then the doctor must explain that this is a feature of normal binocular vision that is normally not noticed. Some patients are not easily convinced of this physiologic fact about binocular vision because the phenomenon seems counterintuitive. Nonetheless, physiologic diplopia is easy to demonstrate to a patient with normal binocular vision and can be used as a binocular vision screening technique: As a patient fixates a pencil at 40 cm, for example, the clinician asks the patient to hold up an index finger halfway between the fixation object and the patient's nose. If the patient's attention is drawn to the nonfixated finger, then the finger usually appears to be double, like two ghost images. Patients who have active suppression of one eye due to a binocular vision disorder often cannot easily see the diplopic image. Physiologic diplopia is an important tool in vision training, used to help remediate binocular vision in both strabismic and nonstrabismic cases.

PATHOLOGIC DIPLOPIA

Diplopia of a fixated target, or pathologic diplopia, is considered abnormal. It occurs in cases of strabismus in which there is little or no suppression. Figure 1-13 shows one eye (left) fixating the target of regard while the esotropic (right) eye is not fixating the target. In the right eye, the image, rather than falling on the fovea, is nasal relative to the fovea. This produces homonymous diplopia ("uncrossed"), in which the diplopic image is seen on the same side as the strabismic eye. In contrast, in cases of exotropia, pathologic diplopia is heteronymous ("crossed"); that is, the diplopic image is seen on the opposite side of the strabismic eye.

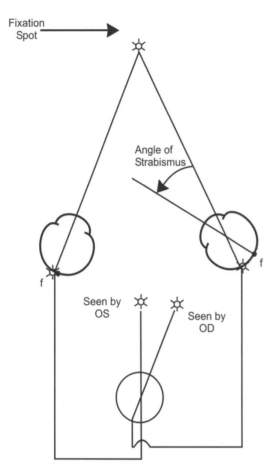

Figure 1-13. Pathologic diplopia in an example of esotropia of the right eye. The diplopia is homonymous (uncrossed), (f = fovea.)

TYPES OF SENSORY FUSION

Binocular fusion of forms occurs within the singleness horopter, whereas diplopia occurs outside the horopter. Fused binocular vision is precious, but it is possible only in a relatively small band of visual space analogous to a vein of gold in the side of a granite mountain.

A common clinical method for classifying fusion was developed by Worth[31] who defined three levels of fusion; first, second, and third degree. Although, this is not a theoretically accurate classification system it does have clinical utility. The ability to perceive two dissimilar target as occupying the same visual direction is classified superimposition or "first degree fusion" This is not true fusion since the targets are dissimilar but allows the clinician to identify the spatial localization of similar retinal points. The importance of superimposition testing is in measuring the subjective angle of directionalization, clinically called angle S, and also assessing the degree of suppression, particularly in strabismic patients.

Worth[31] classified flat fusion as "second-degree fusion." This is true fusion but without stereopsis. Flat fusion is defined as "sensory fusion in which the resultant percept is two-dimensional, that is, occupying a single plane, as may be induced by viewing a stereogram in a stereoscope in which the separation of all homologous points is identical."[17] The most important reason to consider flat fusion is for vision testing and training purposes, as in phorometry measurements, fixation disparity testing, and in amblyoscopic assessment and treatment (i.e., major amblyoscope instrumentation).

Worth[31] classified stereopsis as third-degree fusion. Stereopsis may be defined as "binocular visual perception of three-dimensional space based on retinal disparity."[17]

Figure 1-14 illustrates central or fine stereopsis: The fused, small vertical line is perceived as being closer than the star. Although there is lateral displacement of the vertical line, as seen by each eye, there will be fusion of the two lines into one vertical line which appears centered (but closer) with respect to the star. Lateral displacement of such types of stimuli to produce stereoscopic depth is a feature of many vision therapy targets, such as vectographs (Vectograms), anaglyphs, and stereograms (as in this example).

When the laterally displaced stimuli are located more than 5 degrees from the center of the fovea, peripheral stereopsis is being evaluated. In Figure 1-15, the "Y" appears to be closer to the patient and the "X" farther away in relation to the star. Clinicians also describe stereopsis as "gross" or "fine." Peripheral stereopsis is necessarily classified as being "gross," whereas central stereopsis is considered "fine" if it measures 200 seconds of arc or better.

Stereoscopically fused images appear to be nearer to a bifixated reference point if Panum's areas are stimulated temporally from the center of the foveas. Conversely, if Panum's areas are stimulated nasally from the center of the foveas, an image seems farther from the bifixated reference point. If we think of the temporal retina as having positive values for nearness and of the nasal retina as having negative values, we can more easily understand the concept of stereopsis related to lateral displacement. The greater the distance from the center of the fovea, the greater the value—either positive or negative—for the perception of objects appearing

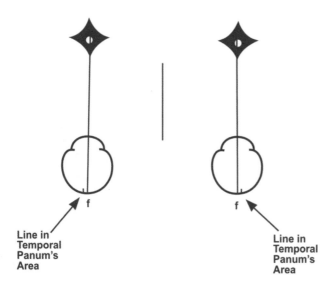

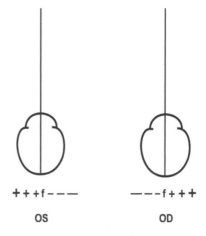

Figure 1-14.Stereogram for central stereopsis induced by laterally displaced vertical lines. The fused vertical line appears closer than the star because the temporal (to the fovea [ff]) Panum's area is stimulated in each eye.

Figure 1-16. Stereopsis values for nearer and farther perception. Plus signs indicate nearness, which is also referred to as "crossed disparity." Minus signs indicate far distance, or "uncrossed disparity." The greater the temporal Panum's area (larger plus signs) the greater the stereopsis effect, as is true also for the nasal Panum's area (minus signs), (f = fovea.)

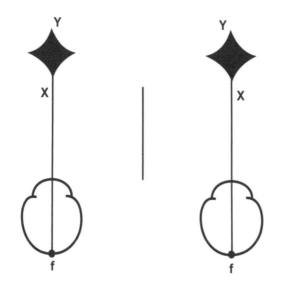

Figure 1-15. Example of target for peripheral stereopsis. (f = fovea.)

nearer or farther, respectively. The detection of stereopsis within Panum's area is called quantitative or patent stereopsis. This concept is illustrated in Figure 1-16 by the increasing sizes of the plus and minus signs toward the periphery of the retina. As the disparity of targets exceeds Panum's area, diplopia will be noticed. At this point, qualitative or coarse stereopsis is available and allows the detection of in front of or behind the target of regard.

Generally speaking, the finer the degree of stereoscopic discrimination, the higher the quality of binocular vision. Conversely, suppression

and excessive fixation disparity tend to decrease stereoacuity; these anomalies often predispose a patient to asthenopic symptoms and reduced visual performance. The main value of stereopsis is as a clue to depth at close viewing distances; its value to the individual is barely significant at far distances.[32] For instance, a surgeon is more likely to need stereoscopic depth perception than is an airline pilot. Monocular clues to depth (e.g., size, linear perspective, texture gradient, and overlap) tend to predominate at far distances. Nevertheless, most passenger airlines require their pilots to have superior stereopsis, because safety and prudence demand that every possible perceptual clue to making accurate depth judgments be available. This stringent criterion is probably imposed because stereopsis is the "barometer of binocular vision."

In contrast to fusion, diplopia is the simultaneous perception of two ocular images of a single object. This sensory phenomenon is important in clinical assessment and vision therapy. As discussed previously, physiologic diplopia testing refers to the perception of diplopic images that lie outside the singleness horopter. Physiologic diplopia training is frequently useful in vision therapy to break pathologic suppression and to increase vergence ranges.

Clinicians use many tests involving pathologic diplopia, particularly as part of strabismus evaluations. In cases of noncomitant strabismus, for example, pathologic diplopia testing is very impor-

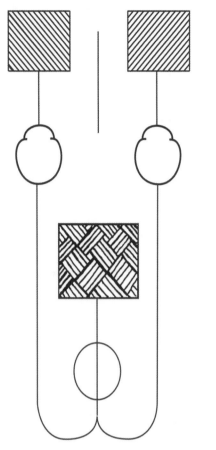

Figure 1-17. Cyclopean projection showing perception of retinal rivalry.

tant in determining the severity of underactions and over-actions of extraocular muscles in various positions of gaze.

Whereas diplopia results from stimulation of non-corresponding retinal points, superimposition of two ocular images (e.g., a bird in a cage) requires stimulation of retinal areas having common visual directions.

THEORIES OF SENSORY FUSION

The salient features accounting for sensory fusion are retinal correspondence, retinal image disparity detection, and neural summation of information from the two eyes. A system of correspondence provides feedback about whether the motor alignment of the eyes is in registry. Retinal image disparity detection is the stimulus to the vergence system to make correctional vergence eye movements.

Within certain limits, retinal image disparities are also necessary for stereopsis. Research has indicated that certain striate cells in areas V1 and V2 (in occipital areas 17 and 18) are sensitive to

horizontal disparity for the perception of stereopsis.[33,34]

Studies of higher mammals have shown that approximately 80% of cells in the striate cortex can be binocularly stimulated.[35] Neural summation of these binocular cells has been demonstrated by single-cell neurophysiologic investigations.[33] The corresponding areas, however, must be in proper registry for maximum responsiveness. When these fields are out of alignment, they mutually inhibit one another.[36] These physiologic features are the basis for the perceptual unification of the two ocular images and represent some of the advantages of normal binocular vision. As discussed previously, contrast sensitivity and visual acuity are enhanced by binocular neural summation.

One of the more popular, older theories of binocular vision, the alternation theory, held that unification of the two ocular images did not, in fact, take place. This theory claimed that retinal rivalry phenomena provided evidence that the binocular field was composed of a mosaic of monocularly perceived patches. Hence, no true fusion occurred; the input for one eye would inhibit the input from the other. Retinal rivalry of dissimilar forms, a common clinical observation, is the primary evidence supporting the alternation theory, which purports that the mosaic pattern of the "fused" image is ever-changing, with certain portions at times being dominated by the left eye's responses and at other times by the right eye's responses (Figure 1-17). This theory left unexplained many features of binocular perception, such as contrast sensitivity enhancement. Moreover, single-cell electrophysiologic evidence has conclusively shown this notion of binocular vision to be essentially incorrect. The more modern theory of neural summation is fundamental to binocular perception. Studies of reaction time to binocular versus monocular vision stimulation and cortical electrophysiology indicate that information from both eyes is available during binocular viewing.[37] Binocular fusion is characterized by summation of information from the two eyes and synchronization of neural activity from each eye's dominance columns in the striate cortex (see Figure 1-17).

BINOCULARLY DRIVEN CELLS & OCULAR DOMINANCE

Ocular dominance is another important physiologic feature of binocularly driven cells. Only approximately one-fourth of these cells respond equally to input from the right and left eye; the others respond more vigorously to the input from either one eye or the other.[35] Ocular dominance of binocular cortical cells is particularly sensitive to the amount of binocular stimulation during development in infancy. Even minor obstacles to sensory fusion can have long-term consequences. Obstacles to sensory fusion, such as anisometropia, aniseikonia, strabismus, and form deprivation (e.g., cataract), can result in a rapid shift in striate cell ocular dominance. When most cortical cells are controlled exclusively by one eye during the sensitive period, the natural consequences are binocular anomalies.[38] These include suppression, amblyopia, anomalous retinal correspondence, loss of stereopsis, and deficient fusional vergences. Such binocular anomalies may become permanent unless timely and appropriate vision therapy takes place.

REFERENCES

1. Barany E. A theory of binocular visual acuity and an analysis of the variability of visual acuity. Acta Ophthalmol 1946;24:63.
2. Horowitz M. An analysis of the superiority of binocular over monocular visual acuity. J Exp Psychol. 1949;39:581.
3. Campbell F, Green D. Monocular vs. binocular visual acuity. Nature 1965;200:191-2.
4. Sheedy J, Bailey I, Muri M, Bass E. Binocular vs. monocular task performance. Am J Optom Physiol Opt 1986;63(10):839-46.
5. Servos P, Goodale MA. Binocular vision and the on-line control of human prehension. Experimental Brain Research 1994;98:119–27.
6. Jackson SR, Jones CA, Newport R, C P. A Kinematic Analysis of Goal-directed Prehension Movements Executed under Binocular, Monocular, and Memory-guided Viewing Conditions. Visual Cognition 1997;4(2):113-42.
7. Michaels D. Visual Optics and Refraction. In. St. Louis: Mosby, 1980:677.
8. Clark R, Miller J, Demer J. Location and stability of rectus muscle pulleys. Invest Ophthalmol Vis Sci. 1997;38:227-40.
9. Clark R, Miller J, Demer J. Three-dimensional location of human rectus pulleys by path inflections in secondary gaze positions. Invest Ophthalmol Vis Sci. 2000;41:3787-97.
10. Demer J, Miller J, Poukens V. Evidence for fibro-muscular pulleys of the recti extraocular muscles. Invest Ophthalmol Vis Sci. 1995;36:1125-36.
11. Moses R. Adler's Physiology of the Eye, 7th ed. In. St. Louis: Mosby, 1981.
12. Gay A, Newman N, Keltner J, Stroud M. Eye Movement Disorders. In. St. Louis: Mosby, 1974.
13. Glaser J. Neuro-ophthalmology. In. Philadelphia: Lippincott, 1990.
14. Fischer B, Biscaldi M, Gezeck S. On the development of voluntary and reflexive components in human saccade generation. Brain Research 1997;754:285-97.
15. Munoz D, Broughton J, Goldring J, Armstrong I. Age-related performance of human subjects on saccadic eye movement tasks. Exp Brain Res 1998;121:391-400.
16. Solomons H. Binocular Vision: A Programmed Text. In. London: Heinemann Medical, 1978.
17. Hofstetter H, Griffin J, Berman M, Everson R. Dictionary of Visual Science and Related Clinical Terms, 5th ed. Boston: Butterworth-Heinemann, 2000.
18. Maas E, Huebner W, Seidman S, Leigh R. Behavior of human horizontal vestibulo-ocular reflex in response to high-acceleration stimuli. Brain Res. 1989;499:153-6.
19. Michaels D. Visual Optics and Refraction: A Clinical Approach. In. St. Louis: Mosby, 1980: 417.
20. Richards J, Holley F. Infant attention and the development of smooth pursuit tracking. Dev Psychol. 1999;35:856-67.
21. Bajandas F, Kline L. Neuro-Ophthalmology Review Manual, 2nd ed. Thorofare, N.J.: Slack Inc., 1987: 51-54.
22. Hoffman F, Bielshowsky A. Über die der Wilkur entzo-genen Fusionsbewegungen der Augen. Arch Ges Physiol. 1900;80:1.
23. Mukuno K. Electron microscopic studies on the human extraocular muscles under pathologic conditions. Jpn J Ophthalmol. 1969;13:35.
24. Dale R. Fundamentals of Ocular Motility and Strabismus. New York: Grune & Stratton, 1982:105.
25. Enright J. Slow-velocity asymmetrical convergence: a decisive failure of "Hering's law". Vision Res. 1996;36:3667-84.
26. Tamler E, Jampolsky A. Is divergence active? An electromyographic study. Am J Ophthalmol. 1967;63:452.
27. Steinman SB, Steinman BA, Garzia R. Foundations of Binocular Vision, First ed. New York: McGraw-Hill, 2000; 345.
28. Ogle K. Researches in Binocular Vision, First ed. Philadelphia: W.B. Saunders, 1950.
29. Panum P. Physiologische Untersuchungen über das Sehen mitzwei Augen. In. Kiel: Schwerssche Buchandlung, 1858.
30. von Noorden G. Binocular Vision and Ocular Motility: Theory and Management of Strabismus, 4th ed. St. Louis: Mosby, 1990.
31. Worth C. Squint: Its Causes, Pathology and Treatment. Philadelphia: Blakiston, 1921.
32. Schor C, Flom M. The relative value of stereopsis as a function of viewing distance. Am J Optom Physiol Opt 1969;46:805-9.
33. Hubel D, Wiesel T. Stereoscopic vision in macaque monkey: cells sensitive to binocular depth in area 18 of the macaque monkey cortex. Nature 1970;225:41.
34. Poggio G, Poggio T. The analysis of stereopsis. Annu Rev Neurosci. 1984;7:379.
35. Hubel D, Wiesel T. Receptive fields, binocular interaction and functional architecture in the cat's visual cortex. J Physiol (Lond) 1962;160:106.
36. Nikara T, Bishop P, Pettigrew J. Analysis of retinal correspondence by studying receptive fields of binocular single units in cat striate cortex. Exp Brain Res. 1968;6:353.
37. O'Shea R. Chronometric analysis supports fusion rather than suppression theory of binocular vision. Vision Res. 1987;27:781-91.
38. Weakly Jr. D. The association between nonstrabimic anisometropia, amblyopia, and subnormal binocularity. Ophthalmology 2001;108:163-71.

Chapter 2 / Visual Skills Assessment Part 1
Case History, Eye Movements, and Accommodation

Background and Rationale for Vision Skills Testing	16	Summary of Pursuit Testing	32
Patient History	17	Fixation	32
Maladaptive Behaviors	18	Symptoms and Differential Diagnosis	32
Educational History	19	Southern California College of Optometry 4+ System	33
Vision Skills and Reading	20	Summary of Fixation Testing	33
Testing For Visual Skills	21	Vestibulo-Ocular Reflexes	33
Ranking Visual Performance	21	Management of Deficits in Saccades and Pursuits	33
Saccadic Eye Movements	21	Accommodation	33
Symptoms and Differential Diagnosis	21	Symptoms and Differential Diagnosis	33
Saccadic Eye Movements and Reading	22	Testing of Accommodation	34
Objective Testing	23	Absolute Accommodation	34
Southern California College of Optometry System	24	Relative Accommodation	35
NSUCO Oculomotor Test	24	Lag of Accommodation	36
Ophthalmography (Visagraph and ReadAlyzer)	25	Nott Method	36
Sequential Fixation Tests	27	Monocular Estimate Method Retinoscopy	37
Subjective Testing	27	Insufficiency of Accommodation	37
Developmental Eye Movement Test	27	Management of Accommodative Insufficiency	38
Summary of Saccade Testing	30	Excess of Accommodation	38
Pursuit Eye Movements	30	Management of Accommodative Excess	39
Symptoms and Differential Diagnosis	30	Facility of Accommodation	39
Testing of Pursuit Skills	31	Ill-Sustained Accommodation	42
Southern California College of Optometry 4+ System	31	Management of Accommodatve Infaciltiy and Ill-Sustained Accommdation	43
NSUCO Oculomotor Test	31	Summary	43

BACKGROUND AND RATIONALE FOR VISION SKILLS TESTING

For any patient being treated for binocular anomalies, the ultimate goal is the achievement of clear, single, comfortable, and efficient binocular vision. Visual skills (VS) is the term applied to the ways in which various ocular systems operate over time and under various viewing conditions. Clinical evaluation of vision skills necessitates the assessment of sufficiency (amplitude), facility (flexibility), accuracy, and stamina of each ocular function.

Practitioners in the nineteenth century were concerned almost exclusively with clearness of eyesight and with lenses that would optimally reduce or eliminate blurred vision. Clearness and singleness of binocular vision became the issue with the advent of orthoptics. Effective therapeutic regimens for strabismus were introduced by Javal[1] and were expanded later by others.

Astute clinicians in the first half of the twentieth century became aware of the relationship between accommodation and vergence. Knowledge of the zone of clear, single, comfortable binocular vision was gained through various models of vision, such as the graphical analysis approach, and through an understanding of fixation disparity (see Chapter 3).

In the latter half of the twentieth century, more and more emphasis was placed on efficiency of vision, implying that efficient visual skills are related to good scholastic abilities (school) and occupational production (work) and to achievement in sports and hobbies (play). As a result, lenses or functional training techniques frequently are applied in clinical practice to help patients attain efficient binocular vision in these activities. (Surgery is not a mode of therapy commonly associated with vision skills therapy.)

Fundamental to having good VS is the optimum correction of any significant refractive error. Clinicians have found that correcting even small errors of refraction can result in large changes in visual comfort, stamina, and performance. If a patient presents with a significant uncorrected refractive error, a vision skills evaluation ideally should be performed after the patient has worn the correction for two weeks. Normative data presented in this chapter assume that refractive error has been corrected.

Dysfunctions of visual skills also result from a mismatch between a patient's oculomotor and binocular physiology and the environmental demands placed on the individual's visual system. As with other neuromuscular abilities, the health and vigor of specific visual-motor skills required for everyday tasks varies considerably among individuals. Normative data collection has indicated that most oculomotor and binocular vision skills are distributed in a population along a normal bell-shaped curve. Some people are well suited for intensive visual activity such as prolonged periods of reading or computer work, whereas others are not. Occupations and recreational activities vary tremendously in their requirements for efficient visual skills. The visual work requirements of an attorney and computer programmer are much more intensive than those of the average farmer and sales clerk. Full-time computer operators have come to expect some eyestrain and discomfort as part of their job. Several studies have shown that the prevalence of visual symptoms increases with increased visual demands.[2,3] Sensitivity to visual and other forms of stress also differs among individuals, so a psychological dimension influences the manifestation of symptoms as well. Hence, at least three factors interact to define a vision skills dysfunction: (1) a patient's physiologic level of visual skills, (2) specific visual requirements (how vision is used), and (3) sensitivity to visual stress. The clinician must evaluate these factors when obtaining a patient's case history and performing the examination.

The oculomotor and binocular visual skills that have been widely implicated in dysfunction are (1) deficient pursuit tracking; (2) deficient saccadic tracking, particularly in reading; (3) overstressed or deficient accommodative skills; (4) excessive heterophoria (esophoria, exophoria, and hyperphoria); (5) deficient or overstressed vergence skills; and (6) deficient sensory integration and stereopsis. The relationships among accommodation, vergence, and sensory fusion skills have been a focus of optometric research and practice since the 1930s and encompass classic heterophoria case analysis and fixation disparity analysis (covered in Chapter 3). These historic approaches are part and parcel of vision skills analysis, but testing and evaluation of oculomotor and binocular visual skills have evolved to include efficiency considerations of how a patient's specific skills respond over time and relative to specific tasks or conditions. In a society of increasing educational, occupational, and recreational demands on vision, the testing and evaluation of VS has taken center stage.

PATIENT HISTORY

The most important and revealing component of the history is the chief symptom. Intense eye pain and prolonged double vision are not symptoms commonly associated with vision efficiency dysfunctions and usually indicate more severe and acute disorders. Instead vision skills dysfunctions, often are associated with symptoms related to visually demanding activities at near distances, such as reading, writing, sewing, and computer use. The symptoms usually increase in intensity with increased time devoted to the task and abate with sleep or rest.

Symptoms associated with reading and close work can be divided into three basic categories; somatic, perceptual or visual, and performance. Somatic symptoms, often called asthenopia are associated with symptoms of ocular fatigue or discomfort. The common symptom of tired eyes with sustained visual activity should be distinguished from reports of general fatigue. Tired eyes do occur as part of chronic fatigue, systemic diseases (e.g., hypothyroidism and other endocrine imbalances), allergy attacks, and general stress reactions. Clinicians are often challenged to make the distinction between ocular fatigue and general fatigue, because each can contribute to manifestations of the other. A carefully obtained, detailed patient history may be necessary but sometimes still is insufficient.

Another common somatic symptom is headaches which can be caused by or exacerbated by dysfunctions of accommodation or vergence or both. However, headaches are attributable to many different medically-related and/or psychological etiologies, and so differential diagnosis is necessary. Ocular headaches usually are described as a dull to moderate ache at the brow line, around the eyes, or emanating from the orbits. Other locations may be implicated, particularly the back of the head and neck, which are also associated with general stress.

Perceptual or visual symptoms are typically associated with reports of intermittent blur, doubling, or "wobbling" of print and are highly associated with disorders of accommodation and vergence. Recent research using analysis of symptom types have found that adults reporting perceptual symptoms typically have the highest scores on surveys measuring somatic, perceptual, and performance symptoms.[4] Thus, when the patient reports symptoms of perceptual distortions the clinician should suspect the presence of a significant visual skills deficit.

Finally, performance symptoms relate to a variety of symptoms including (1) skipping over words, parts of words, or sentences; (2) inadvertent rereading of a line of print; (3) losing one's place; (4) laborious or slow reading; and (5) the need to use a finger or ruler as a place keeper. Performance complaints are usually thought of as a result of poor visual skills and are difficult to pinpoint to isolated deficit in accommodation, vergence, or saccades. However, performance symptoms commonly overlap with several developmental disorders such as dyslexia and attention deficit disorder. Therefore the case history should include questions about the patient's medical and educational histories.

Despite the long history of association between visual skills and symptoms there has been a lack of standardized instruments that assess patient complaints. However, there has been an increased interest in developing survey instruments that measure a range of symptoms of visual discomfort in children and adults. Several survey's, have been developed and include those developed by Conlon et al, COVD quality of life survey, and the Convergence Insufficiency Symptom Survey (CISS).[5-7] All three surveys sample a variety of symptoms associated with visual skills deficit but the CISS is the one survey that was designed to measure directly symptoms associated with a common vergence problem, convergence insufficiency. The CISS is a 15 item survey that uses a 4-point scale to quantify the severity of symptoms and yields scores that range from 0 to 60. (See Table 2-1) The CISS has been researched extensively and has been shown to be reliable, valid, and sensitive to changes following treatment of CI.[7-11] Thus, we recommend using the CISS to evaluate symptoms in children and adults with visual skills deficits.

The CISS can be used for determining whether the patient's symptoms are abnormal and to monitor changes in symptoms following treatment. A score of 16 or higher for children (ages $\geq$ 9 years) and 22 or higher for adults are considered a significant level of symptoms. For example, if a child has a score of 25 then he or she would be considered symptomatic. In addition, the CISS can help the practitioner determine whether a treatment for a visual skills deficit has made a significant difference in the patient level of symptoms. Using an effect size analysis the Convergence Insufficiency Treatment Trial group suggested that a change of 8 would be considered a clinical significant improvement.[8,9,12] For example, if a patient's CISS score changed from 30 to 21 then the improvement is considered significant. It should be remembered that the CISS assesses a broad range of symptoms and that the recommended criteria are not absolutes. Therefore, the clinician still needs to use his or her judgment when assessing symptoms in patients. For example, a patient may focus on a particular symptom, such as, blur occurring fairly often and not report other types of symptoms. In this case the CISS score may be in the clinically normal range but most practitioners would treat the primary complaint of blur.

MALADAPTIVE BEHAVIORS

Preschool and early elementary school children may have difficulty reporting visual symptoms, even in cases of frank visual dysfunction. We have found that children younger than 9 years of age often have difficulty reporting and quantifying symptoms. On careful examination, some are found to have significant dysfunctions by standardized clinical criteria but, when asked, they seldom admit to any vision problem. As observed in cases of early-onset myopia, in which reports of blurred vision are also rare, young children do not have a standard for comparison. They believe that what they are experiencing visually, for better or worse, is normal and expected. Children may also modify their behavior when they do encounter difficulties. With careful questioning of a child, parents, and teacher, the clinician often finds that the child compensates or maladapts by demonstrating avoidance behavior, a short attention span, and distractibility, and develops a dislike for the activity causing discomfort. In fact, a recent study found that parents reported significant avoidance

Table 2-1. Convergence Insufficiency Symptom Survey (CISS)

Doctor instructions: *Read the following questions and instructions to children (≥ 9 years of age) while he or she looks at the survey. Adults can read the instructions and questions to themselves.*

Patient instructions: *Please answer the following questions about how your eyes feel when reading or doing close work. First think about whether or not you have the symptom. If you do, please tell me whether the problem occurs: Infrequently (not very often), Sometimes, Fairly Often, or Always.*

		Never	Infrequently	Sometimes	Fairly often	Always
1.	Do your eyes feel tired when reading or doing close work?					
2.	Do your eyes feel uncomfortable when reading or doing close work?					
3.	Do you have headaches when reading or doing close work?					
4.	Do you feel sleepy when reading or doing close work?					
5.	Do you lose concentration when reading or doing close work?					
6.	Do you have trouble remembering what you have read?					
7.	Do you have double vision when reading or doing close work?					
8.	Do you see the words move, jump, swim or appear to float on the page when reading or doing close work?					
9.	Do you feel like you read slowly?					
10.	Do your eyes ever hurt when reading or doing close work?					
11.	Do your eyes ever feel sore when reading or doing close work?					
12.	Do you feel a "pulling" feeling around your eyes when reading or doing close work?					
13.	Do you notice the words blurring or coming in and out of focus when reading or doing close work?					
14.	Do you lose your place while reading or doing close work?					
15.	Do you have to re-read the same line of words when reading?					

behaviors in children with symptomatic convergence insufficiency.[13] To compensate for a binocular vision problem, a child might hold reading material very close to enlarge the print, shut or cover an eye with a hand, or lay his or her head on the upper arm to disrupt binocular fusion. Some children learn to hold the head up and turned to one side so that the nose can act as an effective occluder. Thus, the clinician should ask the child and parent about possible adaptations the child has made to compensate for the visual skills deficit in addition to a standardized symptom scale such as the CISS.

EDUCATIONAL HISTORY

Visual skills most commonly affect the child when reading and studying and this in turn can result in parents pursuing eye care for their child. Although, visual problems are very common disorders, there are several developmental disorders that affect the child's ability to read and study efficiently. The most common are learning disability, dyslexia and attention deficit hyperactivity disorder (ADHD). Learning disability is characterized by poor school achievement despite normal potential to learn. The most common area of difficulty is reading which is often accompanied by a specific difficulty in the decoding and encoding of individual words, i.e. dyslexia. Another co-morbid disorder ADHD is characterized by either significant hyperactivity or impulsivity or inattention. During the case history it is important to ask the parent about the presence of a learning disability, dyslexia or ADHD. The practitioner can often identify ADHD by medication usage and can identify a learning disability by asking the parent if their child has an ongoing Individualized Education Plan. If the practitioner suspects an undiagnosed problem a referral to a primary care physician or school psychologist may be warranted. If the practitioner wants to determine the reading level or specific deficits in coding language of the child, then the Decoding and Encoding Screening Test for Dyslexia (DESD) can be administered. (See Appendix B.)

VISION SKILLS AND READING

Do visual skill deficiencies adversely affect reading performance? Does vision therapy for visual skill dysfunctions result in improved comfort, reading efficiency, and reading performance on standardized tests? These are important and somewhat controversial questions. The American Academy of Ophthalmology and the American Academy of Pediatrics drafted a position statement denying any relationship between visual conditions (save uncorrected refractive error) and reading disabilities. The implication is that vision therapy is ineffective and a waste of remedial time.[14] This statement is ambiguous in that the term "reading disability" can be interpreted to mean dyslexia, a neurologically based disorder in word decoding, or it can be interpreted to mean any significant reading problem from other causes. The American Academy of Optometry, in collaboration with other optometric organizations, have issued their own position statement arguing that several visual conditions aside from refractive error are associated with poor reading performance and not necessarily dyslexia.[15]

Furthermore, vision therapy is a recognized and effective therapeutic intervention for improving or curing vision efficiency dysfunctions. In cases in which such therapy is applied, improved reading performance often occurs. However, vision therapy techniques for visual skill deficiencies are not intended to cure language based reading disability such as the dyseidetic or dysphonetic types of dyslexia.[16] Both vision specialists and the public at large need authoritative information on these issues, due to the obvious important implications for school vision screening and because of the serious social concern regarding improving students' reading performance across the nation.

Many studies have sought an association between visual conditions and reading performance. As one might expect, these studies vary considerably in their subject groups, tests of reading and vision, and quality of research design and analysis. One statistical approach used to evaluate a large number of studies with varying design features is called meta-analysis. Simons and Gassler[17] used this technique in evaluating the results of 32 controlled studies that used valid tests for vision conditions and reading performance. Good reading performance was found to be associated with uncorrected myopia. The tested students, as a group, read better than did emmetropic students requiring no spectacle correction. In uncorrected myopia, the farpoint of accommodation (the punctum remotum) resides at a near distance, so less accommodative effort is required for reading. Distant vision is impaired, but the eyes are optically in focus at some near distance if the amount of nearsightedness is approximately equal in each eye and is not severe. In contrast, poor reading has been associated with uncorrected hyperopia (i.e., farsightedness). In these cases, hyperopes must use accommodative effort to bring a distant image into clear focus on the retina, thus requiring additional and often excessive accommodation to clear print at the preferred reading distance. These facts suggest that the amount of accommodative effort is associated with poor reading performance—a relationship that we found in our clinical experience.

As part of the meta-analysis, Simons and Gassler[17] found several other conditions associating disorders of fusion with poor reading: Among poor readers, there was a high prevalence of (1) anisometropia, in which different refractive errors in the two eyes presented an obstacle to binocular integration of the images; (2) aniseikonia, in which different image sizes in the two eyes posed as an obstacle to fusion; (3) excessive exophoria and hyperphoria, eye teaming conditions that stress fusion skills; and (4) fusional vergence deficiency or restricted vergence skills. The common feature among these conditions is emphasis on an individual's sensory fusion capacity and vergence system, which keeps the eyes in alignment for nearpoint tasks. Asthenopia and quick visual fatigue usually are the consequences. This association with poor reading skills implies that the symptoms or maladaptive behaviors are severe enough to influence reading progress, although a direct causal relationship has not been established.

Adults with symptoms of visual discomfort have shown poorer reading skills. Conlon et al[6] found a correlation of 0.71 between measures of visual discomfort and reading rate. Grisham et al[2] have found a significant, although weak, correlation between reading test scores and the number of visual symptoms that college students reported. Generally, the more symptomatic the students were, the poorer was the reading performance, and vice versa.

TESTING FOR VISUAL SKILLS

Following the case history, assessment of VS should include both sensory and motor functions of the eyes. We recommend testing of the following systems: (1) saccades, (2) pursuits, (3) position maintenance, (4) accommodation, and (5) vergences (aside from accommodation). Sensory fusion and stereopsis are the final goals of accurate and efficient binocular alignment of the eyes; hence, they should be included in a comprehensive evaluation (see Chapter 5). The remaining portion of this chapter will review assessment of eye movements and accommodation. Testing for non-strabismic vergence disorders will be discussed in Chapter 3.

RANKING VISUAL PERFORMANCE

Tests of visual skills vary in recommended pass and fail criteria, but a standard scoring system is desirable. Griffin[18] reported a common 5-point scale for most visual skills, where each visual skill function can be ordinally ranked from 5 (best) to 1 (worst), with semantic differential descriptions (Table 2-2). Such a ranking system is convenient when comparing strengths and weaknesses among various visual skills. It allows for better understanding and communication to patients and interested third parties (e.g., the patient's health insurance company). This is but one of many possible ways that a practitioner can convert other scoring systems for saccades into a 5-point scale for ordinal ranking.

We have based our ranking system for most tests assuming that values are normally distributed within the population. This applies to most, but not all tests of visual skills. When the population data is available and scores are normally distributed within the population the 1 to 5 ranking system will be based comparing the standard deviation to the mean of the normative sample. A score of 1 or very weak, means the finding is less than or equal to 1 standard deviation below the mean and would be considered dysfunctional in most

Table 2-2. Ranking Visual Performance

Rank	Description
5	Very strong
4	Strong
3	Average
2	Weak
1	Very weak

cases. A score of 2 or weak corresponds to a value that is between 0.5 standard deviations below the mean and 1 standard deviation below the mean and should be considered in the borderline category and may warrant further investigation by the practitioner. A score of 3 or average corresponds to a value that is within 0.5 standard deviations above and below the mean. Scores of 4 or 5 are strong or very strong and usually indicate a healthy system.

SACCADIC EYE MOVEMENTS

Symptoms and Differential Diagnosis

The first differential diagnostic issue for consideration is whether a pathologic etiology is present when deficient saccadic eye movements are found. If voluntary versions are severely restricted, the clinician should suspect neurologic problems affecting the saccadic pathway, such as myasthenia, vascular disease, or tumors that may affect supranuclear control. Other signs of neurologic dysfunctioning would likely be evident in such cases. Many times, however, only subclinical "soft" signs are present, with the patient appearing to be normal in all other respects. Many patients have functional saccadic problems, such as those from poor attention, hyperkinesis, or poor visual acuity due to uncorrected refractive errors, and possibly because saccadic skills never developed adequately.

What are the symptoms of either organic soft-sign or functional saccadic dysfunctioning? Several performance problems may be evident if saccadic eye movements are poor, even though the patient is otherwise considered neurologically normal. Inefficiency in reading is a major problem and is frequently reported in such cases. Words may be omitted, lines may be skipped, or loss of place may occur often during reading. "Finger reading" may indicate the need for hand support due to poor eye movements. Head movement when reading is another common sign of poor saccades. The patient may present with a history of "having

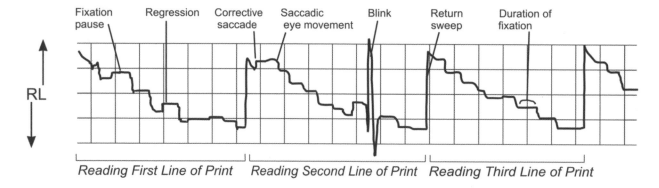

Figure 2-1. Recording of reading eye-movement patterns taken from a photoelectric Eye Track. This illustrates the characteristics of eye movement patterns during reading. From Grisham D, Simmons H: Perspectives on reading disabilities. In Rosenbloom AA, Morgan MW, editors: Pediatric optometry, Philadelphia, 1989, Lippincott.

trouble hitting the ball" or "doing poorly in many athletic events." Job performance may be affected adversely if eye-hand coordination is exceptionally poor due to saccadic eye movement problems.

Saccadic Eye Movements and Reading

Due to the fact the accurate saccades are required for effective reading it is important to understand the basic principles affecting eye movements when reading. Upon entering school the child is faced with different demands on the eye movement system. In preschool the visually based activities include building puzzles, coloring, and block play. In elementary school, learning to read requires smaller and more accurate saccadic eye movements than tasks in the preschool years.[19] An illustration of saccadic eye movement when reading is shown in Figure 2-1. Eye movements during reading are characterized by a series of rightward saccades, which are called "forward fixations." When the end of the line is reached, a large leftward saccade, or return sweep, of about 10 degrees returns the eye to the beginning of the line. This may be accompanied by a small corrective saccade if the return sweep was not accurate. A small leftward movement of the eye is a regression that occurs approximately 5% to 20% of the time.[20] On each fixation, or pause, the fovea processes the linguistic infor-

mation while the retinal periphery directs future saccadic eye movements. The length of time that the eye pauses during a fixation is called the "duration of fixation." The amount of reading material that is processed during a fixation pause is the span of recognition.

In the elementary school years reading eye movements show a steady improvement.[21,22] The number of forward fixations and regression show a sharp reduction from grades 1 to 4. After this point, the decrease is more gradual (Table 2-3). There is also an accompanying increase in the span of recognition and reading rate during this period. Why do young children show an increased number of fixations and regressions when reading? There are probably two principle factors: underdeveloped oculomotor control and limited linguistic processing skills. Before starting school, children have little experience generating the types of eye movements that reading requires. Therefore young children would be expected to have difficulty programming a sequence of small saccades. To test this hypothesis would require measuring eye movement patterns to targets that simulate eye movement patterns made when reading. In this approach the child does not have to comprehend specific text but simply scans a series of targets. Gilbert[19] investigated the ability

Table 2-3. Developmental trends in reading eye movements

Grade	1	2	3	4	5	6	7	8	9	10
Fixations (including regressions) per 100 words	224	174	155	139	129	120	114	109	105	101
Regressions per 100 words	52	40	35	31	28	25	23	21	20	19
Average span of recognition (in words)	0.45	0.57	0.65	0.72	0.78	0.83	0.88	0.92	0.95	0.99
Average duration of fixation (in seconds)	0.33	0.30	0.28	0.27	0.27	0.27	0.27	0.27	0.27	0.26
Rate with comprehension (in WPM)	80	115	138	158	173	185	195	204	214	224

From Taylor EA. The Fundamental Reading Skill. Springfield, ILL: Charles C. Thomas, 1966.

of children in grades 1 through 9 to fixate on a series of digits. The results indicate that fixation and regression patterns in this task are similar to those found in reading. Younger children showed an increased number of fixations and regressions, both of which declined with age.

The ability to process semantic and syntactic information is also a factor that contributes to poorer eye movements in younger children.[20] Improvement in linguistic processing would result in a reduced number of fixations and regressions because the child is better able to process the meaning of the text. That is, eye movement patterns during reading, to a large extent, reflect the ability to understand the reading material. However, this theory does not fully account for the developmental changes in oculomotor control found by studies having children scan a series of letters or numbers that simulate reading.[19,23] When assessing saccades as related to reading it is important to minimize the cognitive and linguistic demands of the test being administered.

In real life situations saccadic eye movements are integrated with the vergence system and both saccadic and vergence eye movements are observed. The integration of saccadic and vergence systems appears to be poorer in children.[24, 25] For example, Yang and Kapoula[25] assessed the binocular coordination of saccades in children and adults. The subjects looked between targets at either a 150 cm or 20 cm distance and made horizontal saccades of 10 or 20 degrees. The study found that binocular coordination of saccades was particularly poor at near for children and could compromise single vision. Children did not reach adult-like levels until 10 to 12 years of age. In addition, a recent study suggested that some poor readers have poor binocular coordination when reading that would adversely impact eye movements occurring during reading.[26] Thus, it is important to diagnose and treat disorders in the vergence system in cases of saccadic dysfunction.

Objective Testing

Clinicians should evaluate saccadic eye movements using both gross and fine tasks. Fine saccades are those involved in reading (approximately 7 degrees or less). Larger saccades than these are considered gross. A patient's saccadic eye movement skills can be evaluated either on an objective or a subjective basis.

Any target, such as small letters on two pencils, can be used to test for gross saccadic ability. The patient is asked to look voluntarily from one target to the other. This usually is done in right- and left-gaze orientations, but vertical as well as oblique orientations can be tested. If one of the patient's eyes is occluded, testing is for saccadic ductions. If both eyes are open, testing is for saccadic versions. It should be noted that even behind an occluder, the covered eye moves conjugately with the uncovered, fixating eye. A difference may be noted, however, in the performance of one eye as compared with the other during duction testing. This possibility is an important consideration in therapy, as the patient should, if possible, have equal saccadic skills in both eyes.

Gross saccades are used in general environmental scanning to direct fixation to a point of interest. They can be initiated by reflex stimuli or by volition, so both stimulus modes can be employed in screening. Because reading requires finer control of saccades than is sampled by such screening tests, these procedures are more appropriate for evaluating saccadic skill in general scanning and in sports performance. The patient is asked to stand free of support in front of the clinician and is instructed to participate in a penlight game: "Look only at the light that is on, not at the light that is off." The clinician then holds two penlights approximately 10 cm apart at a distance of 40 cm from the patient. Directing the beams away from the patient's eyes, the doctor alternately flashes the lights in a random pattern to elicit "reflex" saccades. The patient wins the game if he or she does not make a mistake and look at the "off" light through 10 randomized cycles. Most children, age 6 and older, who follow a normal developmental pattern can complete this task with three or fewer errors, show good saccadic accuracy, and exhibit minimal head and body movement. Children having attentional difficulties often cannot play this game successfully. Children in whom oculomotor coordination development is immature and adults having neurologic conditions show saccadic undershoots or overshoots and excessive head and body movements.

"Voluntary" (volitional) saccades are sampled in a similar way. Still standing, the patient is instructed to look back and forth from one light to the other 10 times and as quickly as possible; both lights are now on. The clinician counts aloud as the patient performs the task. Observations indicating immature or defective voluntary control of saccadic fixation include (1) inaccuracy of saccades (undershoots and overshoots); (2) multiple intervening saccades; (3) slow alternation (longer than 2 seconds per cycle); (4) lack of rhythm in the alternating pattern of fixation; (5) motor overflow, indicated by facial movements, particularly jaw and eye brow movements; and (6) excessive head and body movements (greater than a few degrees). This screening test is quite good at identifying those school-aged children who have immature oculomotor skills and who have not made the developmental shift from making predominantly head movements to eye movements. Immature gross saccadic tracking is a prodromal sign of tracking difficulties in reading and writing. However, just because a child shows good gross saccadic maturity does not necessarily mean that tracking for reading material is also adequate to the task. Furthermore, we have seen deficient gross saccadic tracking even as reading eye movements appear to be normal, although this finding is infrequent.

Southern California College of Optometry System 4+ System

A quick and simple routine used at the Southern California College of Optometry (SCCO) for testing horizontal saccadic eye movements is as follows: A target with a letter printed on it that is approximately equivalent to 20/80 (6/24) acuity demand is placed to the patient's right side. A similar target is placed to the patient's left. The targets are separated by approximately 20 cm and are held at a distance of 40 cm from the patient. (In the past, 25-cm separation was recommended, but separation greater than 20 cm is not always feasible without the need for some head movement.) The patient is asked to move his or her eyes alternately to each target approximately 10 times. The clinician should look for inaccuracies (i.e., either undershooting or overshooting). Scoring the results of observation is on a 4+ basis, as follows: 4+ if movements are accurate, 3+ if there is some undershooting, 2+ if there is gross undershooting or any overshooting, and 1+ if there is either inability to perform the task or an increased latency. A score of 2+ or less

is considered failing, as would be any uncontrolled head movement.

Hoffman and Rouse[27] considered a failure on this basis to indicate a need for referral for vision therapy for saccadic dysfunctioning. Whether or not referral is actually made, failure of the SCCO test, which demonstrates poor saccadic skills, should alert the practitioner at least to consider the possibility of advising vision therapy. In other words, clinical judgment is required; referrals for vision therapy are not automatic merely on the basis of a single poor test result.

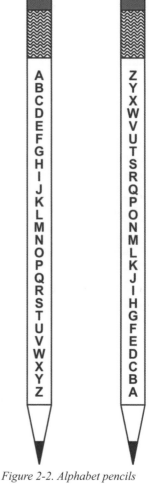

Figure 2-2. Alphabet pencils

Two alphabet pencils may be used in the manner described earlier (Figure 2-2). However, the young child cannot be expected to proceed all the way through the alphabet; rather, the patient should be allowed to read the "A" on each pencil. For an adult, one pencil can be turned to expose the Z, Y, X sequence; such a task is demanding and checks for false reporting as the patient looks from one alphabet pencil to the other. This is because verbalizing the alphabet in reverse sequence without seeing the letters is difficult (see Figure 2.2).

The NSUCO Oculomotor Test

Dr. W. C. Maples[28] has produced, in our opinion, the best standardized and normed set of oculomotor tests based on the clinician's gross observations. The testing protocol and scoring are too elaborate to be presented here, but the test is available from the Optometric Extension Program Foundation. Maples' system comes with an instructional videotape that contains many fine examples of children displaying dysfunctional, but not pathologic,

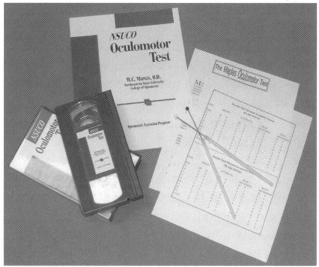

Figure 2-3. The NSUCO Oculomotor Test

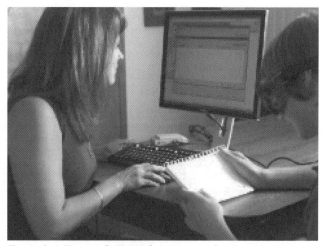

Figure 2-4. Visagraph. View of examiner and examinee wearing goggles to detect eye movements. (Reprinted with permission from Bernell Corp.)

oculomotor behavior. The saccadic test involves rating of gross reflex saccades across the midline in response to the tester's commands.(Figure 2-3) Observations are made of the basic ability to perform the test, accuracy of saccades, and rating of collateral head and body movements. The patient's eight scores are compared with normative data for boys and girls between the ages of 5 and 14+ years; the norms indicate that girls mature faster than boys in these visual skills. According to Dr. Maples, the oculomotor norms for 14-year-olds are adultlike. Inter-rater and test-retest reliability seem acceptable. Interestingly, oculomotor behavior on this test, particularly head and body movement, was found to discriminate between good and poor readers.[29] The authors recommend minimal acceptable scores by age and sex for ability, accuracy, head movement, and body movement.

Ophthalmography (Visagraph and Read-Alyzer)

Advances in technology have provided relatively inexpensive instruments that can be used to record eye movements for a variety of tasks. This is in stark contrast to the older clinical ophthalmographic test for recording reading saccades such as the Eye-Trac. The newer instruments use spectacles containing infrared sensors and allow for head movements that will not interfere with recordings. The two instruments that are currently available are the The Visagraph III and the Readalyzer. Both instruments use similar technologies to record eye movements. (Figure 2-4) These instruments allow for recording eye movement during non linguistic

(such as: dots or numbers) or linguistic tasks (paragraph reading).

The Visagraph III is an infrared eye movement-recording systems used in conjunction with a personal computer for analysis of the eye movement record. Taylor Associates (see Appendix J) designed this instrument for clinicians and educators to evaluate an individual's eye movement characteristics during the act of reading standardized selections of print and for analysis of saccadic control independent of information processing. For the purpose of oculomotor evaluation, patients are asked to stare at a X target for 10 seconds and then alternately to fixate two separated X's for 15 seconds. The record then is evaluated for stability of fixation and saccadic accuracy (i.e., the number of fixations actually made during the test). No normative data are currently available, but gross disorders of fixation (e.g., nystagmus, saccadic intrusions, and lapses of visual attention) can be identified by the computer analysis of the fixation record or by direct inspection of the original graph.

For evaluating sequential saccades (as used in reading) independent of information processing, several lines of digits are presented on a test card (see Figure 2-5). This is called the Visagraph Numbers Test. The patient (or student) is instructed as follows: "Look at each and every number as rapidly as possible as if you were reading a book. Don't say anything, however, even to yourself. Don't miss any numbers; and move from one to the next as quickly as you can." After the test is given, the computer eye movement profile and the original graph can be inspected relative to several

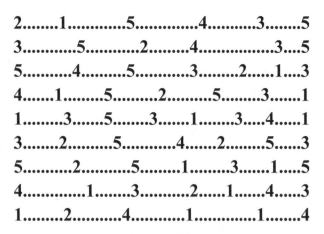

```
2........1.............5..............4............3........5
3.............5.........2.........4..................3...5
5.........4..........5...........3.........2......1...3
4.......1.........5..........2.........5.........3......1
1.........3.....5.........3......1.........3....4......1
3.........2..........5..............4......2..........5.....3
5..........2..........5.......1.......3......1....5
4.............1.......3..........2.....1......4......3
1.........2...........4.............1...............1........4
```

Figure 2-5. The numbers test used with the Visagraph. The purpose is to assess binocular and tracking accuracy. (Courtesy of Taylor Associates.)

detailed oculomotor indices of performance: excessive number of fixations, number of regressions, prolonged average duration of fixation, rate in targets per minute, saccades in return sweeps, and cross-correlation of the two eyes, a possible measure of vergence accuracy (Figure 2-6). Although normative data have not been published to date, Taylor Associates offer clinical guidelines for evaluating oculomotor performance of children and adults.

In an interesting study, Lack[30] compared the Visagraph Numbers Test (VGN), a temporally (timed) scored test, to the Test of New York State Standards which measures students' mastery of English Language Arts (ELA). The most significant correlation was the VGN fixation duration to three of the ELA scores (range: 0.277 to 0.343). These values,

while statistically significant (at the 0.05 level) are small to moderately significant on a clinical level.[31] Although this study measured eye movements in children, the study did not correlate the Visagraph reading paragraph individual measures and grade equivalent score with the ELA test.

Some practitioners advocate having the child read paragraphs to see if the fixation and regression patterns are at an age appropriate level. In this approach the practitioner has the child read a passage at his or her independent or instructional reading level and determines whether the eye movement patterns are consistent with the reading level of the child (see Chapter 16 for detailed explanation). For example, a fifth grade child may have a third grade reading level and would in turn be asked to read a third grade passage on the Visagraph or ReadAlyzer. If the eye movement recordings show fixation or regression patterns that are below third grade then a saccadic dysfunction is suspected. However, if the eye movement patterns are at third grade or higher then no oculomotor deficit would be suspected. One criticism of this approach is that the grade level of the passage chosen may have words that the child cannot decode accurately and this would disrupt the eye movement pattern.

An alternative to the Visagraph is the ReadAlyzer which also objectively measures eye movements. One advantage of this instrument is that longer stories are available. This may be beneficial in cases where the clinician suspects that ocular fatigue is reducing performance over time (see

Numbers Profile Visagraph version 4.1

	Left	Right
Fixations/100 numbers	164	164
Regressions/100 numbers	36	38
Av. Duration of Fixation (sec)	0.28	0.28
Rate (numbers/min)		130

Directional Attack	23%	Countable lines in text	7
Rate adj. for Rereading (numbers/min	281	Lines found	6
		Saccades in Return Sweeps	10
Cross correction	0.990	Anomalies (Fix/Regr/Both)	1/1/0
Name: Test Numbers		Recorded: 11/29/99 09:39	
Class: Sex: M	Grade: 1	Text: 1–0–0.txt	
School:		Title: Numbers	
School:			
Comment:			

Figure 2-6. Example of computerized results of the numbers test.

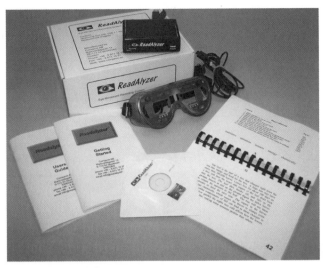

Figure 2-7. ReadAlyzer

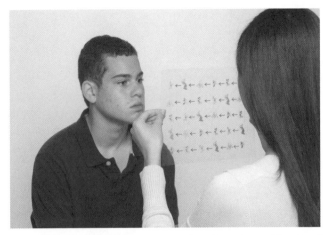

Figure 2-8. Sequential fixation test using clear sheet with printed symbols.

Figure 2-7). If this is the case then it is easy to show the patient or parent the reduction in performance over time.

Sequential Fixation Tests

Another reading saccade test that is objective but much less sensitive than the Visagraph or the Read-Alyzer is the use of printed cards, such as the five-dot test, for which the clinician directly observes a patient's eye movements to evaluate dot-to-dot saccades. These sequential fixation tests come in a variety of forms. The dots (or other symbols such as asterisks, stars, numbers, letters, and words) may be printed on a clear acetate sheet so that the clinician can look directly at the patient's eyes through the printed sheet to observe inaccuracies and head movements (Figure 2-8). Another variation is an opaque card on which the symbols are printed and in which a center hole allows the clinician to observe the patient's eye movements. Obviously, in such a test, assessment of saccadic ability must be performed quickly, as there is no permanent printout for later analysis. Judgments are strictly qualitative and lack precision. Notwithstanding these drawbacks, experience goes a long way in making this procedure useful in the event that either the Visagraph or Read-Alyzer is not available at the time of testing. Sequential fixation tests are colloquially called a "poor person's ophthalmograph." The practitioner can increase clinical acumen with this simple testing procedure by comparing results with those obtained by ophthalmograph recording instruments. In addition, this method can be quite helpful when evaluating patients who have had traumatic brain injury.

Subjective Testing

Saccades may also be evaluated indirectly by subjective means rather than directly by objective observations. The older subjective tests of sequential saccades include the Pierce and King-Devick tests. Both tests require the child to name a series of laterally displaced numbers with varying levels of difficulty. However, both tests suffer from the problem that the child's verbal naming rate can confound the results. That is, the child may fail the test because they have deficit in verbal retrieval of number names and not a deficit in the programming of sequential saccades.

Developmental Eye Movement Test

The Developmental Eye Movement (DEM) Test by Richman and Garzia further refined the indirect approach to assessment of saccadic eye movements.[32] The DEM test is designed to evaluate both accuracy and speed of fine saccades, as in the act of reading. The principal difference between the older test and the DEM is that a subtest of number naming in a vertical array is included in the DEM test, presumably to determine a patient's rapid automatized naming (RAN) ability (Figure 2-9). As to the vertical columns, the DEM test manual states: "This becomes a test more heavily dominated by the individual's visual-verbal automatic calling skills (automaticity)" (see Appendix J for DEM source information). A horizontal array of numbers is provided, except the horizontal dimension is slightly reduced (to simulate usual reading demands) and the quantity of numbers is increased to 80 digits in the DEM test. This added demand is designed to assess ability for sustained performance (stamina).

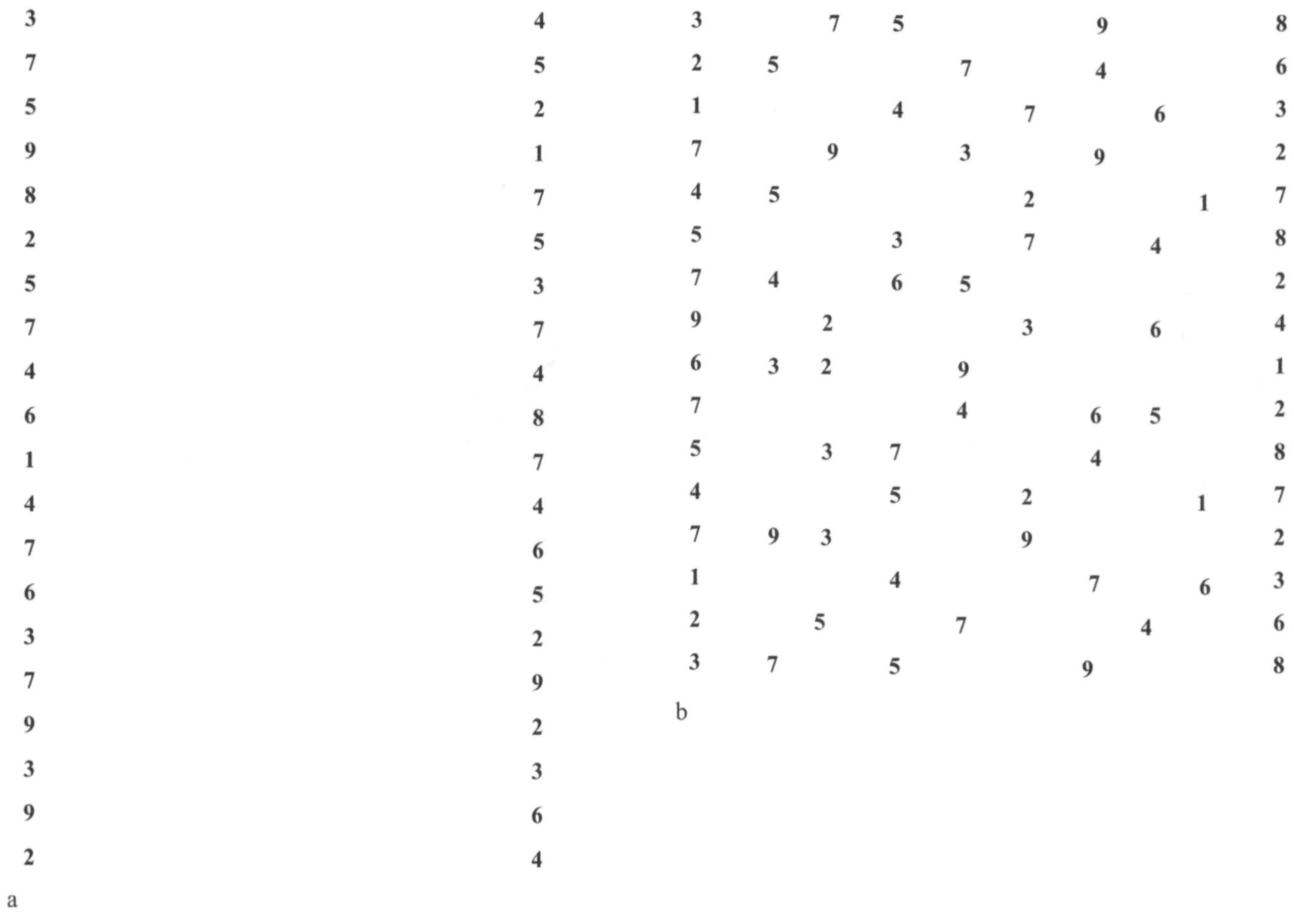

```
3   4        3   7 5       9       8
7   5        2 5       7   4       6
5   2        1       4   7   6   3
9   1        7   9     3   9       2
8   7        4 5           2     1 7
2   5        5       3   7   4     8
5   3        7 4   6 5           2
7   7        9   2       3   6   4
4   4        6 3 2   9           1
6   8        7         4     6 5   2
1   7        5     3 7       4     8
4   4        4       5     2     1 7
7   6        7 9 3       9         2
6   5        1       4     7   6 3
3   2        2   5     7         4 6
7   9        3 7   5       9       8
9   2
3   3      b
9   6
2   4

a
```

Figure 2-9. Developmental Eye Movement Test showing (a) vertical array of numbers and (b) horizontal array of numbers. Similar to the Pierce test, the Developmental Eye Movement Test uses a formula to determine "adjusted" time: Adjusted time = test time x 80/(80 - O + A), where test time = actual time for number calling on the horizontal array; O = omission errors; and A = addition errors (numbers either being repeated or added).

Visual stamina and attention in performing saccadic tests have been found to be important factors in distinguishing those students who fail the DEM test and those who pass.[33] More errors were made in the second half of the horizontal test by the failing students.

Similar to the Pierce test, the DEM test uses a formula to determine "adjusted" time:

Adjusted time = test time x 80 / (80 - O + A)

where test time is the actual time for number calling on the horizontal array, O represents omission errors, and A indicates addition errors (numbers being either repeated or added).

The essence of the DEM test is to compare the test results of vertical time with horizontal time. Four outcomes are possible:

1. Both the vertical time and the adjusted horizontal time are normal. This is considered normal performance.

2. The vertical time is normal but the adjusted horizontal time is abnormally increased. This indicates "oculomotor dysfunction" and, presumably, poor horizontal fine saccadic eye movements.

3. Both the vertical time and the adjusted horizontal time are abnormally increased but are approximately the same. This indicates a problem in automated number calling rather than a saccadic deficiency (i.e., RAN problem).

4. Both the vertical and horizontal times are abnormal, but the horizontal is much worse. This indicates both a RAN problem and a saccadic eye movement deficiency.

In evaluating symbol tracking using the DEM test, both the speed of tracking (the ratio index) and accuracy (the number of additions and omissions) must be considered. Normative data are provided for subjects 6-13 years of age. Children should have a good knowledge of numbers 1-9, which most do by age 6 years. However, attention skills and ability to deal with detail seem to be lacking in many 6-year-old children. Therefore, we recom-

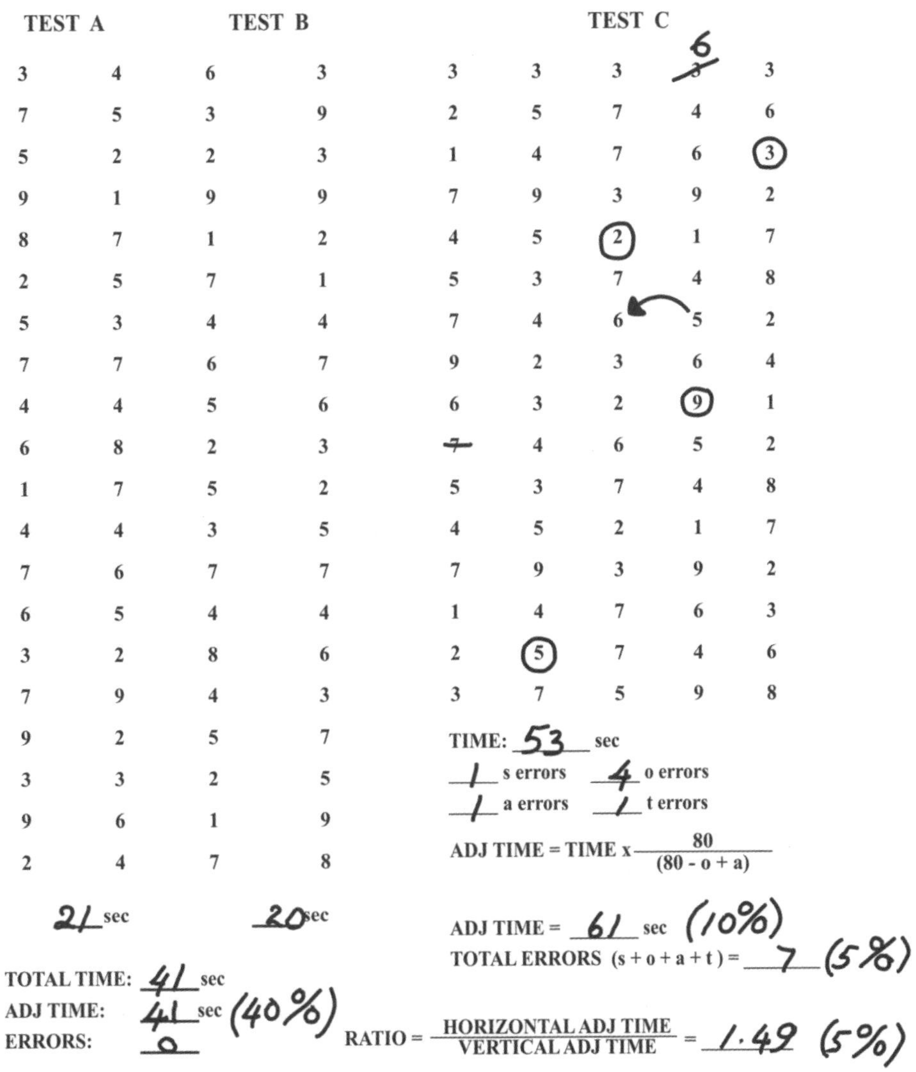

TEST A   TEST B   TEST C

TEST A		TEST B		TEST C				
3	4	6	3	3	3	3	6/5	3
7	5	3	9	2	5	7	4	6
5	2	2	3	1	4	7	6	(3)
9	1	9	9	7	9	3	9	2
8	7	1	2	4	5	(2)	1	7
2	5	7	1	5	3	7	4	8
5	3	4	4	7	4	6←5		2
7	7	6	7	9	2	3	6	4
4	4	5	6	6	3	2	(9)	1
6	8	2	3	7̶	4	6	5	2
1	7	5	2	5	3	7	4	8
4	4	3	5	4	5	2	1	7
7	6	7	7	7	9	3	9	2
6	5	4	4	1	4	7	6	3
3	2	8	6	2	(5)	7	4	6
7	9	4	3	3	7	5	9	8
9	2	5	7					
3	3	2	5					
9	6	1	9					
2	4	7	8					

TIME: __53__ sec

__1__ s errors   __4__ o errors

__1__ a errors   __1__ t errors

$$\text{ADJ TIME} = \text{TIME} \times \frac{80}{(80 - o + a)}$$

ADJ TIME = __61__ sec (10%)

TOTAL ERRORS (s + o + a + t) = __7__ (5%)

$$\text{RATIO} = \frac{\text{HORIZONTAL ADJ TIME}}{\text{VERTICAL ADJ TIME}} = \underline{1.49}\ (5\%)$$

__21__ sec   __20__ sec

TOTAL TIME: __41__ sec

ADJ TIME: __41__ sec (40%)

ERRORS: __0__

Figure 2-10. Example of results from a 10-year-old patient who passed the vertical subtest of the Developmental Eye Movement Test (36% or higher is passing) but failed as to errors (5%), horizontal time (10%), and ratio (5%). This suggests poor saccadic eye movements but reasonably good automaticity.

(Figure 2-10 shows an example of DEM test results for a patient, with percentile ranks for vertical and horizontal tests, ratio, and errors.) We have presented a 1 to 5 ranking scheme for the DEM based on the percentile rank of the child's performance (see Table 2-4).

The results of the DEM should be correlated with patient symptoms. A recent study by Tassinari[36] using a retrospective analysis of charts showed that children with low DEM scores reported more symptoms related to eye movements disorders and the disorders tended to persist over time when not treated. However, a recent study by Ayton et al[37] did not find significant differences in scores on the CISS in children who passed or failed the DEM.

mend that such subjects be asked to complete only half the vertical and horizontal tests and that the examiner then double the times and errors before applying the normative analysis. Furthermore, the DEM test is too difficult for most kindergartners.[34] Nonetheless, the DEM test, specifically the ratio index, can be used reliably with Spanish- as well as English-speaking students.[35]

Accuracy can be evaluated by noting the pattern of errors a child makes. Whole lines skipped or added usually reveal saccadic inaccuracy. Omission errors within a line of numbers also suggest inaccuracy, but verbal errors can also explain additions, transpositions, and substitutions (e.g., miscalling a 9 for a 6). The clinician must use judgment when evaluating saccadic accuracy rather than relying entirely on the total error norms listed in the test manual.

The practitioner should be somewhat cautious when interpreting DEM results due to studies that have found only good to fair reliability for this test. For example, a study by Rouse et al[38] found that the vertical and horizontal scores had good reliability but the ratio score had poor reliability and the ratio score could vary up to +/- 0.39.

Table 2-4. Ranking of Saccadic Performance on the Developmental Eye Movement Tests

Description	Results for Ratio or Error Score
Very strong	86th to 99th percentiles
Strong	69th to 85th percentiles
Average	32nd to 68th percentiles
Weak	17th to 31nd percentiles
Very weak	0 to 16th percentiles

The validity of the DEM as an indirect measure of saccadic eye movements has been called into question. Ayton et al[37] compared performance on the DEM to objective measures of eye movements, visual processing and reading. The researchers found no significant correlations between any component of the DEM test and quantitative eye movement parameters including gain, latency, and corrective saccades. However, there were significant correlations between DEM and tests of reading and visual processing speed. The highest correlations were found between the horizontal sub-test and reading and a test of visual processing. The authors argue that the horizontal sub-test may be a measure of visual processing and cognition and not a direct measure of eye movements. Thus, the DEM test may be more appropriate for measuring visual processing as related to reading and not a direct measure of saccadic functioning. We hope that future studies will provide more valid techniques for measuring functional deficits in fine saccades.

Summary of Saccade Testing

The clinician should attempt objective testing of saccadic eye movements even when electro-ophthalmography (e.g., Visagraph or Read-Alyzer) is not available. This can be accomplished, for example, with the SCCO 4+ system or the NSUCO Oculomotor Test. When subjective and indirect assessment is performed, the DEM test accounts for deficiencies in RAN skill, which must be distinguished from poor saccadic skills. Unless the RAN is known, the practitioner is unable to ascertain whether poor horizontal saccades are due to RAN problems or are due to actual saccadic deficiencies. It is desirable to convert scores into a ranking system so that there is a common denominator for each visual skill function. We propose a 5-point ordinal ranking system that is easy to understand and convenient for patient communication purposes.

Most of the testing procedures described in this section are appropriate for patients 7 years and older. Some children between the ages of 5 and 6 are able to respond to some of these tests, but in patients younger than 5 years, the clinician must rely on gross and objective methods, such as the SCCO 4+ system.

PURSUIT EYE MOVEMENTS

Symptoms and Differential Diagnosis

A pursuit eye movement is defined as a "movement of an eye fixating a moving object."[39] Pursuits are a form of duction eye movements when only one eye is being tested (monocular viewing conditions), whereas binocular viewing conditions allow for testing of pursuit versions. (Versions, as with ductions, may be saccades, pursuits, or nonoptic eye movements.) Regardless of the fact that an eye may be occluded, the covered eye moves conjugately with the fixating eye under most normal circumstances.

Defective pursuit eye movements, seen in many elementary school children, may be attributable to lack of development (immaturity), lack of experience (untrained), or lack of attention. In many cases, pursuit exercises seem appropriate and effective in remediating this oculomotor dysfunction. Inattentive children may benefit also from vision therapy, but other treatments maybe necessary. In adults, however, the absence of smooth pursuit tracking is predominantly an indication of neurologic dysfunction. Deficiencies in pursuits, for example, have been found in patients experiencing schizophrenia,[40,41] cerebellar degeneration,[42] Parkinson's disease, and many other neurologic degenerative conditions. Interestingly, Thaker et al[40] reported poorer predictive pursuits in schizophrenic subjects than in normal control subjects, even when effects of antipsychotic medications were taken into account.

There may be neurologic "soft signs" in the case of jerky pursuits. Problems may be so subtle that no lesion can be found (by radiology or other means) along the occipitomesencephalic pathway. In some cases, functional training techniques may help. In many others, however, not much can be done to improve pursuits when a neurologic organic etiology exists. Nevertheless, differential diagnostic testing should be considered. For example, assume a patient has normal voluntary saccades but pursuit movements that are significantly restricted and jerky: A supranuclear lesion affecting the occipitomesencephalic pathway would be suspected. In contrast, if saccades are inaccurate and restricted but pursuits are normal, a frontomesencephalic pathway lesion is suspected.

It is always wise to check both pursuits and saccades on a routine basis, not only to determine gross organic defects but to detect subtle problems that can handicap individuals because of resulting inefficiencies of vision. Additionally, drugs, fatigue, emotional stress, and test anxiety may adversely affect pursuit performance. For example, we have examined many children with reading difficulties in whom we found a "midline hesitation" during confrontation pursuit testing using a penlight, although no irregularity in pursuit function was found using laboratory electronic tests. On follow-up clinical testing, our initial findings were repeatable. This mystery was solved when we discovered that if we moved to the patient's side, the "hesitation" also moved toward that side. The children evidently were making eye contact with the examiner, possibly because of being apprehensive in the clinical testing environment. This example points out the importance of distinguishing between true pursuit dysfunction and poor tracking induced by inattention, lack of cooperation, or test anxiety.

Patients who have poor ocular pursuit skills may also have histories of various inefficiencies. Poor readers may have poor pursuits, although the cause-and-effect relationship is not as great as with saccadic dysfunction and poor reading. Reading road signs from a moving vehicle would present problems in a case of poor pursuit skills. Patients with poor pursuit eye movements also tend to have significant problems participating in sports. It is conceivable, for example, that tracking a tennis ball accurately would be much more difficult if head movements were necessary, because the gross neck muscles are not as efficient as the finely tuned extraocular muscles. However, we saw a patient who had Duane retraction syndrome involving both eyes, which severely restricted ocular activity. This patient reported being able to play tennis "fairly well," despite the fact that head turning was necessary for the patient to see the approaching ball. Therefore, statements relating to pursuit skills and athletic skills should be made with caution and with other factors (e.g., athletic prowess) kept in mind.

Testing of Pursuit Skills

As was the case for saccadic testing, the SCCO 4+ system and the NSUCO Oculomotor Test are both appropriate for testing pursuit eye movements.

Southern California College of Optometry System 4+ System

A quick and convenient testing and rating system for pursuits on a 4+ scale is used at SCCO.[27] A fixation target approximately the size of a 20/80 (6/24) letter is moved in front of a patient at a distance of approximately 40 cm to extents of nearly 20 cm from primary gaze. The target is moved left-right-left (one cycle), up-down-up (one cycle), and in two diagonal orientations (one cycle each), as in the lines of a British flag, with the patient being instructed to track the target (Figure 2-11). A 4+ is given if pursuits are smooth and fixation is always accurate, 3+ if there is one fixation loss, 2+ if there are two fixation losses, and 1+ if there are more than two fixation losses. The patient is considered to have pursuit problems if the score is 2+ or less. If there is any obvious head movement during testing after the patient has been instructed not to move the head, performance is considered to be inadequate. The right eye, the left eye, and then both eyes should routinely be tested for pursuits by eye care practitioners, whether by this or another method. However, the SCCO method lends itself to testing of patients of all ages, including infants and young children.

NSUCO Oculomotor Test

The NSUCO Oculomotor Test[28,29] evaluates the ability to perform two clockwise and counter clockwise rotations while fixating a colored bead.

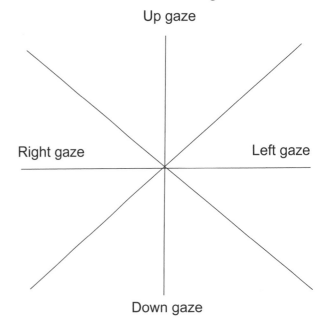

Figure 2-11. British flag pattern from clinician's view (lines indicating movements of penlight) for testing pursuits with the Southern California College of Optometry 4+ test.

The examiner looks for noticeable re-fixations for pursuits and whether the patient needs to use head movements to accomplish the pursuit. The testing is done binocularly at 40 cm or the Harmon distance (distance from the patient's middle knuckle to the elbow). Observations are made of the basic ability to perform the test, accuracy of pursuits, and rating of collateral head and body movements. The patient's scores are compared with normative data for boys and girls between the ages of 5 and 14+ years; the norms indicate that girls mature faster than boys in these visual skills. Inter-rater and test-retest reliability seem acceptable. The authors recommend minimal acceptable scores by age and sex for ability, accuracy, head movement, and body movement.

Summary of Pursuit Testing

Clinical assessment is important for identifying neurologic problems and dysfunctional visual tracking (particularly relevant to sports performance). The SCCO 4+ test or the NSUCO Oculomotor Test is recommended for assessment of pursuits in routine cases. Pursuit tests should usually include monocular (duction) as well as binocular (version) testing. Functional and organic causes should be differentiated. Some patients may require "diagnostic therapy" to determine whether the identified problem abates as a result of vision training.

Because pursuits are mainly involuntary and many of the neurologic soft signs are likely incurable, one must ask how functional training techniques might help patients with pursuit problems. As mentioned previously, the testing procedures for pursuits encompass some voluntary aspects (e.g., head movement, automation, and stamina). These aspects can be improved and made more reflexive, starting from volition and progressing to automation. In many cases, accuracy and smoothness are improved as a result of functional training techniques. In patients in whom the pursuit problem is of functional etiology (e.g., due to inattention), the prognosis for improvement is favorable.

FIXATION

Symptoms and Differential Diagnosis

Fixation (known also as position maintenance) involves all four eye movement systems—saccades, pursuits, nonoptic (e.g., VOR) system, and vergences. Fixation evaluation usually is accom-

plished toward the beginning of an eye examination (e.g., during the unilateral test). Assessment is made as the patient fixates on a target in primary gaze.

True position maintenance is actually a misnomer, in that very small movements are occurring all the time during so-called steady fixation: The eyes are not motionless during fixation. Ocular micromovements consist of rapid flicks and slow drifts of very small amplitude that are not observable without special equipment. These small movements are believed to be useful for the purpose of correcting fixational errors, to keep the fixated target precisely on the fovea, and possibly preventing retinal adaptation (fatigue).

Position maintenance can be assessed by asking the patient to fixate (monocularly) on a target. There should be no noticeable drifting or eye movement from the target of regard. If the patient cannot maintain steady fixation, he or she should be instructed to hold a thumb at 40 cm to determine whether the proprioceptive input from the "hand support" is helpful in maintaining steady eye positioning. The problem may persist (e.g., due to congenital nystagmus). If the problem is psychological (e.g., lack of attention) or from other known causes (e.g., fatigue or drug effects), improvement of position maintenance often is possible through appropriate environmental changes and the efforts of functional training techniques.

The vast majority of patients show steady fixation ability with each eye. Unsteady fixation of one eye can be seen in some cases of amblyopia or decreased monocular visual acuity from other causes. Saccadic intrusions are unconscious, rapid, bidirectional flicks of fixation off a target and back on. These intrusions may be a presenting sign of a neurologic disorder. They look like square-wave, to-and-fro "darting" movements of the eyes on attempted fixation. Small saccadic intrusions, from 1 to 5 degrees, can be seen in the elderly; in patients with dyslexia, strabismus, or schizophrenia; and in patients who are extremely fatigued. However, larger saccadic intrusions, 5 to 20 degrees, can be associated with degenerative conditions such as multiple sclerosis.

Southern California College of Optometry 4+ System

The SCCO 4+ system is a quick and easy test for position maintenance.[27] The patient is instructed to fixate a target approximately the size of a 20/80 (6/24) letter E at a distance of 40 cm. The left eye is occluded for testing of the right eye; afterward, the left eye is tested and, then, binocular testing is undertaken. Testing time is at least 10 seconds per eye. The quality of steadiness is assessed as follows: 4+ if steady for at least 10 seconds, 3+ if steady for at least 5 seconds, 2+ if steady fewer than 5 seconds or if hand support is needed, and 1+ if fixation is unsteady almost continuously. A 2+ or 1+ is considered failing as criteria for possible referral.

Summary of Fixation Testing

An ophthalmographs instrument such as the Visagraph is desirable for assessment of position maintenance. When this is not practical, as in very young children, a quick objective test, such as the 4+ system for direct observation, is recommended. Therapy to improve position maintenance is discussed in Chapter 16.

Vestibulo-Ocular Reflexes

The eyes maintain gaze on a target with rotation of the head through the neurologic control of VOR. Head position and acceleration are sensed by the semicircular canals and otolith apparatus and are communicated to the oculomotor centers in the midbrain. The effect of this process is that a head movement in any direction is accompanied by an equal and opposite eye movement, thus stabilizing the eyes relative to a target. Vestibulo-ocular, neck, and body reflexes combine with optokinetic reflexes to stabilize the retinal image as an individual moves through the environment. Developmental disorders of VOR tracking are relatively rare; most deficiencies are acquired by trauma or neurologic disease.

A complete assessment of VS should include a screening of VOR tracking. The patient is directed to hold gaze on a discreet fixation target at far or near, while either he or she moves or the clinician gently moves the patient's head up and down for several cycles at the rate of 1 cycle per second. This procedure then is repeated moving the patient's head from side to side—the so-called "doll's-head" maneuver. Smooth tracking is the rule. The presence of either saccadic intrusions ("catch-up" saccades) or nystagmus indicates a failure in VOR tracking and should be further assessed. In children, intervening saccades may indicate simply lapses of attention to the task, which should be taken into consideration.

Further assessment can include challenging VOR tracking through head shaking that is greater than 1 cycle per second. Immediately after 10 to 15 seconds of head shaking by the patient in the vertical or horizontal plane, the practitioner should look for nystagmus using a magnifier or ophthalmoscope. Another technique is to measure binocular visual acuity before and during head shaking, both horizontal and vertical. Snellen visual acuity should not decrease more than one line (e.g., 20/20 to 20/25) during head shaking if there is good VOR tracking. Patients having signs or symptoms of a VOR disorder should be referred for further neurologic testing.

MANAGEMENT OF DEFICITS IN SACCADES & PURSUITS

The management of functional deficits in saccades and pursuits is through vision therapy. Although, there has not been extensive research looking at the effectiveness of treating eye movement problems, our clinical experience, indicates that many cases respond well to treatment. In Chapter 16 a comprehensive treatment strategy is presented for treating dysfunctions of both saccades and pursuits

ACCOMMODATION

Symptoms and Differential Diagnosis

Functional disorders of accommodation are common in clinical practice and can be separated into four types of problems: (1) insufficiency, (2) excess, (3) infacility, and (4) ill-sustained accommodation (poor stamina). Patients can present with an accommodative dysfunction that falls into any one or all of these categories, as the categories are not mutually exclusive. In fact, many patients who can be described as having an accommodative insufficiency also show signs of infacility and poor stamina. Two additional categories of accommodative dysfunction are (5) unequal accommodation and (6) paresis or paralysis of accommodation. The etiology of these last two disorders is not functional. In cases of accommodative dysfunction stemming from neurologic disease or trauma, patients are best served by a prescription

Table 2-5. Possible Causes of a Reduction of Accommodation

Functional etiology
Binocular: deficient accommodation due to biological variation in the population, excessive nearpoint work, low illumination, low oxygen level, ocular and general fatigue or stress, vergence problems.
Monocular: strong sighting-eye dominance resulting in poor accommodation in the nondominant eye

Refractive etiology
Binocular: manifest and latent hyperopia, myopes who do not wear spectacles at near, pseudomyopia, premature and normal presbyopia
Monocular: uncorrected anisometropia, poor refractive correction, unequal lens sclerosis

Ocular disease
Binocular: internal ophthalmoplegia, bilateral organic amblyopia, premature cataracts, bilateral glaucoma, iridocyclitis, ciliary body aplasia, partial subluxation of lens
Monocular: same as for binocular condition, but affecting one eye more than the other, anterior choroidal metastasis, trauma, rupture of zonular fibers

Systemic diseases or conditions affecting binocular accommodation
Hormonal or metabolic: pregnancy, menstruation, lactation, menopause, diabetes, thyroid conditions, anemia, vascular hypertension, myotonic dystrophy
Neurologic: myasthenia gravis, multiple sclerosis, pineal tumor, whiplash injury, trauma to the head and neck, cerebral concussion, mesencephalic disease, including vascular lesions
Infectious: influenza, intestinal toxemia, tuberculosis, whooping cough, measles, syphilis, tonsillar and dental infections, encephalitis, viral hepatitis, polio, amebic dysentery, malaria, herpes zoster, many acute infections

Drugs, medications, and toxic conditions affecting binocular accommodations
Residual effects of cycloplegic drops, alcohol neuropathy, marijuana, heavy metal poisoning, carbon monoxide, botulism, antihistamines, central nervous system stimulants, large doses of tranquilizing drugs (phenothiazine derivatives), parkinsonism drugs, many other systemic medications

Emotional, usually binocular: stress reactions, malingering, hysteria

for reading glasses rather than vision training.[43] The first four categories described above do not imply an organic etiology, as they often arise from functional causes (e.g., deficient physiology, overwork, or inattention). Besides describing the characteristics of an accommodative dysfunction, the clinician must determine, insofar as possible, the specific etiology and must seriously consider the many nonfunctional factors (Table 2-5) before the condition is assumed to be functional in origin.

Symptoms of accommodative dysfunction are typically somatic, perceptual, or performance related. Common complaints include asthenopia, eye fatigue, blur, and reduced performance with extended near work.[44-46] Because the symptoms of accommodation dysfunction often overlap with vergence disorders, we recommend using the CISS to quantify the frequency and severity of symptoms associated with a dysfunction in accommodation. In our experience, the four types of accommodative deficits are not associated with a unique symptom pattern.

A review of accommodative conditions and appropriate testing follows. We have divided the accommodation testing and conditions into two broad categories based on the tests used for diagnosis and diagnostic strategy. Testing and diagnosis for accommodative insufficiency and excess are discussed first and then the testing the accommodative facility and accommodation ill-sustained are discussed second.

TESTING OF ACCOMMODATION
Absolute Accommodation

The amplitude of accommodation is measured monocularly using the push-up method for one eye and then the other. This is absolute accommodation. The print size should be equivalent to 20/20 (6/6) at 40 cm, or smaller or larger depending on the patient's maximum visual acuity. The maximum farpoint visual acuity lenses with most plus power (also called CAMP lenses [corrected ametropia most plus]) should be worn for testing. If the patient does not give reliable responses, the clinician should move the target from near to far by starting at the spectacle plane and pushing it away until the designated line of print is read aloud correctly. Then testing reverts to the push-up method until first blur is reported. This technique is the method-of-adjustment (method-of-limits) research technique, referred to as bracketing in clinical parlance.

Table 2-6 is an abridged table of the amplitude of accommodation according to age.[47] A formula to calculate the minimum expected amplitude of accommodation was introduced by Hofstetter.[47] The minimum amplitude is calculated as $A = 15 - 0.25(x)$ where x is the patient's age in years. For example,

TABLE 2-6. Donders' Table of Amplitude of Accommodation

Age (yrs)	Amplitude (D)
10	14.0
20	10.0
30	7.0
40	4.5
50	2.5

TABLE 2-7. Ranking of Accommodative Amplitude

Rank	Description	Amplitude
5	Very strong	1.00 D or more above average
4	Strong	0.50 D above average
3	Adequate	Average for age
2	Weak	2.00 D below average
1	Very weak	4.00 D or more below average

if a patient is 10 years old, the expected amplitude is 15 -0.25(10), or 12.5 D. An amplitude of only 8.5 D in the right eye would be very weak, as this is 4 D below average. Table 2-7 gives accommodative ranking. The Hofstetter formula may not hold true for very young children because their clinically measured amplitudes are often lower than would be predicted theoretically.[48, 49] In a recent study, Sterner et al [49] measured amplitude of accommodation in a group of children ages 6 to 10 years of age. They found that the measured value was 3.5 diopters less than predicted by Hofstetter's expected amplitude formula (18.5 – 0.3 [age]). In addition, 50 percent of children failed to meet Hofstetter's minimum expected formula. Practitioners should consider this when testing children younger than 10 years of age and we recommend using 2 diopters below the minimum expected formula as the initial criteria for determining whether the amplitude of accommodation is weak.

An alternative approach for measuring the amplitude of accommodation is the minus lens technique. In this test, a reduced Snellen target is placed at 40 cm and minus lenses are introduced monocularly in 0.25 increments until the patient notices sustained blur. This technique typically results in lower amplitudes of accommodation (1 to 4 D) when compared to the push up test described above. Two factors may help to explain the lower amplitude; 1) minification of the near target with increasing lens power and 2) a lack of proximal cues to the accommodative system. In a recent study Anderson et al[48] measured the minus lens amplitude of accommodation objectively using an open field auto-refractor in children and adults. The results showed that minus lens measured amplitude of accommodation is stable in children with a mean value of 7 D up to almost 20 years of age.

The reliability of measuring the accommodative amplitude has been investigated in children and adults. Rouse et al[50] evaluated the within and between session reliability of the accommodative push up test for measuring accommodative amplitude. Each examiner measured accommodative amplitude three times at session 1 and then the child returned one week later and the tests were repeated. This method allowed evaluation of both within session (same day) and between session (one week later) reliability. The within session repeatability was good to excellent for the push up test. However, the 95% limits of agreement for the between session reliability, showed that the amplitude of accommodation could vary up to +/-5 D. Measures of repeatability in adults have tended to show better reliability when compared to children. Rosenfield and Cohen[51] measured accommodative amplitude over five sessions separated by a minimum of 24 hours, in 13 adult subjects and found 95% limits of agreement of approximately +/-1.5 D. A recent study compared the reliability of the push up and minus lens methods of measuring the accommodation in young adults.[52] The 95% limits of agreement for the push up test were similar to the Rouse et al findings with values varying up to +/-4 D. In contrast, the minus lens method showed 95% limits of agreement of +/-2.5 D which was significantly better than the push up method.

Relative Accommodation

Another form of accommodative insufficiency is that of poor positive relative accommodation (PRA). Positive relative accommodation is tested with minus-power lenses to first sustained blur under binocular viewing conditions at 40 cm while the patient looks through CAMP lenses for baseline reference. The patient is instructed to maintain clearness and singleness while looking at a designated line of letters (20/20 [6/6] equivalent or smaller if visible) as the plus or minus lens stimulus is increased (Table 2-8). The rate of stimulus increase is approximately every 3 seconds in 0.25-

Table 2-8. Ranking of Relative Accommodation (in which Dioptric Powers Represent the First Sustained Blur)

Rank	Description	PRA (-) and NRA (+)
5	Very strong	>2.50 D*
4	strong	2.25 D
3	Adequate	1.75-2.00 D
2	Weak	1.50 D
1	Very weak	<1.50 D

NRA = negative relative accommodation; PRA = positive relative accommodation.

*The clinician should be skeptical of an NRA finding exceeding +2.50 D at a 40-cm testing distance. If NRA exceeds +2.50 D, the patient maybe over-minused or there is latent hyperopia (i.e., corrected ametropia most plus [CAMP] lenses not being worn). Theoretically, 40 cm is the farpoint (optical infinity) with +2.50-D lenses. The patient's vision should be blurred when +2.50-D power is exceeded. CAMP lenses, therefore, are absolutely necessary for reliable baseline clinical data.

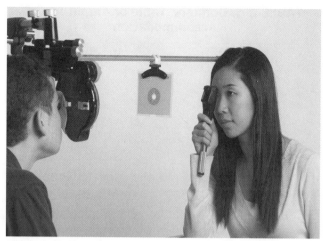

Figure 2-12. Nott method of dynamic retinoscopy to measure lag of accommodation.

D steps. A momentary blur is allowed. Approximately 5 seconds should be allowed to determine whether the blur is sustained. The PRA recording represents the first sustained blurpoints. Failure on the PRA test is a sustained blur for 5 seconds with lens powers weaker than -1.75 D (relative to CAMP lenses). In other words, passing requires clear and sustained vision with -1.50 lenses. Clinicians should bear in mind that relative accommodation often is limited by deficient vergence ranges. For example, an esophoric patient with a high accommodative convergence-accommodation ratio and with poor fusional divergence will likely have a reduced PRA (see Chapter 3).

In contrast to the PRA, the negative relative accommodation (NRA) is tested with plus-power lenses to first sustained blur under binocular viewing conditions at 40 cm. while the patient looks through CAMP lenses for baseline reference. The test is done in a similar manner to the PRA test described above. Failure on the NRA test is a sustained blur for 5 seconds with lens powers weaker than +1.75 D (relative to CAMP lenses). In other words, passing requires clear and sustained vision with +1.50 lenses. Clinicians should bear in mind that relative accommodation often is limited by deficient vergence ranges. For example, an exophoric patient with a low accommodative convergence-accommodation ratio and with poor fusional convergence will likely have a reduced NRA. Table 2-8 presents the 1 to 5 ranking scheme for PRA and NRA.

Lag of Accommodation

Although it does not necessarily imply insufficient amplitude of accommodation, lag of accommodation can be thought of as a clinical form of accommodative insufficiency for a particular nearpoint target. Accommodative lag can also be thought of as accommodative inaccuracy, just as fixation disparity can be considered to be an inaccuracy in vergence. Lag of accommodation can be measured in several ways, but two of the most reliable clinical methods are described here.

Nott Method

The Nott dynamic retinoscopy method is based on the linear difference between the fixation distance (usually 40 cm) and the distance of the retinoscope from the patient. This distance is converted into diopters to determine the accommodative lag.[53] The patient fixates reading material at 40 cm (2.50-D accommodative stimulus) while retinoscopy is performed through a hole in a card (Figure 2-12). The clinician physically moves away from the patient until a neutralized reflex is observed, say, at 67 cm (1.50D accommodative response). The accommodative lag, according to the Nott method, would be 1.00 D in this example. This test is done while the patient is behind the refractor.

With the Nott method, the accommodative stimulus does not change, because the testing distance is kept constant, and no dioptric changes are made by the intervention of additional lenses. The nearpoint rod of the refractor can be used to measure directly the dioptric distance between the fixation distance and the retinoscopic neutralization distance (i.e., the distance representing the accommodative lag).

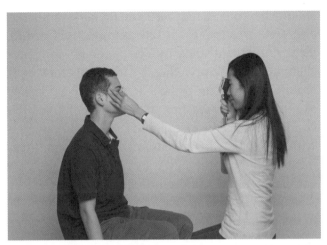

Figure 2-13. Monocular estimate method retinoscopy (dynamic) to assess accommodative accuracy (i.e., lag or lead of accommodation).

Monocular Estimate Method (MEM) Retinoscopy

When testing is performed outside the refractor, monocular estimate method (MEM) retinoscopy may be more convenient than the Nott method. The MEM is called "monocular" despite the fact that the patient has both eyes open and testing is conducted under binocular viewing conditions. The MEM of Haynes[54] is similar to the Nott method except that the retinoscopic distance is kept constant. This is often at the Harmon distance (distance equal to that from the tip of one's elbow to the middle knuckle of the clenched fist measured on the outside of the arm).[39] Distances, however, may vary, as the patient's habitual reading distance is recommended. The binocularly viewing patient is instructed to read appropriate material (for his or her age or cognitive level) mounted on the retinoscope. A trial lens is quickly interposed in the spectacle plane of one eye to neutralize the retinoscopic reflex (Figure 2-13). The lens is removed from the eye within a second, because latency of accommodation response is short. Tucker and Charman[55] found a mean reaction (latency) time of 0.28 second for one subject and 0.29 second for another. Therefore, the neutralizing lens must be quickly removed once it is introduced before an eye. The stimulus to accommodation might be changed if the lens is before the eye for a longer duration. The possibility of changing accommodative responses by changing accommodative stimuli must always be kept in mind when one is conducting the MEM test.

The lens power (addition of plus) necessary to achieve retinoscopic neutralization is the estimated accommodative lag of the eye being tested at the moment. If minus power should be required for neutralization, accommodative excess would be indicated.(see following section on Accommodative Excess)

Using the Nott or MEM procedure, we believe an accommodative lag of 1.00 D or greater is cause for further investigation. This concern was shared by Bieber.[56] A high lag of accommodation suggests the possibility of anomalies of insufficiency of accommodation, infacility of accommodation, and ill-sustained accommodation, any of which can be adverse factors in vision efficiency. Ranking of either Nott or MEM results is shown in Table 2.9. A rank of 2 or 1 is failing, and referral for vision therapy may be recommended.

In a study comparing Nott and MEM retinoscopy, Goss et al[57] looked at both the repeatability of each procedure as well as comparing Nott to MEM. The interexaminer repeatability showed little mean difference between examiners for either Nott or MEM and the 95% limits of agreement were +/- 0.17 for Nott and +/- 0.31 for MEM. When comparing Nott to MEM there the two methods agreed with each other, within 0.5 D, for 95% percent of cases. Thus, both Nott and MEM appear to be reliable measures of accommodative posture.

Insufficiency of Accommodation

The diagnosis of accommodative insufficiency is typically based on the assessment of the amplitude of accommodation, lag of accommodation, and relative accommodation. Patients diagnosed with accommodative insufficiency have difficulty with one or more tests that stimulate accommodation and will tend to have receded accommodative

Table 2-9. Ranking of Accommodative Lag (Insufficiency or Inaccuracy of Accommodation)

Rank	Description	Nott or MEM Retinoscopy Lag of Accommodation (OD or OS)
5	Very strong	+0.25 D
4	Strong	+0.50 D
3	Adequate	+0.75 D
2	Weak	+1.00 D
1	Very weak	+1.25 D or greater

MEM = monocular estimate method; OD = oculus dexter; OS = oculus sinister.

amplitude, weak relative accommodation, or high lag of accommodation.

In practice, the most prevalent cause of accommodative insufficiency is functional (i.e., a mismatch between a patient's physiologic accommodative capability and his or her work requirements). A study by Borsting et al[45] compared scores on the CISS with accommodative amplitude in school aged children ages 8 to 15 years of age. As the amplitude of accommodation receded the CISS scores increased. They concluded that a decrease in the amplitude of accommodation increases the risk of becoming symptomatic. In an attempt to clarify the diagnostic criteria for accommodative insufficiency in children, Sterner et al,[44] measured the accommodative amplitude in school aged and related the results to self-report of symptoms. The authors concluded that a monocular amplitude of accommodation of 8 D or less predicted the presence of symptoms in 90% of cases. Chrousos et al[58] described 10 detailed cases of healthy young people who reported intermittent blur at near. They demonstrated amplitudes of accommodation considerably lower than those expected for their respective ages (an average reduction of 6 D). No organic etiology for the diminished accommodation was suggested by history or could be identified by careful examination. All patients were successfully managed optically with bifocals or reading glasses, although three required the addition of base-in (BI) prisms because of exophoria at near.

Convergence insufficiency is commonly associated with accommodative insufficiency. Two recent studies have found the approximately 80% of children with CI had an associated reduction in the amplitude of accommodation.[45,59] Thus, the clinician should always evaluate the vergence system in children who have reduced amplitude of accommodation.

Management of Accommodative Insufficiency

Prior to treating a patient with AI, it is important to rule out latent hyperopia with cycloplegic refraction. Patients with AI respond well to plus lenses for reading by either correcting hyperopia or by prescribing additional plus lenses for near. In cases of fully corrected hyperopia or other ametropia, where the additional plus lens prescription creates distance blur, then a bifocal correction should be considered. Vision therapy is also an effective treatment for accommodative insufficiency. A recent study by Sterner et al[60] compared sham accommodative therapy to real therapy in 20 children. They used the NRA and PRA findings as the outcome measure. The results showed that children receiving accommodative facility therapy with a +/-2.00 flipper lenses showed a significant increase in both the NRA and PRA findings when compared to the children receiving sham therapy. A sequential approach to managing accommodative dysfunction is presented in Chapter 16.

Excess of Accommodation Characteristics

Another inaccuracy is accommodative excess, sometimes called spasm of accommodation, hyper-accommodation, hypertonic accommodation, or pseudomyopia. Accommodation may be excessive in focusing on a stimulus object or the patient may have difficulty relaxing accommodation. The same three tests, amplitude of accommodation, relative accommodation, and near point retinoscopy, can be used to diagnose an excessive accommodative response. In addition, the excessive accommodative response can be seen at distance and retinoscopy can identify this problem.

Latent hyperopia is another variation of accommodative spasm (i.e., accommodation fails to relax using noncycloplegic ["dry"] refractive techniques); cycloplegic ("wet") refraction may be indicated. Causes of spasm may be overstimulation of the accommodative system as a result of prolonged near work, emotional problems, focal infections, or other unknown etiologies. Numerous symptoms may be associated with accommodative excess, such as asthenopia, blurring of distant vision, headaches, diplopia (if excessive accommodative convergence is brought into play), and inefficient performance at nearpoint (e.g., a person may hold reading material at an exceptionally close range).

Maintaining or sustaining accommodation in the absence of a dioptric stimulus is another form of accommodative excess. This form is physiologic in that it is not abnormal for accommodation of approximately 1.00 D to be in play in a formless field, as in "night myopia." There is no specific training technique for night myopia; rather, the affected individual must become familiar with the set of circumstances in which the anomaly occurs and must make appropriate adjustments to it (e.g., temporarily wearing minus overcorrective lenses, if necessary, for nighttime driving).

Retinoscopy is necessary for reliable diagnosis of accommodative excess. Static retinoscopy with the aid of cycloplegia can determine ametropia (i.e., farpoint). At nearpoint, however, dynamic retinoscopy is important; cycloplegia must not be used in nearpoint testing. Either Nott or MEM dynamic retinoscopy can be used to determine whether there is a lag (i.e., insufficiency), but MEM is applicable for lead (i.e., excess) of accommodation. If accommodative response leads the accommodative stimulus by 0.25 D or more, we believe accommodative excess exists at that moment of testing. This observation should be verified on repeated testing. If -0.25 D is consistently required for neutralization, the patient is considered to have accommodative excess (Table 2-10).

Another form of accommodative excess is that of difficulty relaxing accommodation. This can be seen when doing the NRA test where the patient needs to relax accommodation as plus lenses are added binocularly in 0.25 D increments. The patient will have a low finding (below +1.50 D) in the absence of high exophoria or low positive fusional vergence.

Accommodative excess can also occur when excessive accommodative convergence is required to maintain fusion, as in patients with exophoria in whom positive fusional convergence is insufficient. Such a patient may overaccommodate in order to have sufficient accommodative convergence to maintain single (but blurred) vision.

Although objective means for determining accommodative accuracy (with Nott or MEM methods) are reliable, especially for young patients, subjective testing may also be performed. This can be accomplished with the binocular crossed-cylinder test at near. However, we do not believe this subjective method is as reliable as objective testing with either the Nott or MEM method.

Management of Accommodative Excess

As with accommodative insufficiency the management of excess cases can be vision therapy or optical management with plus lenses. However, with the tendency to over-accommodate, these patients may initially reject a plus lens correction for near work. We highly recommend trial framing the tentative

Table 2-10. Ranking of Accommodative Excess Using the Monocular Estimate Method of Retinoscopy

Rank	Description	Lens Power Indicating Lead of Accommodation
5	Very strong	+0.25 D
4	NA	NA
3	Adequate (borderline)	0.00 D
2	Weak	-0.25 D
1	Very weak	-0.50 D or greater

NA = not applicable.

prescription prior to dispensing spectacle lenses. Vision therapy is often a more effective treatment approach for patient with accommodative excess. A sequential approach to managing accommodative dysfunction is presented in Chapter 16.

Facility of Accommodation

Another aspect of accommodation is facility. An infacility of accommodation, also known as inertia of accommodation, is the inability to change focus rapidly. Accommodative infacility can cause discomfort and reduced vision efficiency. For example, such patients typically report slow clearing of vision, most often noting blurring when looking from the "book to the board." The standard testing procedure is to use ±2.00 D lenses. The recommended optotype is the equivalent of a 20/30 (6/9) line of Snellen letters at 40 cm while the lens power is changed from plus to minus, and so on, for 1 minute. Lenses are usually put in a flipper arrangement. Testing is done monocularly (OD then OS) and then binocularly. Suppression for the binocular assessment can be monitored with vectographic targets (Figure 2-14). Although clinicians may ask the patient to say "clear" with each stimulus change, a better technique is to instruct the patient to read each letter aloud as quickly as possible with the introduction of each lens flip. This allows monitoring of correct or incorrect responses. The number of accurate calls is recorded and converted into cycles per minute by dividing that number by 2. For example, if the number of correct calls for an eye is 8, there are 4 cycles per minute.

The standard flipper lens test is contaminated by a number of factors of which the clinician must be aware.[61] Because a patient verbally reports when a target appears to be clear, the measurement depends to some unknown extent on the speed or automa-

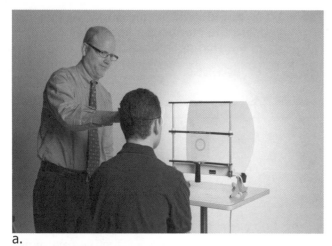
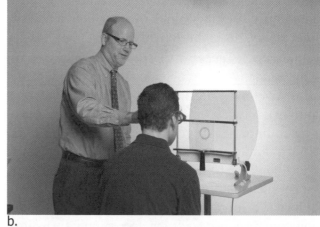

a.

b.

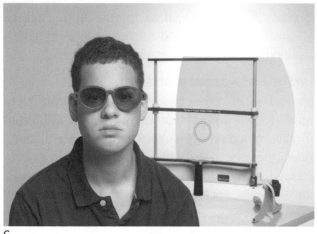
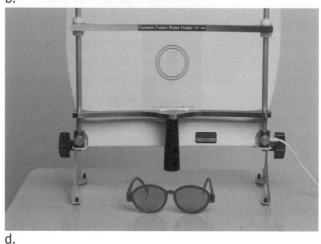

c.

d.

Figure 2-14. Accommodative facility testing: The test is performed at 40 cm with +/- 2.00 flipper lenses, a. Monocular testing; right eye is being tested in this figure, b. Binocular testing, c. View of crossed-polarizing filters worn by the patient, d. Vectographic target (Vectogram 9). Line 4 is seen by the left eye, line 5 by both eyes, and line 6 by the right eye.

ticity of verbal expression. The plus and minus lenses noticeably magnify and minify the optotype stimulus, possibly confounding the perception of blur. Furthermore, time and manual dexterity are involved in mechanically changing the lenses. Until better instrumentation is developed, the clinician should attempt to mitigate these factors when possible. For example, a patient can be instructed to ignore the apparent change in image size and to respond only when the optotype is perfectly clear regardless of size. The practitioner can also test the patient with a plano lens flipper and compare the performance to the +/- 2.00 flipper test to control for automaticity of verbal expression. The clinician should handle the lenses and flip the lenses in a consistent manner for each patient. Currently, normative data are available for most patients using the traditional lens flipper testing modality; the variance in norms from one study to another may be due in part to some of the factors just cited.

The reliability of the +/- 2.00 flipper test has been investigated in children by McKenzie at al[62] and Rouse et al[63] in children 8 to 12 years of age. One principle finding is a practice effect where the patient improves the rate of facility on the second session of testing. This practice effect may occur over a long time frame. In a recent study,[64] 22 adults were tested two times separated by 1 year and showed a significant improvement in accommodative facility at the second visit. Thus, the clinician may want to re-check the facility test in patient who fails the test to insure that the finding is repeatable.

A summary of norms of facility by several investigators is included in Table 2-11. Borish[47] stated that monocular accommodative facility, when tested at the patient's habitual nearpoint distance, should have a range of lenses from +1.50 to -2.00 D with clear vision, with the normal response time being less than 5 seconds.

Liu et al[65] suggested that the criterion for passing be 20 cycles per 90 seconds, allowing each cycle to take 4.5 seconds or each flip to last 2.25 seconds.

Griffin et al[66] studied monocular accommodative facility in 14 subjects ranging in age from 20 to 35 years. They found ±2.00-D rock to have an average value of 17 cycles per minute. The average response time to clear the minus lens was 2 seconds, whereas 1.4 seconds were needed to clear the plus lens.

Griffin et al[67] determined monocular facility as compared with binocular facility. They wanted to eliminate the possibility of guessing and ensure that patients were actually seeing clearly rather than reporting "clear" with each lens flipping. Instead of manually changed targets (which were double-digit numbers), an electrical mechanism introduced random numbers (of six-point type size at a distance of 40 cm) in synchrony with the lens flipper mechanism. Rock of ±2.00 D was conducted for 1 minute to determine the average number of cycles in a young adult population, ages 20-23 years. Monocular facility was approximately 17 cycles per minute. Binocular facility was approximately 13 cycles per minute, without monitoring of suppression. To monitor suppression, a vectographic plate was arranged so that the leftward (first) digit was seen only by the left eye and the right eye saw only the second digit. For example, the number 53 that appeared with the new lens change would be presented so that only the number 5 could be seen by the left eye and the number 3 by the right eye. There were only six cycles per minute as an average for this group of subjects when suppression was monitored. The investigators reviewed the 27 records of complete vision examinations and selected 16 subjects who showed evidence of poor visual skills and 11 who showed good visual skills. Monocular rock for the subjects with good visual skills averaged 18 cycles per minute, as compared with 15 cycles per minute for the subjects having poor visual skills. Binocular rock without suppression monitoring gave averages of 17 and 9 cycles per minute for the same two groups, respectively. When binocular rock was tested using suppression monitoring, there was an average of nine cycles per minute for the subjects with good visual skills but only four cycles per minute for those having poor visual skills. The authors concluded that binocular accommodative facility testing can be definitive in the assessment of a patient's binocular status.

Burge[68] used a practical clinical method to study binocular facility using suppression monitoring. He used a Spriangle Vectogram (see Appendix J) target with crossed polarizing viewers and ±2.00-D lens flippers. The mean value results were 12 cycles per minute monocularly, 10 cycles per minute binocularly without suppression monitoring, and 7 cycles per minute with suppression monitoring. Burge's value for monocular facility was lower than those obtained by Griffin et al[66,67] However, Burge[68] included younger subjects among his test group (ranging in age from 6 to 30 years). These findings are in agreement with Zellers et al.[69]

Grisham[70] and Pope et al[71] established monocular accommodative facility norms for elementary school children and validated these norms by objective accommodative testing. They tested second, fourth, sixth, and eighth graders using ±2.00-D flippers at 33 cm. The target was a 20/30 optotype, and each child was asked to report when the print appeared to "clear" with each lens. The norms proved to be the same for all children except for the second graders, whose responses were often inaccurate, presumably due to lapses of attention. Scheiman et al also found that younger children have difficulty with the facility task and suggested lower norms for younger children (see Table 2-11).[72] Grisham measured the time the subjects took to complete 10 cycles and 20 cycles on the test. Because no significant difference in cycles per minute was found, they recommended using 10 cycles for testing children age 8 years and older. The mean time was 52 seconds, with a standard deviation of 24 seconds. A unique feature of this study was the objective verification of the clinical procedure. The properties of accommodative facility (latency, velocity, and completion time) were objectively measured using a dynamic optometer in randomly selected subjects. The rank correlation between the clinical and objective measurements was high ($r = 0.89$), indicating good concurrent validity. (Other studies are shown in Table 2-11.)

There is no consensus on developmental norms from childhood to adulthood for accommodative facility. As to referral criteria for facility, Hoffman and Rouse[27] recommended the following: flipper test of ±2.00 D monocularly and binocularly

Table 2-11. Partial List of Norms for Accommodative Facility

Study	Results	Age Group
Burge[68]	±2.00 D; 12 c/min monocular; 10 c/min binocular; 7 c/min binocular, with suppression being monitored	Children and young adults
Griffin et al[66]	±2.00 D; 17 c/min monocular	Young adults
Griffin et al[67]	±2.00 D; 17 c/min monocular; 13 c/min binocular; 6 c/ min binocular, with suppression being monitored	Young adults
Liu et al[65]	±1.50 D; 20 cycles in 64 secs with 26 sec SD	Adults
Grisham et al[70] and Pope et al[71]	±2.00 D; 10 cycles in 52 secs with 24 sec SD	Children
Zellers et al[69]	+/- 2.00 D Monocular 11 c/m with 5 SD; binocular 7 c/m with 5 SD	Adults
Scheiman et al[72]	Monocular 6 years of age 5.5 c/m with 2.5 SD 7 years of age 6.5 c/m with 2.5 SD 8 to 12 years of age 7 c/m with 2.5 SD Binocular 6 years of age 3.0 c/m with 2.5 SD 7 years of age 3.5 c/m with 2.5 SD 8 to 12 years of age 5 c/m with 2.5 SD	Children

SD = standard deviation.

showing less than 12 cycles per minute, with the patient viewing a 20/30 line at 40 cm, or a difference of more than 2 cycles per minute between the two eyes. In light of the results shown in Table 2-11, these referral criteria may be too stringent, especially for young children. Retesting or lowered initial standards should be considered during the routine testing of new patients. We recommend the following cutoff criteria for failing such a test:[69] A subject is considered to be at risk for a dysfunction if monocular facility is less than 10 cycles per minute or if the difference between the eyes is greater than 2 cycles per minute; at risk also is recognized if binocular facility with suppression monitoring is less than 6 cycles per minute. A more definitive problem occurs when the monocular facility is 6 cycles per minute or less or when the binocular facility is 3 cycles per minute of less. Table 2-12 provides clarification and ranking of accommodative facility. These criteria do not apply to children younger than 8 years of age. Professional judgment must be used when evaluating accommodative facility in very young children.

An alternative to the +/- 2.00 flipper test is the amplitude based facility test proposed by Wick et al[73] who criticized the standard facility testing especially for adults because the test does not account for individual differences in accommodative amplitude. They proposed that the test distance should be 45% of the binocular amplitude of accommodation and the lens power range should be 33% of the binocular amplitude of accommo-

dation. For example a patient with an amplitude of 10 diopters would be tested at a distance of 22 cm with +/- 1.50 powered lenses. A study of 152 children ages 9 to 16 and 52 optometry students found a mean cycles per minute rate of 13 cycles per minute which was much higher than the 8 cycles/min found with the +/- 2.00 D flipper test. Additionally, the results showed that amplitude based was significantly better at differentiating symptomatic from asymptomatic in children and adults. However, the results did show that the +/- 2.00 binocular flipper test was able to differentiate between symptomatic and asymptomatic children. This confirms previous research that has found poorer correlation between symptoms and performance on the +/- 2.00 facility test, especially in adults.[73-75] We would recommend using the amplitude scaled facility measure in adult patients with suspected accommodative facility disorders.

Ill-Sustained Accommodation

Testing for ill-sustained accommodation is similar to that for facility of accommodation. Ill-sustained accommodation relates to stamina, or the power to endure fatigue.[76] It is easily detected in most routine accommodative facility testing, which is why clinicians should carry out facility testing over a period of at least 1 minute. Speed and sufficiency may be normal in the beginning but may be maintained only with effort and will decrease with time. The time during which stamina diminishes may be short, often within 1 minute. For example, a patient with ill-sustained accommodation may

TABLE 2-12. Ranking of Accommodative Facility with ±2.00 Diopters

		Cycles per Minute	
Rank	Description	OD or OS	Binocular*
5	Very strong	>18	>10
4	Strong	14-18	8-10
3	Adequate	10-13	6-7
2	Weak	7-9	4-5
1	Very weak	<7	<4

Suppression monitoring with vectographic targets.

Table 2-13. Ranking of Accommodative Stamina

Rank	Description	Monocular (secs)	Binocular (secs)*
5	Very strong	>108	>60
4	Strong	84-108	48-59
3	Adequate	60-83	36-47
2	Weak	36-59	24-35
1	Very weak	<36	<24

*Note: Testing is at the rate of 6 secs/cycle (i.e., 3 secs per each correct response) with ±2.00-D lenses. The cutoff point is designated as a response time exceeding 3 secs on any lens flip or whenever there is an incorrect response.
Suppression should be monitored using either anaglyphic or vectographic targets when binocular testing is done.

begin ±2.00-D lens rock quickly and sufficiently, but the responses may become inadequate after a few flips of the lenses. If the clinician tests for only one or two cycles, the patient's lack of accommodative stamina may not be discovered.

Ill-sustained accommodation can affect performance and result in various visual symptoms. Individuals vary widely in their ability to meet and sustain accommodative demands for a variety of reasons (e.g., physiologic variation, medication, visual demands, and general health). Clinical experience has shown, however, that accommodative stamina can be improved in most cases in which the cause is functional in nonpresbyopic patients. (Therapy is discussed in Chapter 15.)

For testing of accommodative stamina, we recommend using the ranking shown in Table 2-13. These are clinical empiric observations; fully researched norms await further reports. The clinician flips the lenses at a constant rate, 6 seconds per cycle. If this rate is maintained for 36 seconds under binocular conditions, the patient passes this recommended standard for accommodative stamina. Stability is emphasized, as opposed to frequency of correct calls as in facility testing. It is one thing to be fast

for a while but, in real life, an individual will not do well if he or she lacks stamina. This is as true for the accommodative system as it is for saccades, pursuits, and position maintenance (discussed previously).

If a patient meets the recommended criteria for accommodative facility testing with a consistently good rate of responses throughout the test, there is no need for stamina testing.

Management of Accommodatve Infaciltiy and Ill-Sustained Accommodation

Both accommodative infacility and ill-sustained appear to respond well to vision therapy in our clinical experience. If the patient is not good a candidate for vision therapy, then a plus add for near work is also a viable treatment option. Again, it is important to trial frame the tentative prescription to insure that the lenses help relieve visual discomfort prior to dispensing lenses. Bifocal corrections may be necessary in patients who have distance blur with the appropriate near correction. A sequential approach to managing accommodative dysfunction is presented in Chapter 16.

Summary

In this chapter we have emphasized visual skills diagnosis and management for eye movements and accommodative disorders. The first step is to conduct a comprehensive case history from the patient and of parents when examining children. We recommend using the CISS for quantifying the frequency and severity of symptoms associated with vision skills deficits. Testing for eye movements relies on the doctor's interpretation of eye movements for saccades, pursuits, and fixations. Testing for eye movements used in reading can be assessed objectively with newer eye movement recording systems or inferentially from the Developmental Eye Movement Test. The next vision skill assessed is accommodation. We recommend testing the amplitude or range of accommodation, relative accommodation, accommodative posture, and facility of accommodation. Based on these test results the practioner can make an appropriate diagnosis and treatment plan. In the next chapter we discuss assessment and management of nonstrabismic vergence disorders. This is the final phase of visual skills assessment.

REFERENCES

1. Revell MJ. Strabismus: A History of Orthoptic Techniques. In. London: Barrie and Jenkins, 1971.

2. Grisham J, Sheppard M, Tran W. Visual symptoms and reading performance. Optom Vis Sci. 1993;70:384-91.

3. Iribarren R, Fornaciari A, Hung G. Effect of cumulative near-work on accommodative facility and asthenopia. International Ophthalmology 2002;24:205-12.

4. Borsting E, Chase C, Ridder WH. Measuring visual discomfort in college students. Opt Vis Sci 2007;84: 745-51.

5. Farrar R, Call M, Maples W. A comparison of the visual symptoms between ADD/ADHD and normal children. Optometry 2001;72:441-51.

6. Conlon E, Lovegrove W, Chekaluk E, Pattison P. Measuring visual discomfort. Visual Cognition 1999;6:637-63.

7. Borsting E, Rouse M, Mitchell G, Schieman M, Cotter S, Cooper J, Kulp M, London R, CITT Group. Validity and reliability of the revised convergence insufficiency symptom survey in children ages 9-18. Opt Vis Sci 2003;80:832-38.

8. Scheiman M, Cotter S, Rouse M, Mitchell G, Kulp M, Cooper J, Borsting E, The Convergence Insufficiency Treatment Trial (CITT) Study Group. Randomised clinical trial of the effectiveness of base in prism reading glasses versus placebo reading glasses for symptomatic convergence insufficiency in children. Br J Ophthalmol. 2005;89:1318-23.

9. Scheiman M, Mitchell L, Cotter S, Cooper J, Kulp M, Rouse M, Borsting E, London R, Wensveen J, The Convergence Insufficiency Treatment Trial (CITT) Study Group. A Randomized Clinical Trial of Treatments for Convergence Insufficiency in Children. Arch Ophthalmol. 2005;123:14-24.

10. Borsting E, Rouse M, Deland P, CIRS group. Prospective comparison of convergence insufficiency and normal binocular children on the CIRS symptom survey. Optom Vis Sci 1999;76:221-8.

11. Rouse M, Borsting E, Mitchell G, Schieman M, Cotter S, Cooper J, Kulp M, London R, Wansveen J, (CITT) Study Group. Validity and reliability of the revised convergence insufficiency symptom survey. Ophthal and Physiol Opt 2004;24:384-90.

12. Convergence Insufficiency Treatment Trial (CITT) Study Group. Randomized clinical trial of treatments for symptomatic convergence insufficiency in children. Arch Ophthalmol.;126(10):1336-49.

13. Rouse M, Borsting E, Mitchell G, Kulp M, Scheiman M, Amster D, Coulter R, Fecho G, Gallaway M. Academic behaviors in children with convergence insufficiency with and without parent-reported ADHD. Optom Vis Sci. 2009:1169-77.

14. Policy statement. Pediatrics 1998;102:1217-19.

15. Vision, learning and dyslexia. J Am Optom Assoc. 1997;68:284-86.

16. Griffin J, Christenson G, Wesson M, Erickson G. Optometric Management of Reading Dysfunction. Boston: Butterworth-Heinemann, 1997.

17. Simons H, Gassier P. Vision anomalies and reading skill: a meta analysis of the literature. Am J Optom Physiol Opt. 1988;65:893-904.

18. Griffin J. Visual skills: ranking scores of clinical findings. Optom Monthly 1984;75:451-4.

19. Gilbert L. Functional motor efficiency of the eyes and its relationship to reading. Univ. of Calif publications in Education 1953;11(3):159-232.

20. Grisham D, Simons H. Perspectives on reading disabilities. In: Rosenbloom AA MM, ed. Principles and practices of pediatric optometry. Philadelphia: JB Lippincott, 1989.

21. Taylor E. The fundamental reading skill, 2 ed. Springfield: Charles C Thomas, 1966.

22. Taylor SE. Visagraph Eye Movement Recording System. Huntington Station, N.Y.: Taylor Associates, 1997.

23. Vurpillot E. The visual world of the child. New York: International Universities Press, 1976.

24. Fioravanti F, Inchingolo P, Pensioro S, Spanio M. Saccadic eye movement conjugation in children. Vision Research 1995;35:3217-28.

25. Yang Q, Kapoula Z. Binocular coordination of saccades at far and at near in children and in adults. J Vis 2003;3(8):554-61.

26. Bucci M, Bremond-Gignac D, Kapoula Z. Poor binocular coordination of saccades in dyslexic children. Graefes Arch Clin Exp Ophthalmol. 2008;246:417-28.

27. Hoffman L, Rouse M. Referral recommendations for binocular function and/or developmental perceptual deficiencies. J Am Optom Assoc. 1980;51:119-25.

28. Maples W. Oculomotor Test Manual. Santa Ana, Calif.: Optometric Extension Program Foundation, 1995.

29. Maples W, Atchley J, Ficklin T. Northeastern State University College of Optometry's Oculomotor Norms. J Behav Optom. 1992;3(6):143-50.

30. Lack D. Comparison of the Developmental Eye Movement Test, the Visagraph Numbers Test with a test of the English Language Arts. J Behav Optom 2005;16:63-7.

31. Hopkins W. A scale of magnitudes for the effect statistics. A new view of statistics. http://www.sportsci.org/resource/stats/effectmag.html, 2002.

32. Garzia R, Richman J, Nicholson S, Gaines C. A new visual-verbal saccade test: the Developmental Eye Movement Test (DEM). J Am Optom Assoc. 1990;61:124-35.

33. Coulter R, Shallo-Hoffman J. The presumed influence of attention on accuracy in the Developmental Eye Movement (DEM) test. Optom Vis Sci. 2000;77:428-32.

34. Kulp M, Schmidt P. The relation of clinical saccadic eye movement testing to reading in kindergartners and first graders. Optom Vis Sci. 1997;74:37-42.

35. Fernandez-Velazquez F, Fernandez-Fidalgo M. Do DEM test scores change with respect to language? Norms for Spanish-speaking population. Optom Vis Sci. 1995;72(12):902-6.

36. Tassinari J. Untreated oculomotor dysfunction. Optom Vis Develop 2007;38:121-4.

37. Ayton L, Abel L, Frick T, McBrien N. Developmental eye movement test: What is it really measuring? Optom Vis Sci 2009;86:722-30.

38. Rouse M, Nestor E, Parrot C, DeLand P. A reevaluation of the Development Eye Movement (DEM) test's reliability. Optom Vis Sci. 2004;81:934-38.

39. Hofstetter H, Griffin J, Berman M, Everson R. Dictionary of Visual Science and Related Clinical Terms, 5th ed. Boston: Butterworth-Heinemann, 2000. (Available from Richmond Products)

40. Thaker G, Ross D, Buchanan R, Adami H, Medoff D. Smooth pursuit eye movements to extra-retinal motion signals: deficits in patients with schizophrenia. Psychiatry Res. 1999;88:209-19.

41. Lee K, Williams L. Eye movement dysfunction as a biological marker of risk for schizophrenia. Aust N Z J Psychiatry 2000;34(suppl):S91-S100.

42. Moschner C, Crawford T, Heide W, et al. Deficits of smooth pursuit initiation in patients with degenerative cerebellar lesions. Brain Res. 1999;122:2147-58.

43. Russell G, Wick B. A prospective study of treatment of accommodative insufficiency. Optom Vis Sci. 1993;70:131 - 5.

44. Sterner B, Gellerstedt M, Sjostrom A. Accommodation and the relationship to subjective symptoms with near work for young school children. Opthal Physiol Opt 2006;26:148-55.

45. Borsting E, Rouse M, DeLand P, Hovett S, Kimura D, Park M, Stephens B. Association of symptoms and convergence and accommodative insufficiency in school-age children. Optometry 2003;74(1):25-34.

46. Daum K. Accommodative insufficiency. Am J Optom Physiol Opt 1983;60:352-9.

47. Borish I. Clinical Refraction, 3rd ed. Chicago: Professional Press, 1975.

48. Anderson H, Glasser A, Stuebing K, Manny R. Minus lens stimulated accommodative lag as a function of age. Optom Vis Sci 2009;86:685-94.

49. Sterner B, Gellerstedt M, Sjostrom A. The amplitude of accommodation in 6-10-year-old children- not as expected! Ophthalmol Physiol Opt 2004;24:246-51.

50. Rouse M, Borsting E, Deland P, CIRS group. Reliability of binocular vision measurements used in the classification of convergence insufficiency. Opt Vis Sci 2002;79:254-64.

51. Rosenfield M, Cohen A. Repeatability of clinical measurements of the amplitude of accommodation. Opthal Physiol Opt 1996;16(3):247-9.

52. Antona B, Barra F, Barrio A, Gonzalez E, Sanchez I. Repeatability intraexaminer and agreement in amplitude of accommodation measurements. Graefes Arch Clin Exp Ophthalmol. 2009;247:121-7.

53. Nott I. Dynamic skiametry: accommodation and convergence. Am J Physiol Opt. 1925;6:490-503.

54. Haynes H. Clinical observations with dynamic retinoscopy. Optom Wkly 1960;51:2306-9.

55. Tucker J, Charman W. Reaction and response times for accommodation. Am J Optom. 1979;56:490-503.

56. Bieber J. Why nearpoint retinoscopy with children? Optom Wkly 1974;65:54-7.

57. Goss D, Groppel P, Dominguez L. Comparison of MEM Retinoscopy & Nott Retinoscopy & Their Interexaminer Repeatabilities. J Behav Optom. 2005;16(6):149-55.

58. Chrousos G, O'Neill J, Lueth B, Parks M. Accommodation deficiency in healthy young individuals. J Pediatr Ophthalmol Strabismus. 1988;25:176-8.

59. Rouse M, Borsting E, Hyman L, Hussein M, Cotter S, Flynn M, Scheiman M, Gallaway M, Deland P, CIRS, group. Frequency of convergence insufficiency among fifth and sixth graders. Optom Vis Sci 1999;76:643-9.

60. Sterner B, Abrahamsson M, Sjostrom A. The effects of accommodative facility training on a group of children with impaired relative accommodation--a comparison between dioptric treatment and sham treatment. Opthal Physiol Opt 2001;21(6):470-6.

61. Kedzia B, Pieczyrak D, Tondel G, Maples W. Factors affecting the clinical testing of accommodative facility. Opthal Physiol Opt 1999;19(1):12-21.

62. McKenzie M, Kerr S, Rouse M. Study of accommodative facility testing reliability. Optom Vis Sci 1987;66:72-7.

63. Rouse M, DeLand P, Chous R. Binocular accommodative facility testing reliablity. Optom Vis Sci. 1992;69:314-9.

64. Borsting E, Chase C, Tosha C, Ridder WH 3rd. Longitudinal study of visual discomfort symptoms in college students. Optom Vis Sci 2008;85:992-8.

65. Liu J, Lee M, Jany J, et al. Objective assessment of accommodation. Orthoptics: I. Dynamic insufficiency. Am J Optom Physiol Opt 1979;56:285-94.

66. Griffin J, Britz D, Zundell M. A Study of Variables Influencing the Facility of Accommodation. On file in the M.B. Ketchum Library. Fullerton, Calif.: Southern California College of Optometry, 1972.

67. Griffin J, Clausen D, Graham G. A New Apparatus for Accommodative Rock. On file in the M.B. Ketch um Library. Fullerton, Calif.: Southern California College of Optometry, 1977.

68. Burge S. Suppression during binocular accommodative rock. Optom Monthly 1979;79:867-72.

69. Zellers J, Alpert T, Rouse MW. A review of the literature and a normative study of accommodative facility. J Am Optom Assoc 1984;55:31-7.

70. Grisham J. Treatment of Binocular Dysfunctions. In: Schor C, Ciuffreda K, eds. Vergence Eye Movements. Boston: Butterworth-Heinemann, 1983.

71. Pope R, Wong J, Mah M. Accommodative Facility Testing in Children: Norms and Validation. OD thesis, School of Optometry. Berkeley, Calif.: University of California, Berkeley, 1981.

72. Scheiman M, Herzberg H, Frantz K, Margolies M. Normative study of accommodative facility in elementary schoolchildren. Am J Optom Physiol Opt 1988;65:127-34.

73. Wick B, Gall R, Yothers T. Clinical testing of accommodative facility: Part III. masked assessment of the relation between visual symptoms and binocular test results in school children and adults. Optometry 2002;73(3):173-81.

74. Siderov J, DiGuglielmo L. Binocular accommodative facility in preprebyopic adults and its relation to symptoms. 1991;68:49-53.

75. Levine S, Ciuffreda K, Selenow A, Flax N. Clinical assessmeny of accommodative facility in symptomatic and asymptomatic individuals. J Am Optom Assoc 1985;56:286-90.

76. Duke-Elder S, Abrams D. System of Ophthalmology: V. Ophthalmic Optics and Refraction. In. London: Henry Kimpton, 1970.

Chapter 3 / Visual Skills Assessment Part II
Vergence Testing and Heterophoria Case Analysis

Vergence Symptoms and Differential Diagnosis	46
Tonic Vergence and Accommodative-Convergence/Accommodation Ratio	47
Calculated Accommodative-Convergence/Accommodation Ratio	47
Gradient Accommodative-Convergence/Accommodation Ratio	48
Absolute Convergence	49
Testing Techniques	49
Functions of Norms for Absolute Convergence	50
Developmental Consideration	51
Relative Convergence	52
Testing and Norms	52
Fusional Vergence at Far	52
Fusional Vergence at Near	54
Vergence Facility	54
Summary of Vergence Testing	55
Diagnosing Vergence Disorders Using Case Analysis (Graphical Analysis)	56
Zone of Clear, Single Binocular Vision	57
Morgan's Normative Analysis	59
Integrative Case Analysis	60
Fixation Disparity Analysis	60
Definition and Features	60
Measurement	62
Fixation Disparity and Case Analysis	67
Criteria for Lens and Prism Prescription	68
Morgan's Expected Criterion	68
Clinical Wisdom Criterion	69

Sheard's Criterion	69
Percival's Criterion	70
Fixation Disparity	70
Effectiveness of Prism Prescriptions	70
Recommendations for Prism Prescription	72
Vergence Anomalies	73
Convergence Insufficiency	74
Characteristics	74
Management	74
Basic Exophoria	75
Characteristics	75
Management	75
Divergence Excess	75
Characteristics	75
Management	75
Divergence Insufficiency	75
Characteristics	75
Management	75
Basic Esophoria	76
Characteristics	76
Management	76
Convergence Excess	76
Characteristics	76
Management	76
Basic Orthophoria with Restricted Zone	76
Characteristics	76
Management	77
Normal Zone with Symptoms	77
Bioengineering Model	77

VERGENCE SYMPTOMS & DIFFERENTIAL DIAGNOSIS

Vergences are disjunctive eye movements (rather than conjugate movements, as in the three other movement systems). The occipitomesencephalic neural pathway for vergences, at least for convergence, extends from area 19 to the third nerve nuclei. Vergence movements are slow (as compared with saccades) and mainly involuntary. According to the traditionally used Maddox classification, there are four components of convergence: tonic, accommodative, fusional (disparity), and proximal (psychic). Although authorities may disagree about whether this classification is the only true classification, the consensus is that the Maddox concept is useful for clinical purposes. Nevertheless, factors other than those considered in the Maddox classification (e.g., prism adaptation) must be taken into account in vision therapy. These are discussed in relation to case examples (along with the Maddox components) in this chapter and also later in this book.

Symptoms of vergence dysfunction are typically somatic, perceptual, or performance related. Common complaints include asthenopia, eye fatigue, diplopia, and reduced performance with extended near work. In addition, recent studies have found that loss of place when reading, distractibility, and slow reading are common in convergence insufficiency.[1,2] We recommend using the CISS to quantify the frequency and severity of symptoms associated with a dysfunction in vergence (see Table 2-1).

When determining the diagnosis of a vergence disorder the relationship between the far and near ocular deviation is the critical first step. By comparing the phoria at far and near the practitioner can identify whether convergence or divergence is excessive or insufficient. For example, a patient with orthophoria at far and high exophoria at near would have insufficient convergence. The next step in diagnosis is determining the relationship between the phoria and the opposing relative vergence ability. In the previous example, the exophoria at near would be compared with the positive fusional vergence ability. Finally, in cases where the phoria is in the normal range at distance and near the practitioner can look at both the relative vergence ability as well as investigating the stamina of the vergence system.

TONIC VERGENCE & ACCOMMODATIVE-CONVERGENCE/ACCOMMODATION RATIO

Tonic vergence position of the eyes is indicated by the farpoint heterophoria measurement. The alternate cover test at far (6 meters) with corrected ametropia most plus (CAMP) lenses is the standard method of establishing this position. Unless otherwise specified, this rule of testing with CAMP lenses in place applies to all testing procedures involved in the investigation of binocular anomalies.

In some cases of excessive heterophoria or intermittent strabismus, prolonged occlusion of an eye is necessary to reveal the full magnitude of the tonic deviation. This is because the effects of fusional vergence responses do not always immediately decrease on momentarily covering one eye.

Measurement of the farpoint heterophoria position through a phoropter can introduce other sources of error through psychic and accommodative vergence effects. Nevertheless, phorometry measurements of heterophoria are usually valuable, because these data are compared with other clinical data obtained under similar testing conditions.

Nearpoint heterophoria is conventionally measured at 40 cm in the primary position. It is measured with either the alternate cover test (objectively) or by phorometry (subjectively). During testing, controlling the influence of accommodation is extremely important. The patient should be instructed to fixate a detailed nearpoint target requiring precise focus while keeping the target perfectly clear. For small children, precise focus can be ensured by asking them to identify a small letter or figure as the measurement is taken. Proper dissociation of the eyes and relaxation of fusional vergence are necessary to measure the angle of deviation at near. When fusional vergence is completely inhibited, the near

heterophoria measurement represents a combination of tonic vergence and accommodative convergence being stimulated at the near testing distance. There may also be proximal vergence effects that are stimulated by testing at a near distance, but these are usually small and essentially ignored during routine clinical evaluation.

Most studies of reliability of phoria measurements have assessed adult subjects. Morgan[3] found that tests for the farpoint phoria showed high reliability even when the interval between tests was many years. Rainey et al[4] measured within session reliability of the von Graefe near phoria in optometry students and reported fair to good reliability (r=0.75). However, the 95% limits of agreement were fairly large +/- 3Δ. Most standard clinical tests of far and near heterophoria have acceptable reliability and concurrent validity, with the exception of the Maddox rod test at nearpoint.[5] The reliability may be improved, as Saladin suggested,[5] by having the patient hold or touch the penlight to stabilize accommodation at the 40-cm test distance. Thus, the reliability of the clinical measure needs to be accounted for when applying case analysis principles discussed later in the chapter.

The relation between accommodative convergence and accommodation is known as the *ACA* or, more commonly, *AC/A ratio*. The ratio means that for every diopter of accommodative response, a certain amount of accommodative convergence (depending on the value of the AC/A ratio) is brought into play. For instance, if the AC/A is 6Δ per 1.00 diopter (D) of accommodation, a patient who accommodates 2.50 D will have an increased convergence of the visual axes of 15Δ.

Calculated Accommodative-Convergence/Accommodation Ratio

There are several ways to calculate the AC/A ratio from far and near deviations. The general formula is

AC/A = IPD (in centimeters) + ([*Hn* - *Hf*]/ [*An-Af*])

where *An* - accommodative demand at near in diopters; *Af* - accommodative demand at far in diopters; *Hn* = objective angle of deviation at near (Δ); and *Hf*= objective angle of deviation at far (Δ). Note that eso deviations have positive (+) values, whereas exo deviations have negative (-) values.

This formula assumes that the CAMP lenses are in place and that the AC/A ratio is linear. Any

Table 3-1. Calculated Accommodative-Convergence/Accommodation Ratio Depending on Far and Near Magnitudes of the Angle of Deviation for an Interpupillary Distance of 60 mm

Angle H at Near	Exo 35	Exo 30	Exo 25	Exo 20	Exo 15	Exo 10	Exo 5	0	Eso 5	Eso 10	Eso 15	Eso 20	Eso 25	Eso 30	Eso 35
35	34	32	30	28	26	24	22	20	18	16	14	12	10	8	6
30	32	30	28	26	24	22	20	18	16	14	12	10	8	6	4
25	30	28	26	24	22	20	18	16	14	12	10	8	6	4	2
20	28	26	24	22	20	18	16	14	12	10	8	6	4	2	0
15	26	24	22	20	18	16	14	12	10	8	6	4	2	0	
10	24	22	20	18	16	14	12	10	8	6	4	2	0		
5	22	20	18	16	14	12	10	8	6	4	2	0			
0	20	18	16	14	12	10	8	6	4	2	0				
5	18	16	14	12	10	8	6	4	2	0					
10	16	14	12	10	8	6	4	2	0						
15	14	12	10	8	6	4	2	0							
20	12	10	8	6	4	2	0								
25	10	8	6	4	2	0									
30	8	6	4	2	0										
35	6	4	2	0											

Eso = either esophoria or esotropia; Exo = either exophoria or exotropia; H = the objective horizontal angle of deviation of the visual axes

two viewing distances can be used, but they are customarily 6 m and 40 cm. Flom[6] offered the most clinically useful form of this general formula:

$$AC/A = IPD + M (Hn - Hf)$$

where M is the fixation distance at near in meters. In this case, the distant fixation (Hf) must be at 6 m or farther. For example, assume that a patient with a 60-mm IPD has 15Δ of exophoria at far and is orthophoric at the near fixation distance of 40 cm. The AC/A would be 12Δ/1 D, which is calculated as follows:

$$AC/A = 6 + 0.4 (0-[-15])$$
$$= 6 + 0.4(15)$$
$$= 12 \text{ (i.e., } 12Δ/1 D)$$

An AC/A ratio of this magnitude is considered very high. Normal calculated AC/A ratios range from 4/1 to 7/1. An AC/A ratio greater than 7/1 is high and less than 4/1 is low. If another patient has 15Δ exophoria at near as well as at far, the AC/A ratio is 6/1. Note that the size of the IPD directly affects the magnitude of the calculated AC/A ratio; the larger the IPD, the larger is the AC/A ratio.

Table 3-1 gives the calculated answers for various angles of deviations at far and near. Looking at this table makes two useful rules readily apparent. First, the AC/A ratio is equal to the patient's IPD when the deviations at far and near are the same. For instance, orthophoria (0) on both scales for

angle H intersects at 6/1. The AC/A ratio is 6/1 on the chart wherever the angles of deviation are equal. Also, a zero AC/A ratio is very improbable, and a negative ratio is probably impossible. The table indicates those spurious combinations that could produce either a zero or negative AC/A ratio. If these questionable combinations occur, the measured magnitudes of deviation for far and near should be rechecked. For example, if the patient has an IPD of 60 mm and a measurement of 0Δ at far and 15Δ exo deviation at near, the combination indicates an AC/A ratio of zero, which suggests an error in clinical testing. However, this deviation of 0Δ at far and 15Δ exo deviation at near is possible if the IPD is larger. If, for instance, the IPD is 70 mm, instead of 60 mm, the AC/A ratio would be 1/1, which is possible.

Gradient Accommodative-Convergence/Accommodation Ratio

The magnitude of the AC/A ratio may also be determined by measuring the effect of spherical lenses on vergence. At far, minus lenses are used for this purpose; at near, either plus or minus lenses will give the value. Regardless of the testing distance, the AC/A ratio should be determined with the patient wearing CAMP lenses.

The following is an example of how the gradient method may be used. Assume that a patient has exophoria of 15Δ at far, as determined by objective means such as the cover test or, possibly, by subjective diplopia testing (e.g., Maddox rod). A spherical lens of -2.00 D is placed before each eye. The patient is instructed to focus and clear the fixation target while looking through the lenses. When the patient reports that the target is clear, another measurement of the angle of deviation is made. If the lenses cause the angle to change—for example, from 15Δ exo deviation to 5Δ exo deviation, the gradient AC/A ratio is 5/1. This is determined by dividing the change in the deviation by the change of accommodative stimulus (i.e., the power of the added lenses). Thus, 10 divided by 2.00 equals 5Δ/1 D.

Clinically, the gradient AC/A ratio is most often determined at near by using a phoropter. The near-point heterophoria is measured subjectively by either the von Graefe method or Maddox rod. Spheres of +1.00 D are added, and the heterophoria is remeasured. The magnitude change of the angle of deviation indicates the gradient. Greater precision is gained by using -1.00 D, than +1.00 D added lenses to evaluate the amount of deviation change. If there is a large depth of focus, either +1.00 D or -1.00 D may be an insufficient stimulus to elicit a sufficient accommodative response. In such cases, larger increments of lens power might be required.

The gradient method will usually give a lower AC/A ratio than will the near-far calculation method. A gradient value of more than 5/1 is considered high. The depth of focus causes the reduced AC/A magnitude, particularly if low-powered lens additions are used. The calculation method usually yields a higher value, because proximal convergence is a factor when fixation is shifted from far to near. Both methods are useful, however. In general, the calculated AC/A ratio is more reliable than the gradient method, but the gradient value may be more useful for prognosis, because it directly shows the effect of added lenses on the angle of deviation. Added lenses often are used in vision therapy to change the magnitude of deviation, in cases of both phoria and strabismus. For example, in cases of esotropia, it is often useful to measure the AC/A ratio in children by the gradient method using large lens changes such as +3.00 D and -3.00 D to observe the effect of added lenses on the angle of strabismus at near.

ABSOLUTE CONVERGENCE

The total amount of convergence of the visual axes (lines of sight) from parallelism at far to a bifixated target at near is called absolute convergence, often also called "gross" or nearpoint of convergence. Absolute convergence may involve all four components of Maddox.

Testing Techniques

The clinical test for absolute convergence is performed with a small target, traditionally a pencil tip, for measuring the nearpoint of convergence (NPC). The patient views a target in the midline as it is moved closer to the spectacle plane. Any object for fixation can be used, but a target requiring accurate accommodation is recommended. A small isolated letter "E"of approximately 20/30 (6/9) size at 40 cm (1.5 minutes of arc) has become a clinical standard. The examiner moves the target steadily at a rate of approximately 3-5 cm per second toward the bridge of the patient's nose. The patient is asked to look at the letter and report when it first becomes blurred and then when it appears doubled. Despite blurring, some patients may be able to maintain bifixation on the target all the way to the bridge of the nose (i.e., approximating the spectacle plane). Most patients, however, will have a breakpoint several centimeters from the spectacle plane. (Refer to Table 3.2 for ranking criteria.) After the blurpoint is reported (although not reported by many patients) and the breakpoint is measured, the target is withdrawn in a similar manner and at the same speed to determine the point of recovery. Supplementary testing in upgaze and down-gaze may be included as warranted (e.g., in cases of A or V patterns). (See the discussion on comitancy in Chapter 4.)

These clinical measurements usually are recorded in centimeter values, although they may alternately be expressed in prism diopter (Δ) units. If, for example, the breakpoint is 7 cm from the spectacle plane, the magnitude in prism diopters of absolute convergence can be calculated trigonometrically. The following formula, however, is convenient for clinical purposes:

$$\text{Prism diopters} = \text{IPD} \times \frac{100}{X + 2.7}$$

where IPD is the interpupillary distance. If, for example, the IPD is 60 mm (6 cm) and the NPC in breakpoint is 7 cm, then

Table 3-2. Ranking of Results of Nearpoint of Convergence Testing

Rank	Description	Breakpoint (cm)	Recovery to Singleness (cm)
5	Very strong	<3	<8
4	Strong	3-4	8-9
3	Adequate	4-6	10-11
2	Weak	7-10	12-18
1	Very weak	>10	>18

$$\Delta = 6 \times \frac{100}{7 + 2.7}$$

$$\Delta = 62$$

Note that the 2.7-cm distance is the approximate distance from the center of rotation of the eyes to the spectacle plane (Figure 3-1).

Functions and Norms for Absolute Convergence

NPC testing allows assessment of three functions of absolute convergence: sufficiency (amplitude), facility (flexibility), and stamina. Norms listed below are from Griffin,[7] Hoffman and Rouse,[8] Hayes et al,[9] and our clinical experience.

Sufficiency of absolute convergence is determined by the usual testing method of pencil pushups, as described earlier, although a small detailed target is recommended rather than a pencil tip. The blurpoint is dependant, in part, on the monocular amplitude of accommodation. Ideally, however, blurring should not occur until the target approaches a distance in the range of 10-15 cm. In contrast, the breakpoint should be much less remote, normally 6 cm or closer. Either diplopia of the target (as reported by the patient) or loss of bifixation (as observed by the examiner) at a distance exceeding 6 cm is considered "weak," which can be used as a cutoff point for referral considerations (see Table 3-2). In a population based study, Hayes et al[9] measured near point of convergence in 292 school children in Kindergarten, third, and sixth grade. An analysis of the data indicated that 85% of children had an NPC value

of 6 cm or less and they recommended that NPC values greater than 6 cm was outside the normal range. The Convergence Insufficiency Treatment Trial Group[10, 11] has used an NPC of greater than 6 cm. along with reduced positive fusional vergence as a criterion for diagnosing convergence insufficiency.

The reporting of diplopia is a subjective test. Subjective NPC results should be corroborated with objective test results (observation of examiner). Ordinarily, direct observation of the patient's eyes will suffice, but greater accuracy is possible by observing the corneal reflexes from an auxiliary penlight source held a few centimeters above the letter E fixation target, a modified Hirschberg test. (See Chapter 4 for discussion of Hirschberg testing.) Suppression may be indicated if there is no report of diplopia and the clinician observes a lack of bifixation.

Facility of absolute convergence can be assessed indirectly by the patient's ability to recover bifix-

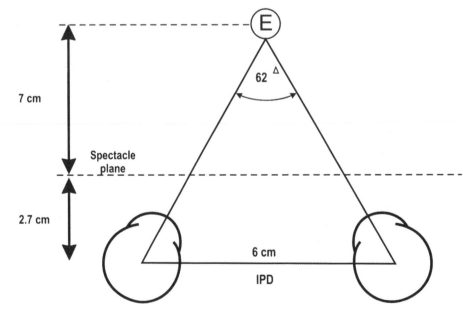

Figure 3-1. Example of nearpoint-of-convergence conversion from centimeters to prism diopters. (E = fixation target; IPD = interpupillary distance).

ation. Only singleness, not necessarily clearness of the target, is demanded for normative evaluation purposes. The patient should be expected to recover singleness (and recurrence of bifixation should be objectively observed by the examiner) at a distance of 10-11 cm or closer as the target is withdrawn. Poor vergence recovery is indicated if the distance is more remote. In other words, a recovery beyond 11 cm is considered "failing," and referral for vision therapy should be considered (see Table 3-2).

Stamina of absolute convergence is assessed by repeating the break and recovery testing four times, for a total of five routines. Poor stamina is indicated if the endpoints are more remote on repetition. Any decrement in performance over this period is considered failing or, at least, is suggestive of a dysfunction of gross convergence. Note that the training effect of repeated NPC testing may result in prism (vergence) adaptation, which theoretically should help the patient to converge more sufficiently. If, however, sufficiency is reduced on repetition because of lack of stamina, the patient most likely has significant binocular problems, and referral for vision therapy should be considered. In summary, the evaluation of stamina, as well as facility and sufficiency of absolute convergence, is important.

Although NPC normative data are not well established for infants and preschoolers, practitioners of vision therapy are well aware that infants of 1 year of age can converge their eyes to view a target at very close distances. Wick[12] reported this in a patient not quite 1 year old.

Rouse et al[13] investigated the reliability of NPC, in fifth and sixth grade children. Each examiner measured NPC three times at session 1 and then the child returned one week later and the tests were repeated. This method allowed evaluation of both within session (same day) and between session (one week later) reliability. The within session repeatability was good to excellent for NPC. The between session reliability showed that NPC can vary up to +/- 5.0 cm.

Developmental Considerations

Absolute convergence, as measured during NPC testing, is composed of Maddox's four components: tonic, accommodative, proximal, and fusional vergence. The developmental period of each of these components differs and should be taken into account by clinicians examining infants and toddlers.

Schor[14] summarized that tonic vergence is stimulated by intrinsic innervation, accommodative vergence responds to blur, and psychic vergence depends on perceived distance. These are "open-loop" responses that do not demand much of visual feedback mechanisms. For example, one eye may be occluded, but convergence will occur if the unoccluded eye responds to the accommodative demand of a minus lens, which would cause accommodative convergence. Fusional (disparity) vergence, on the other hand, is a "closed-loop" response requiring sensory feedback from retinal image disparity. Tonic vergence can be measured at birth and is often a "low tonic" convergence resulting in an exo deviation. Accommodative vergence is evident, to some extent, within a few weeks after birth. Proximal convergence is evident in the neonate as shown by the difference between the deviation in lighted surrounds (usually exo deviation) and the deviation of the visual axes in darkness (usually eso deviation).

According to Schor,[15] however, "It is clear that the binocular disparity vergence system is the last of the oculomotor functions to develop. Little is known about the age at which the response is adultlike." The following section on disparity vergences, therefore, presents established norms for adults. We believe these are applicable also to older children and perhaps to those as young as 7 years. Although children are physiologically capable of responding to testing, attentional problems may cause unreliable results in many cases. Nevertheless, our clinical impression is that a 7-year-old child should have approximately the same magnitudes of sufficiency, facility, and stamina of vergence functions as do older children and adults, assuming that attention is good and optimal performance is attained during testing. In general, testing of very young children must be objective to a large extent.

RELATIVE CONVERGENCE
Testing and Norms

Convergence is the term traditionally applied to both convergence and divergence. However, in discussions of relative vergences, the general term vergence probably is preferable to inclusion of the semantically restrictive prefix con-. Use of vergence would avoid the need for awkward or superfluous denotations such as negative fusional convergence and positive fusional convergence. The terms relative vergence, fusional vergence, and disparity vergence may be used interchangeably for most clinical purposes. The stimulus for fusional vergence eye movements is retinal disparity, with other intervening variables excluded: This means that a constant testing distance is maintained during increasing prismatic stimuli. Relative vergence is conveniently measured from the orthophoric demand point, which simplifies clinical recording. For example, a patient views a target at 40 cm while base-out (BO) demand is increasingly introduced with Risley prisms. The blurpoint, breakpoint, and recovery point are recorded directly from the scale on the instrument as though the patient (and every patient) is orthophoric. The actual magnitude of the disparity vergence response, however, must take into account the fusion-free position of rest, which involves the effects of tonic, accommodative, and proximal vergence. If, for example, a patient has exophoria of 6Δ at 40 cm and the blurpoint with BO demand is 10Δ, the total fusional (disparity) vergence response would be 16Δ. Suppose another patient has an esophoria at 40 cm of 4Δ: The total fusional (disparity) vergence response would be only 6Δ for the 10Δ BO demand. This method of measurement complicates establishment of norms for clinical usefulness. Conveniently, however, relative vergences measured from the common-denominator orthophoric position allow for standardization of norms. Hence, relative vergence is the preferred term and testing procedure for clinical purposes. We will use the term positive fusional vergence (PFV) and negative fusional vergence (NFV) when discussing relative vergence.

Clinical testing of relative vergence should begin with divergence testing. This is so because prism adaptation to BO is relatively strong and prism demands may contaminate the BI findings, making the fusional divergence response appear falsely much weaker than otherwise. According to the hypothesis of Schor,[15] ". . . The stimulus to vergence adaptation is the effort, or output, of the fast fusional vergence controller.' In other words, the reflex-disparity-vergence output resulting from Risley BO prisms can induce prism adaptation during actual clinical testing. Therefore, fusional divergence testing should precede testing of fusional convergence. By tradition in clinical practice, however, farpoint BI and BO vergence testing precedes nearpoint BI and BO vergence testing. The clinical sequence is (1) fusional divergence at far, (2) fusional convergence at far, (3) fusional divergence at near, and (4) fusional convergence at near. Despite the possible contaminant of prism adaptation (especially with BO prism), clinicians find it more convenient to finish farpoint testing before moving on to nearpoint testing. Therefore, we recommend maintaining the traditional sequence, for the sake of clinical ease and expediency.

We have based our ranking of fusional vergence ranges on a 1 to 5 scale using Morgan's norms and assuming the values for vergence ranges are normally distributed within the population (see Tables 3-3 through 3-6, and 3-9). A score of 1 or very weak, means the finding is more than 1 standard deviation below the mean and would be considered dysfunctional in most cases. A score of 2 or weak corresponds to a value that is from 0.5 standard deviations below the mean to 1 standard deviation below the mean. These findings should be considered in the borderline category and may warrant further investigation by the practitioner. A score of 3 or average corresponds to a value that is within 0.5 standard deviation above and below the mean. Scores of 4 or 5 are strong or very strong and usually indicate a healthy relative vergence system. However, in cases where the patient manifests a significantly high phoria, the opposing vergence range may have to be very high for clear, comfortable, single binocular vision to be present.

FUSIONAL VERGENCES AT FAR

Fusional divergence at far is also, known as negative fusional vergence, negative fusional convergence, and negative disparity divergence, among other designations for this function. For the sake of consistency and historical precedent in this text, we adhere to negative fusional vergence (NFV) at 6 m as the clinical nomenclature of choice. The stimulus to fusional divergence is retinal image disparity (which is BI demand). The responses of tonic, accommodative, and proximal vergences must be minimized, to the extent possible, so that only fusional vergence is measured.

Table 3-3. Ranking of Results of Negative Fusional Vergence Testing at 6 m (Base-In). Based on Morgan's norms

Rank	Description	Breakpoint (Δ)	Recovery to Singleness (Δ)
5	Very strong	>11	>6
4	Strong	9-11	5-6
3	Adequate	6-8	4
2	Weak	3-5	2-3
1	Very weak	<3	<2

Fusional divergence can be measured by several clinical methods. The most common method for measuring NFV is by the use of Risley prisms in a phoropter. From a distance of 6 m, the patient is instructed to view a vertical column of letters, normally of 20/20 (6/6) acuity demand, but the letter size may vary depending on the best attainable acuity of the patient. If, for example, the patient's best corrected visual acuity is 20/40 (6/12), that particular minimum angle of resolution for letters should be used for testing. For reliability of all visual skills testing, CAMP lenses for maximum visual acuity at far must be used for all baseline testing.

When vergence ranges are tested with Risley prisms, the speed of prism induction should be standardized. If the rate is too slow, the patient may have an excessive degree of prism adaptation and may falsely pass the test. In contrast, if the prism demand is introduced too rapidly, the patient may falsely fail the test. Most clinicians have found that the best overall rate of introduction of Risley prism power is approximately 4Δ per second. We recommend this rate for all sliding vergence testing, whether with Risley prisms, Vectograms, anaglyphs, or targets in stereoscopes. As Grisham[16] pointed out, "Test results are markedly influenced by such procedural factors as speed and smoothness of prism power induction, amount of contour in the fixation target, and phrasing of instructions (i.e., 'Tell me when the target 'doubles' as opposed to 'Try to keep the target single')."

We recommend the following standard routine:

1. Have the patient view a column of 20/20 (6/6) letters (or the patient's minimum angle of resolution if acuity is worse).

2. Instruct the patient to try to keep the letters clear and report whether there is any blurring. The Risley prisms are rotated symmetrically. Note: Be skeptical if a blur is reported on BI testing at far. Blurring could be due to an incorrect refractive status, such as latent hyperopia, or the patient may be over-minused. Therefore, it is vital to perform vergence testing with the patient looking through CAMP lenses. The first sustained blur exceeding 2 seconds is recorded. Blurring should be that amount of degraded form acuity that would be caused by +0.25-D overcorrection at 6 m. Demonstrate this to the patient, if necessary, for reliable reporting for "blur." Again, blurring should not normally occur with BI prism testing at 6 m.

3. Instruct the patient, "Try to keep the target single but tell me when the target doubles." The first sustained diplopia is recorded. If the patient reports a momentary diplopia that does not exceed 5 seconds, that is disregarded. The amount of prism causing a "sustained" diplopia is recorded for "breakpoint."

4. After the endpoint of sustained diplopia is reached, reduce the prismatic demand (at the rate of 4Δ per second) until sustained singleness (but not necessarily clearness) is reported. A good instruction is, "Tell me when the double images join again into one." This endpoint is recorded for the recovery value.

Once the breakpoint and recovery values for NFV are recorded, these findings may be evaluated in terms of their normalcy. Table 3.3 shows a ranking system whereby ranks of 2 or less are suspicious or failing. Ranks of 3 or higher are passing. This indicates that 6Δ break and 4Δ recovery are passing, which is in accord with Morgan's norms (see Table 3-3).

Positive relative vergence (PFV) at 6 m is tested in a manner similar to that used for NFV. The difference is that BO rather than BI prism demands are given. Unlike NFV at 6 m, a blurpoint usually is expected when BO prism demand (PFV at 6 m) is increased. Some patients, however, do not report blurring, only breakpoint and recovery. We have found that with proper instruction and demonstra-

Table 3-4. Ranking of Results of Positive Fusional Vergence Testing at 6 m (Base-Out)

Rank	Description	Blurpoint (Δ)	Breakpoint (Δ)	Recovery to Singleness (Δ)
5	Very strong	>13	>27	>14
4	Strong	11-13	23-27	12-14
3	Average	8-10	16-22	9-11
2	Weak	5-7	11-15	6-8
1	Very weak	<5	<11	<6

Table 3-5. Ranking of Results of Negative Fusional Vergence Testing at 40 cm (Base-In)

Rank	Description	Blurpoint (Δ)	Breakpoint (Δ)	Recovery to Singleness (Δ)
5	Very strong	>17	>25	>19
4	Strong	15-17	23-25	16-19
3	Average	12-14	20-22	11-15
2	Weak	9-11	17-19	7-10
1	Very weak	<9	<17	<7

Table 3-6. Ranking of Results of Positive Fusional Vergence Testing at 40 cm (Base-Out)

Rank	Description	Blurpoint (Δ)	Breakpoint (Δ)	Recovery to Singleness (Δ)
5	Very strong	>23	>27	>19
4	Strong	20-23	24-27	15-19
3	Adequate	15-19	19-23	8-14
2	Weak	11-14	15-18	3-7
1	Very weak	<11	<15	<3

tion, more than 90% of non-presbyopic patients are able to appreciate the blurpoint at 6 m with BO prism demand. A blur-point of 6Δ is "weak"; it should be at least 8Δ (Table 3-5). The breakpoint should be at least 16Δ, and recovery should be at least 9Δ; otherwise, the cutoff criteria for passing are not met for breakpoint and recovery.

FUSIONAL VERGENCES AT NEAR

The nearpoint testing procedure for fusional divergence is similar to that at farpoint, except a blur-point is expected. It is known simply as NFV, the 40-cm testing distance being implied. Ranking standards are shown in Table 3-5. All nearpoint testing of fusional divergence is conducted at 40 cm. The BI demand is presented to the patient in the same manner as was discussed previously for other fusional vergence testing. The blurpoint should be at least 12Δ for passing, the breakpoint should be at least 20Δ, and recovery should be at least 11Δ.

Positive fusional vergence at 40 cm is conducted as discussed earlier. BO prism demand is increased gradually until the endpoints of blur, break, and recovery are reached. The blurpoint is PFV. Pass-fail criteria are shown in Table 3-6, along with rankings from very strong to very weak. A blurpoint of less than 15Δ is suspicious, as is a breakpoint

of less than 19Δ and a recovery of less than 8Δ. These findings are entered in the patient's record. If a blur is not reported, place an X to denote this (e.g., X/18/7).

An alternative measurement technique for relative vergence is the use of a prism bar to introduce incremental step vergence demand until the patient notices blur or break.[17] The use of a prism allows the doctor to observe the patients eyes and notice fusional vergence movements. When fusion breaks down and the patient starts to look between the two targets using saccadic eye movements. This is especially helpful when working with young children who may not have reliable subjective responses. The normative values, instructions, and the rate of increasing prism power is similar to the Risley prism technique described above.

The reliability of NFV and PFV in children and adults has been studied in short term and long term studies. Rouse et al[13] measured within and between session reliability in children. The within session reliability was good to excellent, however, the between session reliability for PFV ranged up to +/- 12 Δ. Antona et al[18] measured the reliability of NFV and PFV in young adults, using rotary prism in the phoropter and in free space using a prism bar at distance and near. The authors measured

Table 3-7. Partial List of Studies on Vergence Facility

Study	Fusional (Disparity) Vergence Facility (c/min)	Comments
Kenyon et al.[22]	None in strabismics	Also none in some amblyopic subjects without strabismus
Pierce[23]	8^Δ BI and 8^Δ BO, 10 c/min (median); screening criterion of 7.5 c/min	Median for children; 7.5 c/min recommended as cutoff for "normal" versus "learning-disabled" children Mean for sixth graders
	8^Δ BI and 8^Δ BO approx. 7 c/min	
Stuckle and Rouse[24]	8^Δ BI and 8^Δ BO approx. 5 c/min	Mean for third graders
Mitchell et al.[25]	8^Δ BI and 8^Δ BO, 6.53 c/min	Mean for sixth graders
	8^Δ BI and 8^Δ BO 5.05 c/min	Mean for third graders (cutoff criterion of 3 c/min recommended)
Moser and Atkinson[26]	8^Δ BI and 8^Δ BO, 8.14 c/min	Young adults
Rosner[27]	Screening: 6^Δ BI and 12^Δ BO, 3c/0.5 min	At farpoint
	12^Δ BI and 14^Δ BO, 3 c/0.5 min	
	Goals	At nearpoint
	6^Δ BI and 12^Δ BO, 18 c/1.5 min	
	12^Δ BI and 14^Δ BO, 18 c/1.5 min	At farpoint
		At nearpoint
Jacobson et al.[28]	5^Δ BI and 15^Δ BO in relation to the phoric position of each subject, 8.6 c/min	Young adults with no vision problems; jump vergences with two sets of vectographic targets
Delgadillo and Griffin[29]	5^Δ BI and 15^Δ BO or 8^Δ BI and 8^Δ BO	Approximately same results (adult subjects)
Gall and Wick[21]	3^Δ BI and 12^Δ BO, 16 c/m for asymptomatic and 12 c/m for symptomatic group	Young adults with normal hetereophoria

BI = base-in; BO = base-out.

both within and between session reliability. The authors found only fair agreement between the two methods and NFV was more reliable than PFV for both methods. One interesting finding was that the 95% limits of agreement for PFV at near was 8 prism diopters which was better than reported by Rouse et al[13] in children but is still quite large. Ciuffreda et al[19] investigated the stability of PFV and NFV over ten consecutive weeks in three experienced adult subjects and found good stability in both measures over time. Thus, the practitioner should be cautious when measuring PFV at near due to larger variability on this test in children and adults.

VERGENCE FACILITY

Vergence facility depends on both amplitude and speed of vergence movements. The quantity and quality of disparity vergences should be evaluated. (Discussion will be limited to horizontal vergence facility of fusional divergence and convergence.) Grisham[16, 20] studied the vergence tracking rate, using 2^Δ jump-vergence steps in eight subjects, four of whom had "normal vergence characteristics" and four of whom had "abnormal" heterophoric or vergence characteristics, based on clinical data. Grisham found that the group with normal vergence characteristics had an average minimum stimulus duration of 0.84 seconds per step, whereas the group with abnormal character-

istics had a significantly longer duration of 1.67 seconds per step. Grisham[47] cited the observation of Rashbass and Westheimer "that normal disparity vergence eye movements take on the order of 1 sec to complete independent of step stimulus amplitude" and claimed that his study "compares well with the observation of Rashbass and Westheimer." Grisham also found that the two groups of subjects could be differentiated according to other dynamic properties of fusional vergence response, including percentage of completion of step responses, response velocity, and divergence latency (but not convergence latency).

Testing of vergence facility is analogues to accommodative facility testing discussed in the previous chapter. However, in vergence facility only the binocular testing with monitoring of suppression is performed. The two commonest approaches are using 8Δ BI and 8Δ BO prism flippers or 3Δ BI and 12Δ BO prism flippers at near (see Table 3-7). Studies investigating the 8Δ BI and 8Δ BO prism flippers have found mean cycles per minute ranging from 5 to 8. In contrast, a recent study by Gall and Wick[21] found a mean vergence facility of 16 cycles per minute in normal subjects using the 3Δ BI and 12Δ BO prism flippers. They recommended using a cut off value of less than 15 c/m as a suspected

**Table 3-8. Vergence Facility Tested
with 3Δ BI and 12Δ BO at 40 cm**

Rank	Description	Cycles per Minute
5	Very strong	>21
4	Strong	18-21
3	Average	13-17
2	Weak	9-12
1	Very weak	<8

BI = base-in; BO = base-out
Note: Suppression should be monitored with anaglyphic or vecto-graphic targets with targets equivalent to 20/30 being clear and single with each prism flip. The Vectograms, as used for accommodative facility, are recommended for testing at 40 cm.

problem. We would agree with using the 3Δ BI and 12Δ BO prism flippers because the higher mean flipper rate would appear better at separating normal from abnormal patients. Pass-fail criteria are shown in Table 3-8, along with rankings from very strong to very weak.

SUMMARY OF VERGENCE TESTING

As with accommodation, vergences are classified as either absolute or relative and testing helps to determine sufficiency, facility, and stamina. Accuracy of vergence is assessed with cover test or phoria measurements. Fixation disparity testing, discussed later in the chapter, is another method to assess the accuracy of the vergence system.

DIAGNOSING VERGENCE DISORDERS USING CASE ANALYSIS (GRAPHICAL ANALYSIS)

Most clinical systems used in the analysis of vergence disorders are conceptually based on the interaction of the four Maddox components of vergence: tonic, accommodative, fusional, and proximal. Graphical analysis, with roots extending from Donders[30] and Maddox[31] in the nineteenth century, uses a cartesian coordinate system to illustrate relations between accommodation and vergence. To this day, clinicians may find it helpful to draw a graph of phorometry measurements (i.e., heterophoria, relative vergence, and relative

accommodation) to visualize better the interactions. A graph can readily reveal various clinical syndromes and alert the clinician to inconsistencies in the data. The analysis implies relation between accommodative response and vergence eye position, in which changes in accommodation affect vergence and, conversely, changes in vergence affect accommodation.

By convention, the graph is plotted with accommodative stimulus, in diopters, on the ordinate (y axis) and vergence stimulus, in prism diopters on the abscissa (x axis). A diagonal line (Donders' line) is drawn representing convergence for all points in space along the midsaggital plane, with no prism or lens addition. This is also called the *demand line* (Figure 3-2). The exact positioning of the demand line on the graph is influenced by the interpupillary distance (IPD) of the patient but, for standard diagrammatic purposes, the graph is traditionally scaled for an IPD of 60 mm. In cases of a large IPD (e.g., 70 mm), the convergence demand for binocular eye alignment becomes greater with increasing accommodative stimuli for nearpoint targets. Conversely, the convergence demand is less for a small IPD (e.g., 50 mm). For fixation distances beyond 20 cm, however, the error is small and can be ignored for clinical purposes.

In graphical analysis, the far and near heterophoria measurements taken through a phoropter are plotted; then a straight line is drawn to connect

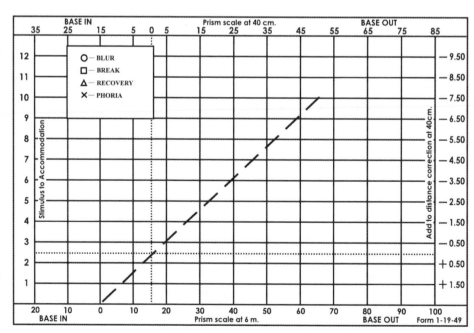

Figure 3-2. Graphical illustration of the demand line (dashed line).

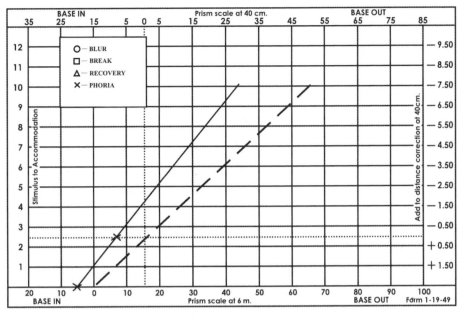

Figure 3-3. Phoria line (solid line). The X marks represent direct measurements of the phoria.

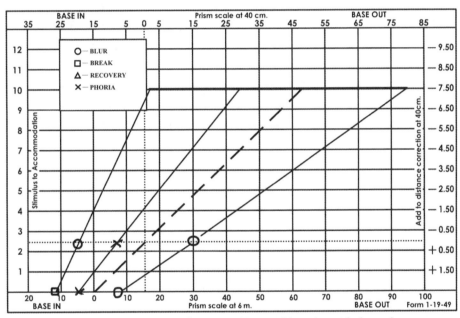

Figure 3-4. Zone of clear, single binocular vision. Vision is blurred outside the enclosure.

dation and vergence that can be elicited while maintaining clear, binocular fusion. The vertical limits of the zone are traditionally defined by the absolute amplitude of accommodation. (Monocular testing results are used because of well-established norms.) This monocular amplitude is determined by the push-up accommodation test. At each particular viewing distance, the horizontal limits of the zone represent the base-in (BI) and base-out (BO) blur-points, usually measured with Risley prisms. Ideally, the divergence limit is measured before the convergence limit (at each viewing distance), to reduce the effect of prism adaptation. Relative vergence blur-points are indicated by circles. They are plotted for at least two viewing distances, customarily at 6 m and 40 cm. At 40 cm, they are designated by circles for negative fusional vergence (NFV), which is BI to blur, and positive fusional vergence (PFV), which is BO to blur; at 6 m, they are the BI to break (designated by a square, as blur should not normally occur) and the BO to blur findings (a circle represents blur, which can happen at far with PFV) (Figure 3-4).

During prism vergence testing, it is customary to record the blurpoint (and the breakpoint and recovery point) in a particular vergence direction, convergence or divergence, at each viewing distance. If no blurpoint is reported by the patient, the breakpoint (diplopia) is charted; this is symbolized by a square. The blurpoints of negative relative accommodation (NRA) and positive relative accommodation (PRA) also are designated by

them. This line is called the *phoria line*. The AC/A ratio can be determined by direct inspection by noting the change in the deviation per unit change in accommodative stimulus. The phoria line is clinically useful because it predicts the magnitude of the heterophoria at various testing distances (Figure 3-3).

ZONE OF CLEAR, SINGLE BINOCULAR VISION

The zone of clear, single binocular vision (ZCSBV) is a graphical representation of the functional relations between accommodation and vergence. The ZCSBV is enclosed by the extremes of accommo-

circles and often are added to the charting of the ZCSBV (not illustrated in Figure 3-5 but shown in Figure 3-6).

The zone of *single* binocular vision can also be plotted (Figure 3-5). This enclosure is formed by connecting the break-points, and it is larger than the ZCSBV. The area difference between these two zones represents the use of accommodative vergence to maintain a single image (at the expense of clarity). As BO prisms are introduced, alignment of the eyes is maintained by fusional convergence. Similarly, the accommodative posture of the eyes is stimulated through the convergence-accommodation/convergence (CA/C) reflex. A normal accommodative *lag* can often become a small *lead* of accommodation without the patient reporting accommodative blur, due to the effect of an eye's depth of focus. At some point of increasing prism demand, however, fusional

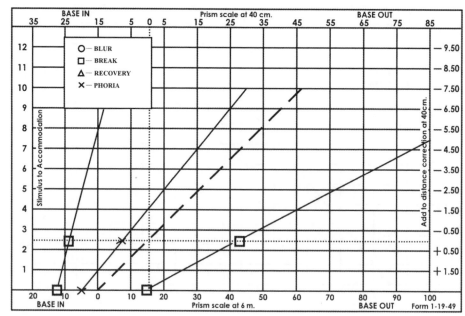

Figure 3-5. Zone of single binocular vision. Vision is diplopic outside the enclosure.

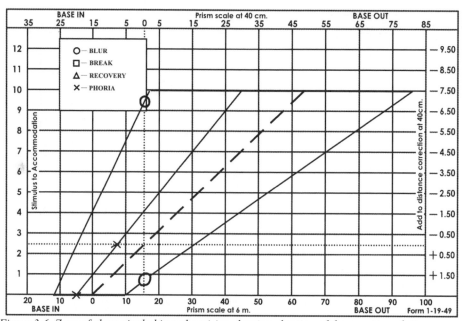

Figure 3-6. Zone of clear, single binocular vision showing charting of the negative relative accommodation (lower circle) and the positive relative accommodation (upper circle).

convergence is exhausted; the only way a patient can then maintain binocular alignment and fusion is to recruit accommodative convergence. This results in excessive accommodation for the fixation distance. Target blur then is reported when the depth of focus is exceeded. As BO prism induction is continued, a point is reached at which even accommodative vergence is inadequate. At this point (i.e., the breakpoint), binocular fusion is lost and diplopia is reported (see Figure 3-6).

A number of characteristics of the ZCSBV can be useful in clinical interpretation. A plot of the zone allows the clinician to predict how a patient will respond to various prisms, lenses, and viewing distances. Some of the important attributes of charting a ZCSBV are illustrated in Figure 3-4 and are listed here:

1. The ZCSBV approximates a parallelogram slanting toward the right, owing to the influence of the AC/A. The AC/A line serves as the axis of the zone. If there is a large deviation from a parallelogram, then spurious data points should be suspected, and retesting is indicated.

2. The slope of the zone is influenced by the slope of the AC/A. The slope of the zone often deviates slightly from the demand line. Large devi-

ations, however, probably are associated with binocular anomalies (e.g., very steep slope indicating excessive esophoria at near).

3. The vertical limits of the zone represent the amplitude of accommodation, which can be judged as either sufficient or insufficient for the patient's work requirements.

4. The horizontal limits of the zone represent the ranges of fusional divergence and convergence, which can be judged as either sufficient or insufficient for the patient's work requirements.

5. The BO blur limit of the zone is steeper (i.e., fans out) from the BI to blur line and the phoria line, primarily owing to the influence of proximal (psychic) convergence for nearpoint targets but also possibly related to convergence ("prism") adaptation with nearpoint stress and during testing with BO prism demands.

6. Normally, there is no blurpoint for fusional divergence at far. That limit is indicated by a breakpoint (diplopia). If a blurpoint is found, then the most likely explanation is that the refractive error is not fully corrected with most plus for hyperopia or is overcorrected with minus in a case of myopia. Such blurring usually indicates a spasm of accommodation.

The horizontal limits are the same as were drawn previously in this example, but the limits of *relative* accommodation are added (Figure 3-6). (Refer to Chapter 2 for discussion of NRA and PRA.)

The clinically relevant features of the ZCSBV are the relations between its constituent parts (i.e., demand line, phoria line, range of fusional vergence, and amplitude of relative accommodation). Custom dictates specific names for each of these features. PFV and NFV are the ranges of fusional (disparity) vergence to the blurpoint that are measured relative to the demand line (see Figure 3-4). These are the values directly measured using the Risley prism vergence method in both convergence and divergence directions. Another way to describe the horizontal extent of the ZCSBV is to refer to the vergence ranges relative to the *phoria* line. Positive fusional convergence is the amount of convergence measured between the phoria at any particular viewing distance to the BO blurpoint (or breakpoint, if no blurpoint is found). Similarly, NFV is represented by the amplitude between the

phoria line and the BI to blur line (divergence blur limit).

Sheard[32] emphasized the relation between the phoria direction and the compensating fusional (disparity) vergence range. When discussing Sheard's concept, the term *reserve* vergence is used. For example, if there is an exophoria as represented in Figure 3-4, then *positive fusional reserve convergence* is the distance between the phoria and the opposing blurpoint. Similarly in an esophoric case, the *negative fusional reserve convergence* is the distance from the phoria line to the BI to blur line. It is the relation between the phoria position and the compensating vergence range that has clinical relevance according to Sheard.[32] The significance and utility of these relations will be discussed later.

Gross convergence (nearpoint of convergence, or NPC) is not usually charted but may be calculated. (See Figure 3-1 and formula on pages 49 and 50.)

MORGAN'S NORMATIVE ANALYSIS

Morgan, a principal founder of binocular vision case analysis, accumulated and analyzed clinical phorometry data on 800 nonpresbyopic adults, ages 20-40 years.[33] He established clinical norms for his patient group, suggested expected values for clinical evaluation (Table 3-9), and recommended using one-half of a standard deviation from the mean to represent clinically suspicious findings. Morgan also evaluated the pattern of clinical findings by determining correlation coefficients for various zone components.[34] His results are presented in Table 3-10. His important contribution demonstrated the quantitative strength of these relations. Other findings also deserve interpretation. For example, the correlation between PFV or BO and NRA was +0.5, a moderate correlation. A direct association exists between these two features of the zone; the larger the PFV, the larger is the NRA. In many cases, accommodation can limit vergence; conversely, vergence can limit accommodation. This relation suggests the possibility of clinical syndromes, as Morgan astutely pointed out.

Morgan demonstrated that certain features of the ZCSBV tend to be congregated. Morgan's group A findings are amplitude of accommodation, PRA, and NFV. Group B findings are NRA and PFV. (Morgan also proposed another classification, group C, which includes the far and near phorias,

Table 3-9. Clinical Norms of Morgan

Test	Mean	0.5 SD	Acceptable Range
Phoria, far	1$^\Delta$ eso	±1	Ortho 2$^\Delta$ exo
BO blur, far	9$^\Delta$	±2	7$^\Delta$ to 11$^\Delta$
BO brk, far	19$^\Delta$	±4	15$^\Delta$ to 23$^\Delta$
BO rec, far	10$^\Delta$	±2	8$^\Delta$ to 12$^\Delta$
BI brk, far	7$^\Delta$	±2	5$^\Delta$ to 9$^\Delta$
BI rec, far	4$^\Delta$	±1	3$^\Delta$ to 5$^\Delta$
Phoria, near	3$^\Delta$	±3	Ortho to 5$^\Delta$ exo
BO blur, near	17$^\Delta$	±3	14$^\Delta$ to 20$^\Delta$
BO brk, near	21$^\Delta$	±3	18$^\Delta$ to 24$^\Delta$
BO rec, near	11$^\Delta$	±4	7$^\Delta$ to 15$^\Delta$
BI blur, near	13$^\Delta$	±2	11$^\Delta$ to 15$^\Delta$
BI brk, near	21$^\Delta$	±2	19$^\Delta$ to 23$^\Delta$
BI rec, near	13$^\Delta$	±3	10$^\Delta$ to 16$^\Delta$
PRA	-2.37 D	±0.62	-1.75 D to -3.00 D
NRA	+2.00 D	±0.25	+1.75 D to +2.25 D

BI = base-in; BO = base out; brk=breakpoint; NRA = negative relative accommodation; PRA = positive relative accommodation; rec = recovery; SD = standard deviation.
Source: Reprinted with permission from MW Morgan. Analysis of clinical data. Am J Optom Arch Am Acad Optom. 1944; 21:477-491.

Table 3-10. Morgan's Correlations among Selected Clinical Findings

Functions	r
Age and amplitude of accommodation	-0.80
PRA and amplitude of accommodation	+0.80
PFV blur and break	+0.70
NFV blur and break	+0.50
NRA and PFV	+0.50
PRA and NFV	+0.50
NRA and PRA	-0.50

NRA = negative relative accommodation; NFV = negative fusional vergence, base-in to blur at near; PRA = positive relative accommodation; PFV = positive fusional vergence, base-out to blur at near

the gradient AC/A ratio, and the calculated AC/A ratio.) When group A findings are low, group B findings tend to be high; Morgan refers to this case type as *accommodative fatigue*. The treatments of choice are often a plus add for reading or vision therapy that would better balance A and B findings. When group B data are found to be low and group A high, then the case type is referred to as *convergence fatigue*. The recommended treatment would be either BI prism to balance the two groups or fusional convergence (BO) vision therapy.

INTEGRATIVE CASE ANALYSIS

Scheiman and Wick[35] have recently advocated an alternative case analysis approach as way to integrate graphical analysis with normative data to arrive at an approach that is more clinically useful. There are three distinct steps in the process: 1) compare individual tests with a table of expected findings; 2) groupings of findings that deviate from expected values; and 3) identification of the syndrome. When applying integrative analysis to vergence disorders, the practitioner first identifies the relationship between the far and near phoria. The next step is looking at the ability to compensate for a phoria that is outside of the normal limits. For example, an exophoria is investigated relative to PFV. Finally, in cases where the phoria is in the normal range at far and near, the practitioner looks at relative fusional vergence and vergence stamina.

FIXATION DISPARITY ANALYSIS

Besides evaluating the relation between heterophoria and vergence ranges, vergence disorders can be identified and managed using the clinical index of *fixation disparity*.

Definition and Features

Fixation disparity is a slight manifest misalignment of the visual axes (minutes of arc) even though there is single binocular vision with central sensory fusion. The misalignment can be horizontal, vertical, or torsional; however, the magnitude of the deviation is within Panum's fusional areas, resulting in a single binocular percept of a target. Ogle[36] suggested that the magnitude of the fixation disparity depends on the amount of the innervation to the extraocular muscles during fusion. This innervation is related to the magnitude of heterophoria, the strength of compensating fusional vergence, and the complexity and detail of the visual target.

Fixation disparity is not always considered to be abnormal. It may represent an individual's physiologic habitual set point from which other binocular disparities are registered (e.g., for stereoscopic depth perception and as a stimulus for vergence eye movements). In fact, for fusional vergence error correction, it serves a useful purpose. Schor and Ciuffreda[37] indicated that fixation disparity may be a purposeful error signal that provides a stimulus to maintain a particular level of vergence innervation. Nevertheless, fixation disparity often indicates stress on the fusional vergence system and can be associated with excessive heterophoria, deficient fusional vergence compensation, and asthenopic symptoms.[38] Both abnormal and normal aspects of fixation disparity can, therefore, occur in the same individual. For example, a heterophoric patient with deficient vergence compensation can have a large fixation disparity, indicating vergence stress but, after vision therapy, there may be only a small residual fixation disparity that indicates a normal set point for that individual.

An example of an exo fixation disparity is illustrated in Figure 3-7, which depicts a posterior view of the eyes. If the error of vergence for the fixated X target is very small and fusion of X is possible because of Panum's areas, the X will appear to be single and not diplopic. The vertical lines (which are seen independently by each eye), however, will not be perceived by the patient as being in vernier alignment. This manifest deviation from exact alignment is too small to be detected by the cover test (i.e., unilateral cover test). For this practical reason, fixation disparity is not considered to be a small-angle strabismus, despite a manifest misalignment of the visual axes. Morgan[3] summed

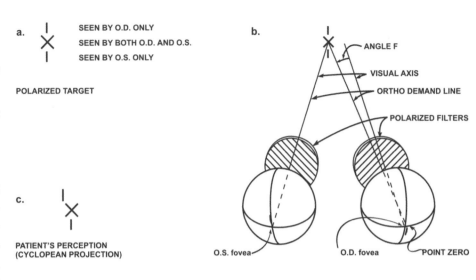

Figure 3-7. Illustrations of fixation disparity, a. Target viewed by patient, b. Theoretical posterior view of eyes illustrating angle F in exo fixation disparity, c. Patient's perception. (OD = oculus dexter; OS = oculus sinister.)

up the quantification of fixation disparity by stating, "Normally, fixation disparity rarely exceeds 10 minutes of arc, although it may be somewhat greater when a substantial degree of heterophoria exists, and probably any deviation approaching 30 minutes should be considered abnormal." Because 30 minutes of arc is regarded as being a limiting value, and it is approximately the magnitude (0.9) of a prism diopter, it is practical to consider any manifest deviation of 1Δ or greater as being a strabismus. If the deviation is less than 1Δ and there is foveal fusion, the condition is considered a fixation disparity.

Clinical evidence suggests that excessive fixation disparity tends to reduce stereopsis. Cole and Boisvert[39] conducted a study and reported that the induction of fixation disparity on otherwise normal binocular subjects caused an increase in stereothreshold (decrease in stereoacuity). In another study, Levin and Sultan[40] neutralized existing fixation disparities in 12 subjects by means of prisms to determine the effect on stereoacuity and found that stereoacuity improved in 10 of the subjects.

Measurement

Fixation disparity testing can be done at both far and near. Instruments for such testing have in common the same general principles. The patient fuses a flat-fusion target under natural lighting conditions. Such tests incorporate vernier fiducials,

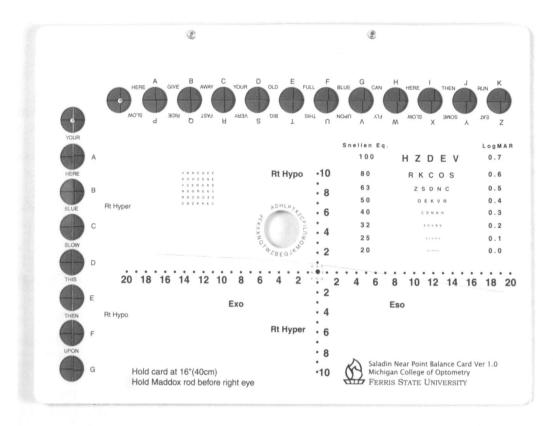

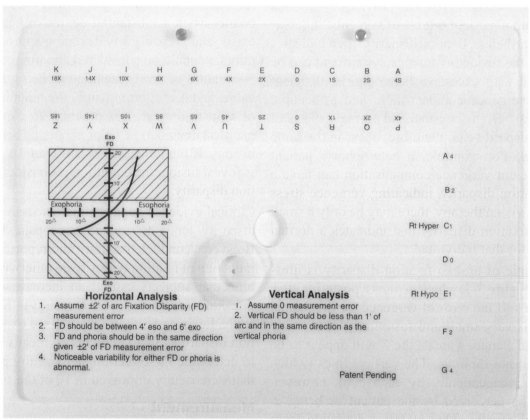

Figure 3-8. Saladin Near Point Balance Card. a. Front or patient view. b. Reverse side of test card. (Courtesy of Dr. James Saladin)

clued to each eye by means of crossed polarizing filters, so that the patient can report any noticeable misalignment. These vernier markings also serve as suppression clues. Central suppression is indicated if one line is not seen. Generally, two types of instruments are used—those that give a direct

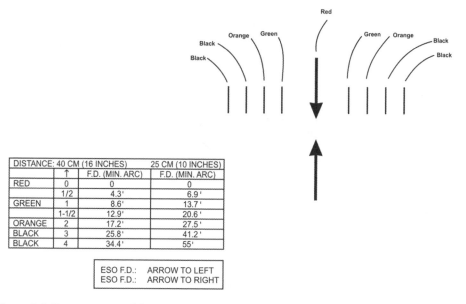

DISTANCE:	40 CM (16 INCHES)		25 CM (10 INCHES)
	↑	F.D. (MIN. ARC)	F.D. (MIN. ARC)
RED	0	0	0
	1/2	4.3'	6.9'
GREEN	1	8.6'	13.7'
	1-1/2	12.9'	20.6'
ORANGE	2	17.2'	27.5'
BLACK	3	25.8'	41.2'
BLACK	4	34.4'	55'

ESO F.D.:	ARROW TO LEFT
ESO F.D.:	ARROW TO RIGHT

Figure 3-9. Representation of the Wesson Card for fixation disparity (F.D.) testing.

measure of fixation disparity (e.g., Saladin Card [Figure 3-8]) and the Wesson Card (Figure 3-9) and those that measure only the associated phoria. The Saladin Near Point Balance Card allows for both dissociated and associated phoria measurements. The numbers 20 exophoria to 20 esophoria are for horizontal phoria testing with the modified Thorington method using a Maddox rod; the 10-10 scale is for vertical measurements. The associated phoria, horizontal or vertical, can be measured using the two targets in the upper left-hand corner, in which a foveal fusion lock appears in each center (see Figure 3-8). The other circles are without a foveal fusion lock and are used for targets to plot a fixation disparity curve (FDC; discussed later). Examples of those tests that indicate only an *associated phoria* are the Bernell test (Figure 3-10) and the Vectographic Slide (Figure 3-11) or similarly designed targets. Vertical associated phoria can be measured with either test; the Bernell test can be rotated 90 degrees to test for vertical fixation disparity (see Figure 3-10b).

The associated phoria is the minimum amount of prism that is necessary to neutralize a fixation disparity. Theoretically, this is the X intercept (XIN, pronounced "zin"). For example, an exo fixation disparity would be neutralized with BI prisms (Figure 3-12). Knowing the direction of fixation disparity and the amount of prism required to reduce it to zero (measurement of the associated phoria) are of clinical importance. The XIN (associated phoria) should not be confused with the magnitude of the fixation disparity, theoretically the Y intercept (YIN, and pronounced as such). The XIN is measured by having the patient focus on the reading portion of the test and then look at the central target when it is illuminated. The vernier perception at that moment is used for clinical purposes. The prismatic power that produces alignment for the patient is the XIN measurement.

Fixation disparity targets similar to the vectographic slide (see Figure 3-11) are good for determining the farpoint-associated phoria. The patient wears crossed polarizing viewers and is instructed to keep fixation on the center of the bull's-eye target and to report any noticeable misalignment of the vertical or horizontal lines. If there is no misalignment, the clinician can conclude that there is foveal fusion with no fixation disparity. If there is misalignment, compensating prisms are used to create vernier alignment. The power of the neutralizing prism is not the magnitude of the fixation disparity (YIN) but, rather, the measurement of the associated phoria (XIN).

A good example of target design for nearpoint fixation disparity testing is the Mallett fixation disparity test.[38] The Mallett Unit is held by the patient at the preferred working distance and position as when reading. The centrally fused target is an X. Two vertical bars (one above and one below the binocularly seen X) are covered with mutually exclusive polarizing filters. One line is seen only by the right eye and the other only by the left eye. As in farpoint testing, any horizontal associated phoria (XIN) should be measured using the minimum amount of neutralizing prism. The fixation target is flashed for each measurement in order to prevent voluntary vergence, and the patient is instructed to look immediately from the reading material to the X. (Some clinicians prefer to have the patient continually fixate the X.) Any vertical associated phoria should also be measured, using a target at another location on the unit for that purpose.

An associated phoria measuring 1Δ or more may be clinically significant if accompanied by heterophoria and deficient fusional vergence ranges, particularly if the patient reports asthenopic symptoms. In contrast, an associated phoria independent of symptoms or other signs may be clinically insignificant. Generally, the direction of the fixation disparity is consistent with the direction of the dissociated heterophoria (e.g., eso fixation disparity often occurs with esophoria). However, as Ogle[36] showed in his classic studies of fixation disparity, the two occasionally occur in opposite directions (e.g., an exophoric patient might exhibit an eso fixation disparity). In such cases, the direction of the fixation disparity is considered to be the more important clinical indicator of the underlying oculomotor stress pattern. In such a case, BO prism may possibly be prescribed to neutralize the eso fixation disparity, even though the patient has an exophoria (under dissociated testing conditions). Vision therapy to improve motor fusion ranges is, however, usually preferred in such rather than prism prescription.

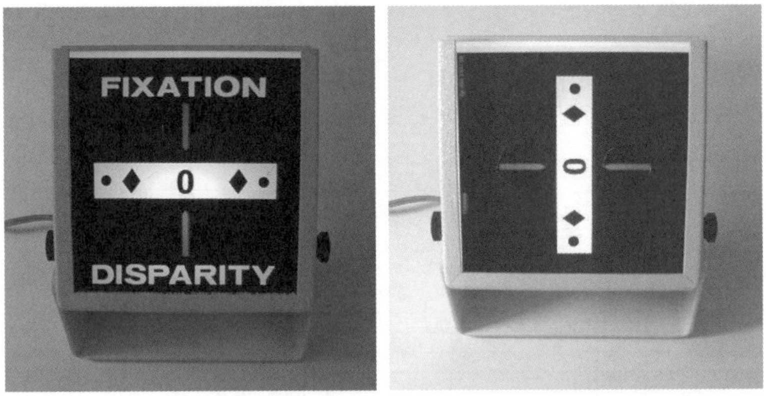

It is sometimes advisable to plot a *fixation disparity-forced vergence curve*, clinically called the *fixation disparity curve (FDC)*. The Saladin Near Point Balance Card can be attached to the nearpoint rod of a phoropter at the 40-cm viewing distance or placed in a light box. Crossed polarizing filters are used to clue the fiducials to the right and left eyes. Fixation disparity is measured by the exam-

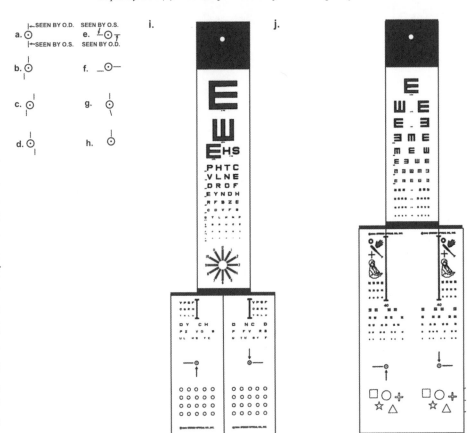

Figure 3-10. Bernell Fixation Disparity Test (a) oriented for horizontal fixation disparity and (b) oriented for vertical fixation disparity.

Figure 3-11. Results of fixation disparity testing with the Vectographic Slide. a. No fixation disparity. b. Eso fixation disparity (oculus dexter [OD] dominant eye). c. Eso fixation disparity (mixed dominance). d. Exo fixation disparity (OD dominant). e. No vertical fixation disparity. f. Hyper fixation disparity (OD dominant). g. Incyclo fixation disparity (OD dominant). h. Foveal suppression of oculus

iner dialing in the particular vernier lines for the patient's perception of exact alignment. The horizontal fixation disparity magnitude (YIN) can be determined to an accuracy of 2 minutes of arc, using the bracketing (method of adjustment) technique. The patient is asked to focus on the letters adjacent to the circular target containing the vernier lines. The vernier lines are transilluminated with a penlight. The examiner illuminates the lines intermittently, and the patient is instructed to look from

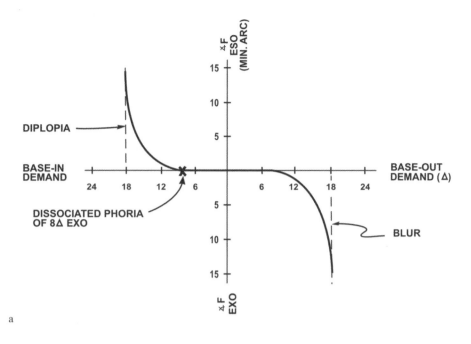

a

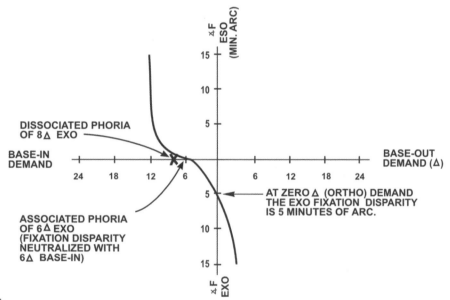

b

Figure 3-12. Fixation disparity curves plotting angle F as a function plotted against horizontal prismatic demand to vergence. a. Good vergence ability in case of 8Δ exophoria. b. Poor vergence ability in case of 8Δ exophoria with Y intercept of 5 minutes of arc (min arc) exo fixation disparity and X intercept of 6Δ exo fixation disparity. This graph could be applicable to available instruments such as the Saladin Near Point Balance Card.

either diplopia of the target or suppression of one fiducial. The instrument is designed for measurement of both horizontal and vertical fixation disparity. The Wesson Fixation Disparity Card (see Figure 3-9) is a relatively inexpensive device but less precise than the Saladin Near Point Balance Card. It can be hand-held or attached to a phoropter nearpoint rod; it also yields an approximate FDC. One study indicated that curves taken with the Wesson Card and the Sheedy Disparometer correlated highly if esophoric and exophoric subjects were analyzed separately.[41] A recent study[42] directly compared the Saladin Near Point Balance Card and Wesson Card and found that the fixation disparity or YIN was more exo for the Wesson card. Consistent with this finding the XIN or associated phoria was more in the base in direction with the Wesson card. The authors speculate that the Saladin card may provide a stronger fusion lock when compared with the Wesson Card.

the letters to the illuminated vernier lines and report any misalignment of a line and its direction.

The FDC is plotted by measuring the magnitude of fixation disparity that corresponds with varying amounts of BI and BO prism. Risley prism increments of 3Δ are advised to produce clinically useful curves. Fixation disparity is measured initially with an ortho demand. Subsequent measurements are taken in the following order: 3Δ BI, 3Δ BO, 6Δ BI, 6Δ BO, and so on. The limit of forced vergence in each direction is indicated when a prism results in

Figure 3-12a illustrates an FDC of a patient with normal binocular vision, whereas Figure 3.12b shows an FDC of a patient with vergence dysfunction reporting asthenopic symptoms. Note the following clinically relevant features of the abnormal curve: (1) the significant fixation disparity at the ortho demand position; (2) the relatively large associated phoria (XIN); (3) the steep slope (exceeding 45 degrees) of the curve at the ortho demand position; and (4) the limited range of fusional vergence. These features of the curve confirm the presence of a vergence dysfunction. Another feature of the FDC that has been suggested to be indicative of a vergence dysfunction is variability of the amount of fixation disparity and the curve over time (i.e., large day-to-day variation). In individuals having normal binocular vision, the FDC appears to be quite stable or reliable over time within a limited range of forced convergence and forced divergence.[43]

Four basic types of FDCs were described by Ogle et al[36] and are believed to have differential diagnostic value (Figure 3-13). The type I curve has a sigmoid shape and is considered to be the most prevalent, found in approximately 60% of the population (64% by Kwan et al[44]). A type I curve having a steep slope (crossing at the ortho demand position) often is associated with visual symptoms. In these cases, vision training often is successful in flattening the slope of the curve while increasing fusional vergence ranges, usually relieving symptoms due to vergence dysfunction. These cases have an excellent prognosis for improvement. Type II and III curves have a flat segment that may or may not cross the x axis (Figure 3-13). Type II is often associated with esophoria (although occasionally exophoria) and is the second most prevalent type, found in approximately 25% of the population. Type III, which is often associated with exophoria (although occasionally with esophoria), is found in approximately 10% of the population. It should be noted that all FDCs should be plotted from break to break (diplopia limits). A type I FDC sometimes is incorrectly labeled as type II or III; this occurs when the examiner takes too few points and fails to find a segment that crosses the x axis.

True types II and III often respond well to prism prescription. Many type III cases that are exo fixation disparities can be treated with fusional convergence training. Type IV cases, the least prevalent (approximately 5%), have the worst prognosis for a functional cure as compared with the other FDC types. Figure 3.13 illustrates type IV exo fixation disparity, but eso fixation disparity is also possible. Individuals with this FDC type seem to adapt to prism so that the fixation disparity can never be neutralized. In other words, there may be no stable XIN. Such binocular dysfunctions are not clearly understood. In type IV curves, sensory and motor fusion disorders may be resistant to therapeutic attempts; the prism adaptation found during testing is characteristic of many strabismic patients. Vision therapy is frequently ineffective in such cases.

It is apparent that establishing the curve type and characteristics aids the clinician in making a diagnosis of a vergence dysfunction and points toward certain therapeutic options. The clinician must be aware that the type of curve can change from far to near fixation in many cases.[36,45] It is important to evaluate the FDC at the distance at which the patient is experiencing binocular vision problems. Ogle et al[36] demonstrated that FDCs can also be generated using lens additions to stimulate forced vergence. By comparing the FDC found with prism stimulation and that found with lens stimulation, a derived AC/A ratio can be computed under associated conditions. Building on this work, Wick and Joubert[46] found four FDC types induced by lens stimulation that are analogous to, but not totally consistent with, the types found by Ogle et al,[36] who used prism stimulation. They suggested that these lens-induced curves have diagnostic value in some cases. Furthermore, the lens power that reduces the near fixation disparity to zero may help to determine the proper near prescription, particularly with prepresbyopic patients. For example, if a +1.25-D addition lens reduces a nearpoint eso fixation disparity to zero, this could be the optimum prescription.

Although generating an FDC is recommended, the clinician can get a general sense of whether the FDC is normal or abnormal merely by measuring the associated phoria and evaluating the total range of fusional vergence. For example, if no fixation disparity is induced over a relatively large range of BI and BO prism demand (e.g., 6Δ BI and 9Δ BO at near), then the clinician can assume the presence of a normal type I FDC. However, if eso fixation disparity and eso associated phoria are present with an ortho demand, the eso fixation disparity increases with small amounts of BI prism, and an exo fixation disparity is induced with relatively small amounts of BO prism, then the clinician can visualize a steep FDC. A three-dimensional model of fixation disparity, vergence, and accommodation can also be conceptualized (Figure 3-14).

Fixation Disparity and Case Analysis

An evaluation of fixation disparity and the attributes of the FDC has become a popular mode of

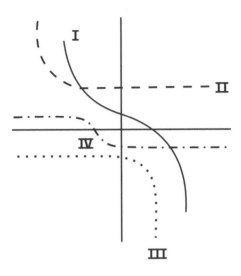

Figure 3-13. Four types of fixation disparity curves.

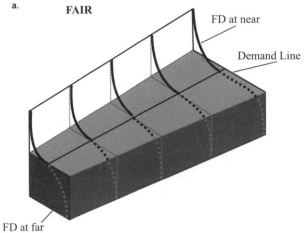

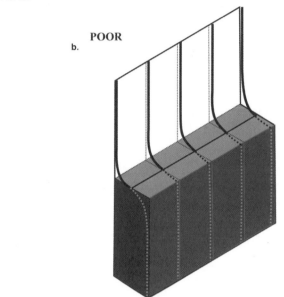

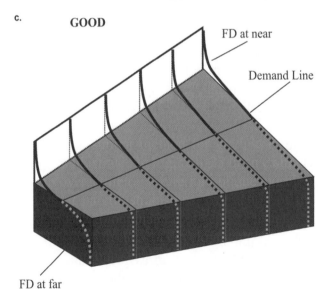

Figure 3-14. Three-dimensional models of binocular vision showing the relations of accommodation, vergence, and fixation disparity (FD). a. Indication of fairly good fusional vergences for clear, single, comfortable binocular vision, b. Poor fusional vergences indicating lack of good, clear, single, comfortable binocular vision, c. Good fusional vergences indicating excellent binocular status as to clarity and comfort.

vergence case analysis. Ogle et al[36] initially reported good reliability of fixation disparity measurements, and subsequent studies of the FDC in individuals having normal binocular vision indicated only a small amount of measurement drift over days and weeks.[43,47] Although increases in convergence or divergence fusional demand (prism demand) may result in some variability of the FDC, the overall shape and type of the FDC remains stable over time. This principle apparently applies to the vertical FDC also. One study found that the shape of the vertical FDC (approximating a straight line) remains stable over time, whereas its slope varied significantly, more so over weeks and months than during the day.[48]

Variability in the FDC in patients with binocular problems has not been adequately studied. There are, however, indications that symptomatic patients with abnormal FDCs show increases in curve slope and magnitude of fixation disparity when reading for short periods.[49] Yekta et a1[50] found that a large fixation disparity (YIN) and associated phoria (XIN) are related to visual symptoms in patients of all ages, including presbyopes. They also reported that by the end of a working day, there is a significant increase in both of these indices that correlates with increased asthenopic symptoms.[51] Although more studies are indicated, it appears that several attributes of the FDC are clinically reliable and valid indicators of vergence dysfunction. In an intriguing study, Karania and Evans[52] added questions about the movement of the nonius lines when determining the presence of fixation disparity using a Mallet Unit. If the patient did report movement, then prism was put in place to neutralize the movement and obtain alignment. They found that adding questions about movement better predicted the presence or absence of symptoms at near.

Dowley[53] has concluded, however, that the associated phoria measured with a Disparometer (and, by implication, the Saladin Card), is not as reliable as the Mallett Unit. The Disparometer has a fusion stimulus, an annulus that is 1.5 degrees in diameter, but no centered foveal binocular stimulus, which the Mallett Unit does have. Studies have demonstrated that the FDC is less variable and the associated phoria has a smaller magnitude if the target contains a foveal fusion stimulus.[54, 55] Agreeing with Dowley, we recommend that clinicians use a Mallett Unit, a Bernell polarized near-point testing unit, or the Saladin Card to measure associated phoria if prisms or adds are to be prescribed by the associated phoria criterion. Our experience indicates that associated phoria prisms identified by the Disparometer are often excessive and rejected by patients. By contrast, the Mallett Unit prism amount usually is accepted by patients and proves to be beneficial if there are asthenopic symptoms and other signs of a vergence dysfunction. The foveal fusion lock prevents the measured XIN from being excessive, but it allows the clinically significant fixation disparity component due to fusional vergence stress to be revealed. Fortunately, the Saladin Card provides a target with a foveal fusion lock for measuring the associated phoria (XIN). In other words, the foveal fusion lock might eliminate the appearance of the physiologic fixation disparity, but it allows the clinically significant fixation disparity component due to fusional vergence stress to be revealed.

Sheedy and Saladin[56] also evaluated the validity of case analysis diagnostic criteria; however, they used the statistical technique of stepwise discriminant analysis to rank the effectiveness of many commonly used clinical criteria in differentiating symptomatic from asymptomatic nonstrabismic subjects. The symptomatic subjects all had clinically determined heterophoric and vergence disorders. Phorias, vergences, and FDCs were measured on all subjects. Sheard's criterion proved to be the best single discriminant variable for the entire population, particularly for the subgroup of exophoric subjects. For esophoric subjects,

Table 3-11. Ranking of Discriminating Factors

Rank	Exophores	Esophores
1	Sheard's criterion	Phoria amount
2	Y intercept	Fixation disparity curve slope
3	X intercept	Recovery range
4	Vergence opposing phoria	Break range
5	Vergence recovery	Vergence opposing phoria

Source: Reprinted with permission from JE Sheedy, J Saladin. Validity of Diagnostic Criteria and Case Analysis in Binocular Vision Disorders. In: Vergence Eye Movements. CM Schor, KJ Ciuffreda, eds. Boston: Butterworths; 1983:517-540

however, the magnitude of the deviation (phoria) was the most discriminating factor (Table 3-11). The power of these individual variables in successfully discriminating between the two subject groups (90% correct) supports the overall validity of binocular vision case analysis as an effective clinical approach.

CRITERIA FOR LENS AND PRISM PRESCRIPTION

Many people have contributed to graphical case analysis over the years. Several researchers and clinicians have recommended various criteria for the prescription of prisms and adds to balance various elements within the ZCSBV. An alternative approach is correcting the amount of prism necessary to correct the fixation disparity. Their clinical popularity of the various prescribing criteria has waxed and waned over the years, depending on the fashion of the time. The selection of one criterion over another usually is based on a particular clinician's training, experiences, and biases. Several criteria currently in use are reviewed here. Recently there has been an increased interest in investigating the effectiveness of prism prescription using acceptable research paradigms and the results of the studies may aid the clinician when prescribing prism correction (see below for summary of studies)

Morgan's Expected Criterion

Morgan's expected ranges for near and far heterophorias have been used as clinical values for the prescription of prism or added lens power. The idea is that if a patient has an excessive phoria falling outside the expected values, a prism or spherical lens addition is prescribed to compensate for the phoria. The lens or prism shifts the demand line relative to the phoria line, so that the measured phoria then falls within expected limits, as can be shown graphically. We will refer to this prism prescription criterion as *Morgan's expected criterion*. For example, if a patient reports eyestrain while reading and has an exophoria of 10Δ at near, the spectacle prescription would be 4Δ BI to reduce the phoria to 6Δ exophoria with respect to the new demand; this is a limiting expected value.

Clinical Wisdom Criterion

Another criterion based on the amount of the heterophoria is called the clinical wisdom criterion. Its origin is obscure, but it seems to be passed from one generation of clinicians to the next. The criterion varies with the direction of the deviation. If a patient has visual symptoms and poor performance associated with an excessive exophoria, then clinical wisdom would recommend prescribing prism in the amount of one-third the angle of deviation to bring symptomatic relief. For example, if the exophoria measures 12Δ by cover test, then 4Δ BI would be prescribed. The prism amount would usually be split between the two lenses (i.e., 2Δ BI each eye), to reduce weight and optical distortion. However, in the cases of esophoria and hyperphoria associated with signs and symptoms, clinical wisdom would recommend neutralizing the entire angle of deviation with prisms or adds, if appropriate. For example, if 4Δ esophoria and 2Δ right hyperphoria were found by cover test in a symptomatic patient, the prism prescription would be: OD 2Δ BO and 1Δ base-down; OS 2Δ BO and 1Δ base-up.

Sheard's Criterion

One of the oldest and most widely used clinical criteria for evaluating lateral phoria imbalance is Sheard's criterion. In 1929, Charles Sheard, a biophysicist at Ohio State University, suggested that the clinically significant relation in assessing vergence dysfunctions is the magnitude of heterophoria as compared with the range of compensatory fusional vergence. He proposed that the compensating vergence "reserve" should be at least twice the demand (heterophoria) to be physiologically sufficient.[32] Therefore, the blur point of the PFV should be at least twice the magnitude of an exophoria, and the blur point of the NFV should be at least twice the amount of an esophoria. Sheard's criterion proposes that if the reserve is less than this amount, a patient is likely to develop asthenopic symptoms with sustained visual activity (e.g., reading a book). If, indeed, a patient does

report visual symptoms and fails to meet Sheard's criterion, then compensating prisms (or a lens addition, in some cases) can be determined. The goal is to prescribe sufficient prism (or added lens) so the compensating relative vergence would be twice the demand. This can be accomplished by either inspection of the graph or by calculation. The formula for calculating Sheard's prism is: Sheard Δ = ([2 x demand] - compensating relative vergence)/3. That is, $\Delta = (2D - R)/3$.

Two examples are offered to demonstrate the use of Sheard's criterion. If a symptomatic patient has a nearpoint exophoria of 9Δ and PFV ranges of 6/10/4 taken through the phoropter, then analysis would indicate that Sheard's criterion at nearpoint is not met. The demand is 9Δ exophoria, and the PFV (blurpoint) is 6Δ. The reserve is much less than twice the demand. The PFV in this case should be 18Δ BO to blur to satisfy Sheard's criterion. A prism can be prescribed to meet the theoretical criterion. Sheard's prism = (2D- R)/3 or ([2 x 9] - 6])/3 - 12/3 = 4Δ BI. With 4Δ BI in place, the measured phoria would be reduced from 9Δ exophoria to 5Δ exophoria, and the reserve of 6Δ would be increased to 10Δ. This prism, therefore, satisfies Sheard's criterion (i.e., 2D = R, or 2 x 5 = 10). In the spectacle prescription, the prism would be split, 2Δ BI each eye. The patient may experience improved visual comfort and efficiency. There is evidence that Sheard's criterion is clinically effective, particularly in exophoric cases.[57] A better approach when feasible, in lieu of prism compensation, is to prescribe convergence vision therapy with the goal of building the PFV to at least 18Δ BO to blur, which would satisfy Sheard's criterion.

The second example is a far and near esophoric patient reporting visually related headaches at the end of a workday. Phoropter findings indicate a far esophoria of 5Δ with 3Δ farpoint BI to break and, at near, esophoria of 7Δ with an NFV of 5Δ (to blur). Hence, Sheard's criterion is not met at either far or near. The Sheard prism at far would be: Δ = (2D- R)/3 = ([10 - 3]/3) = 7/3 -2 1/3Δ BO. The Sheard prism at near would be: Δ = (14 - 5)/3 = 3Δ BO. One approach is to prescribe 3Δ BO in single-vision spectacles, as this prism would satisfy Sheard's criterion at far and near. However, if the symptoms were related primarily to nearpoint work, another approach could be taken using plus added lenses.

The Sheard's prism at near, 3Δ BO, could be satisfied by prescribing a plus add for near, based on the gradient AC/A ratio. If the gradient AC/A ratio measured 4Δ/1 D in this case, then a +0.75-D add would also balance the relationship between the demand and reserve to satisfy Sheard's criterion. (Sheard add = required Sheard prism/gradient AC/A ratio.) This add combined with the lens correction for any existing farpoint refractive error might be prescribed in single-vision lenses for nearpoint (e.g., reading or computer work). A bifocal prescription could also achieve the desired results if appropriate for the work needs of the patient. In addition, fusional divergence training should be considered as either an alternate clinical approach in such cases or in combination with optical treatment.

Percival's Criterion

Percival's criterion differs from the other criteria in that it ignores the phoria position. Percival proposed that the clinically important relationship in the ZCSBV is the position of the *demand line* with respect to the limits of convergence and divergence blur lines.[58] He delineated a *zone of comfort* resting within the middle third of the ZCSBV, limited horizontally by the blur lines on either side and extending vertically from 0 to 3 D of accommodative stimulus. Percival believed that the demand line should ideally fall within or at a limit of this comfort zone. If it did not, then prism, added lens correction, or vision training was indicated. The clinician can assess whether Percival's criterion is satisfied by direct inspection of the plotted ZCSBV and by adding the NFV and PFV findings and dividing by three. This trisects the total range of fusional vergence and defines the zone of comfort, the inner third. Does the demand line fall within the zone of comfort for all viewing distances? If not, the amount of prism necessary to shift the demand line to the nearest limit of the comfort zone can be easily determined from the graph. The amount may necessarily be different for near and far viewing.

Percival's criterion can also be applied by calculation. A useful formula is: Percival's Δ = 1/3 L — 2/3 S, where *L* = larger relative vergence range and *S* = smaller relative vergence range. For example, if the PFV is 24Δ (L) and the NFV is 9Δ (S), the prism necessary would be

Percival's Δ = 1/3 L-2/3 S
= 1/3 (24)-2/3 (9)
= 8-6 = 2Δ BO

A vision therapy approach in this case would call for fusional divergence training (also called *BI training*) to increase the NFV to satisfy Percival's criterion.

Fixation Disparity

Two principal criteria have been recommended for the prescription of prism on the basis of fixation disparity: *Sheedy's criterion*[59] and the *associated phoria criterion*.[38] Sheedy's criterion for the prescription of prism is based on inspection of the FDC. If the curve is steep where it crosses the YIN (ortho demand position) and the patient has fusional problems and symptoms, Sheedy recommends prescribing the least amount of prism that places the ortho demand position on the flattest portion of the curve. If, for example, the FDC is steep at the ortho demand position but flattens out at the 4Δ BO location of the x axis, the prescription would be 4Δ BO prism. This would shift the ortho demand position to the flattest segment of the FDC, if there is no prism adaptation. If there is no completely flat portion, Sheedy would recommend prescribing sufficient prism to place the patient's ortho demand on the flattest portion of the curve. We believe, however, that vision training is of great value in such cases, to flatten the curve near the ortho position.

The associated phoria criterion is the least amount of prism that neutralizes the fixation disparity (XIN). Typically, the targets used to make this clinical measurement are found with instruments similar to the Mallett Unit, Bernell Unit, and Saladin Card with ortho demand target for near testing or the Vectographic Slide for far testing. These targets contain central fusion contours. We believe a central fusion lock is necessary when the associated phoria criterion is used for the prescription of prism. The associated phoria is determined by adding prisms until neutralization occurs. The patient should be instructed to determine whether vernier alignment is achieved with each prism power within a time limit of 20 seconds after the prism has been introduced. Beyond this time, there may be significant prism adaptation to invalidate the measurement of the associated phoria.[37]

EFFECTIVENESS OF PRISM PRESCRIPTIONS

One direct approach for assessing the use of a particular clinical criterion for the prescription of prism is to allow the patient to choose between two comparable spectacle prescriptions, one including the particular prism amount and the other similar in all respects except for the prism. Worrell et al[60] were the first to use this technique when they assessed the prism prescribed by Sheard's criterion in 43 subjects with oculomotor imbalance and asthenopic symptoms. They found that the Sheard prism was accepted at a statistically significant level in preference to no prism in esophoric subjects (particularly for farpoint viewing) and in presbyopic, exophoric subjects. However, nonpresbyopic adults with exophoria did not prefer the prism beyond a chance level. Fortunately, vision training techniques for increasing fusional convergence are very effective in such cases.

Payne et al[61] provided two sets of lenses to 10 patients with asthenopia and fixation disparity at near. The prism amount was determined by measuring the associated phoria using a near-point Mallett Unit, and a double-blind (masked) procedure was employed. By this criterion, all patients (eight nonpresbyopic exophores and two esophores) chose to keep the prism prescription. Grisham[62] reported prism acceptance in a group of symptomatic presbyopic exophores using associated phoria as the prism criterion. Of the 12 patients, 10 chose to keep the prism that neutralized their fixation disparity at near. On the basis of theoretical considerations, some clinicians do not believe in the use of associated phoria alone for prism prescription. However, the preceding evidence suggests that this method has clinical utility, at least when determined by a test that has a central fusion stimulus (i.e., "lock")— for example, the Mallett unit, Bernell fixation disparity slide, or the Saladin Card.

A recent study by Otto et al[63] compared three methods for determining appropriate prism correction in adult patients with a mean age of 26. The researchers used the disassociated phoria, associated phoria and the prism power selected by the patient for most comfort while the subject looked at a near target with a fusion lock. The results of the study found that the prism power selected as most comfortable was significantly different from both prism powers found by phoria measures. In fact, in many cases the subjects with esophoria and eso fixation disparity chose BI prism as most comfortable. This study confirms our clinical experience that trial framing a prism correction is essential for a successful outcome.

There have been two recent clinical trials that have looked at the effectiveness of prescribing prisms in children and adults. Scheiman et al,[64] compared prism correction to placebo reading lenses in children ages 9 to 17 years with symptomatic CI. Sheard's criteria was used to determine the amount of prism correction for prism group and the primary outcome was the CI symptom survey. The prism group had less symptoms following treatment but the placebo group had similar improvements. Thus, this study did not support the effectiveness of Sheard's criteria for determining prism correction in children with CI. Additionally, the significant improvement in the placebo lens group suggests that spectacle lenses may have a large placebo effect when evaluating subjective symptoms associated with vergence disorders.

In contrast to the above study, O'Leary and Evans[65] evaluated the effect of prism correction on reading rate using a placebo controlled masked examiner design. One hundred and sixteen adults (mean age of 43) participated in the study. The study participants read from the Wilken's Reading Rate Test with their habitual correction, a prism that corrected the fixation disparity, and two control lenses. A positive response to the prisms was defined as a 5% or greater improvement in reading rate for the prism when compared with the control lens. For the participants with exophoria and needing 2 or more prism diopters to neutralize the fixation disparity there was a significant improvement in reading rate while wearing the prism correction. One interesting finding was that the patients who responded most to prism correction were not necessarily the ones with the greatest symptoms when reading or studying. O'Leary and Evans advocate looking for improvements in reading rate as opposed to symptoms as the best method evaluating a positive response to the prism correction.

Improvement in reading rate was also reported by Stavis et al,[66] with prism correction in children (ages 8 to 18) with CI using the Gray Oral Reading Test as the outcome measure. In children who initially gave a positive response to prism there was an increase from the 34th to the 66th percentile on the Gray Oral Reading test. The children also reported fewer asthenopic symptoms while wearing the prisms. However, this study was not masked and did not include a control group.

Finally, a recent study by Teitlebaum et al,[67] looked at prism correction in presbyopic adults with CI using a unique prism design. Twenty-nine symptomatic CI presbyopes (ages 45 to 68 years) wore a progressive lens with prism or lenses without prism for three weeks each. The prism prescription was based on the associated phoria measured with a central fusion lock. Following, each three-week wearing cycle the CISS was re-administered. When wearing the prism, the presbyopes showed a greater reduction in symptoms than when wearing only the near correction.

RECOMMENDATIONS FOR PRISM PRESCRIPTION

Based on the above studies there seems to be reasonable clinical support for using either Sheard's criteria or the amount of prism necessary to neutralize the fixation disparity in adults, with exo deviations. There is less clinical evidence for correction of eso deviations. In children, the study by Scheiman et al, casts some doubt on the use of Sheard's criteria for CI cases. Our initial bias in most cases of significant heterophoria, or intermittent strabismus, is to recommend vision therapy for improvement of fusional vergences. Prism compensation may also be necessary as a supplement to therapy. When vision therapy is an unacceptable alternative or training results are unsuccessful, prism therapy may become the treatment of choice. We have summarized our recommendations for the different systems for prescribing prisms in Table 3-12.

We have had good experience using the associated phoria criterion (i.e., the minimum prism that neutralizes the fixation disparity) for the prescription of prism in esophoria, exophoria, and hyperphoria cases, although some clinicians disagree.[68,69] The prism amount we prescribe is derived from clinical testing on fixation disparity targets having both foveal and peripheral fusion stimuli, such as are found on the Bernell slide, Mallett Unit, and the Saladin Card. When a series of prism amounts is found to neutralize the fixation disparity, the minimum amount is prescribed with good effect;

asthenopic symptoms usually are ameliorated and the patient adapts well to the prism spectacles. Care must be taken, however, when prescribing a prism for one distance to ensure that a fixation disparity is not induced at another distance. For example, BI prism may neutralize a fixation disparity at 40 cm for reading but induce a large eso fixation disparity and associated phoria for viewing television at 3 m with that same prism. In this case, the prism spectacles may be unacceptable and rejected for general wear but suffice for sustained nearpoint activity. Therefore, testing of associated phoria should be done at both far and near to judge the effect of a particular prism amount. Sometimes, prism spectacles should be given for a specific viewing distance. This management principle is applicable to prescribing prism by any criterion, but the associated phoria is a convenient criterion, because the prism amount can easily be assessed by testing with far and near targets.

Diagnosis of a binocular vision dysfunction rarely is made on the basis of a single test; likewise, a prism seldom is prescribed unless a number of criteria indicate the necessity for it. The amount of prism power recommended by each criterion often varies, and the clinician must use professional judgment. When there is coherence among criteria, the decision is relative easy, but when there is wide variation, the validity of each criterion should be questioned. Often, retesting or additional testing is required. Particularly in these situations, a *prism confirmation procedure* should be carried out.

We recommend the following procedure to test the suitability of any particular prism: Many patients with an oculomotor imbalance will immediately experience some relief of their symptoms when a compensating prism of appropriate magnitude is introduced. If an esophoric patient's symptoms are related to reading, for example, a reading test card is given to the patient to view. Let us assume that the associated phoria criterion indicates 4Δ BO, so a loose prism of this amount would be used in the confirmation test. With the prism in place, the patient is asked whether the print appears to be clearer or whether vision is more comfortable than without the prism. The prism power that neutralizes a fixation disparity will usually make print appear closer.[70] A valid prism prescription is indicated when there is a strong acceptance response by the patient. To check for a placebo effect, however,

Table 3-12. Clinical Methods for Prescribing Prisms

	Exophoria	Esophoria	Hyperphoria
Clinical wisdom	3	3	3
Sheard's criterion	3	3	NA
Percival's criterion	1	2	NA
Associated phoria	3	3	3
Flat portion of fixation disparity curve (Sheedy's criterion)	2	2	NA
Prism confirmation procedure	3	3	3
Prism adaptation test	1	1	1

3 = best; 2 = good; 1 = fair; NA = not applicable

the prism direction is reversed surreptitiously and again tried. Validity is confirmed if there is strong rejection of the reversed prism. If, however, the patient accepts the reversed prism, further trials with different prisms are necessary. If no prism is accepted by this confirmation procedure, the prescription of prism is often unwarranted. Other approaches to resolving the patient's problem might be recommended (e.g., vision therapy, lens power additions, changing viewing conditions, or referral for a general health examination).

If, after applying these prism-prescribing methods, a question still remains regarding whether a prism is appropriate, a *prism adaptation test* may be helpful in resolving the issue. Heterophoric patients having normal binocular vision with no ocular symptoms typically show strong prism adaptation. After wearing a prism for approximately 10 minutes, they often will have the same, or nearly the same, phoria as originally measured. For example, if a 6Δ exophoric patient with normal binocular vision wears a 6Δ BI prism (which initially neutralizes the angle of deviation) for a short period, the examiner typically finds the phoria to be increasing, resulting in another 4Δ to 6Δ of exo deviation. The prism would be ineffective, because that patient reverts to the habitual phoria through the spectacles. Conversely, symptomatic patients with vergence problems usually benefit from prism compensation and do not typically show significant prism adaptation. If a prism, worn for 10 minutes, continues to neutralize the angle of deviation, then that prism establishes an acceptable physiologic relation between the heterophoria and the compensating vergence, relieving the oculomotor stress. Complete prism adaptation, when it occurs, usually is complete within 24 hours, but most of the adaptation occurs within the first 10 minutes. This test is, therefore, a relatively quick clinical procedure.

The results of this test are not always clear-cut, and interpretation often is difficult. At times, this can be a good backup test of prism acceptance, but professional judgment remains necessary.

Applying Fresnel prisms to spectacle lenses can also be used for prism adaptation testing and, occasionally, for permanent wear. The smooth side of the membrane is placed on the ocular side of a spectacle lens. This is best performed after the membrane and lens are washed and still wet. (Also see Chapter 11, under Optical Therapy, for discussion and illustration.)

VERGENCE ANOMALIES

The predominant classification system for vergence disorders is based on the tonic deviation of the eyes and the AC/A ratio. It is used to describe both strabismic and heterophoric cases and is widely accepted in optometry and ophthalmology and by interested third-parties (e.g., insurance companies). Duane[71] first proposed this model of classification, which clinically is called the *Duane-White classification*. Schapero[72] also used this model as a basis for his 10 case types. Duane proposed that a difference of at least 10Δ between the far and near deviations was necessary before a patient should be classified into one of his four original categories. Other writers have suggested a 15Δ difference between far and near, and many clinicians use 5Δ. We prefer to use a 5Δ difference or greater between the deviations at far (6 m) and near (40 cm) to indicate the presence of an abnormally high or low AC/A ratio.

The larger values typically are used by ophthalmic surgeons, as the desired level of accuracy in surgical procedures is approximately 10Δ. Compensation of the angles of deviation with prisms and added lenses, however, is more refined and often the therapy of choice. For example, if a symptomatic patient with an IPD of 60 mm manifests orthophoria at far and 10Δ esophoria at near, the calculated AC/A ratio is 10Δ/1 D. This convergence excess often is treated with a bifocal add, using the effect of the high AC/A ratio to reduce the near deviation. However, if the same symptomatic patient measured ortho at far and 5Δ esophoria at near, the calculated AC/A ratio would be 8Δ/1 D, which is considered to be high by Morgan's normative data. Added lenses at near remain an ideal management approach. We believe a 5Δ difference between near and far deviations is consistent with optical treatment approaches, and so we prefer this amount for the sake of clinical categories of vergence anomalies. This assumes that there are symptoms and vision inefficiencies resulting from the vergence anomalies. Implicit in any of the Duane-White categories is poor compensatory fusional vergences.

This classification system usually is based on angles of deviation measured by the alternate cover test, not phorometry. The angles of deviation should be measured in an open-space environment. Instrument convergence and accommodation effects may invalidate the measurements of tonic vergence and accommodative convergence. Although the categories apply to cases of strabismus as well as heterophoria, the following discussion of management recommendations is primarily for cases of heterophoria.

Convergence Insufficiency
Characteristics

Convergence insufficiency (CI), or *convergence insufficiency exophoria* as it is sometimes called, is characterized by a low AC/A ratio resulting in an increased exophoria at near viewing distances. The phoria line is shifted to the left of the demand line placing an increased demand on PFV at near. A symptomatic patient showing orthophoria at far and 5Δ exophoria at 40 cm would be an example. Other clinical findings associated with CI include a reduced PFV, a receded NPC (poor gross convergence), and reduced accommodative amplitude.[73, 74] Recently, the Convergence Insufficiency Treatment Trial Group[10, 11] developed a classification scheme for CI. The first criteria dealt with the relationship between the near and far phoria, where the near deviation had to be least 4 more exophoria than the distance phoria. The next step was looking at PFV and the NPC. If only one finding (PFV or NPC) was reduced then the patient had two signs of CI and if both were reduced then the patient had three signs of CI.

Another similar CI case type, usually ignored in most classification systems, is presbyopic exophoria. Most aging presbyopes show increases in their exophoria at near. Often there is reduced PFV, and these patients develop classic symptoms of CI (e.g., tired eyes, sleepiness when reading, and avoidance of near work). Unfortunately, most clinicians and the patients interpret these symptoms as part of the normal aging process. If a young person presented with typical CI symptoms, vision training would likely be recommended. We believe that many symptomatic presbyopic patients are untreated. This neglect is inappropriate

Management

Vision therapy is the treatment of choice for most CI cases (see Chapter 14 for a discussion of therapy for exo deviations). There is abundant evidence in the literature that this is effective.[73] In fact, two randomized masked clinical trials has shown that office based vision therapy is the most effective treatment for CI.[10,75] Both studies indicated that home based therapy, such as pencil push ups, was no better than placebo for children with CI. Because the AC/A ratio is low, added lenses (e.g., minus power) are of little value. Prism prescriptions have the disadvantage in these CI cases by inducing an esophoria at far. Sometimes it is advisable for patients presenting with accommodative insufficiency and CI to have a reading add together with BI prism for nearpoint use only. However, these patients also respond well to vision training. Some CI cases sometimes present with a large exo deviation (low tonic convergence) at far, combined with a low AC/A ratio. These are the cases that most likely benefit from a BI prism prescription (relieving the exo deviation at far) in conjunction with vision therapy to improve fusional convergence at near.

In presbyopic adults, two extensive studies showed very positive outcomes with vision training.[76, 77] Further evidence was supplied by Grisham et al[62] who prescribed two pairs of bifocal spectacles to symptomatic presbyopic individuals with exophoria. One pair had a prism amount equal to the associated phoria at near and the other was identical except there was no prism. The individuals wore the two pairs of spectacles alternately for two weeks and then had to return one pair. Of the 12 subjects, 10 chose to keep the prism spectacles for reasons of visual comfort, a result that illustrates our point. It was also found that the two individuals who returned the prism spectacles were uncomfortable because the prism, although helpful at near, had induced a significant esophoria at far. Those two would have been better managed with single-vision reading lenses that included the BI prism. The effectiveness of prisms in the presbyopics adults has been confirmed in a recent study by Teitlebaum et al[67] outlined above.

Basic Exophoria
Characteristics
Basic exophoria refers to cases in which the tonic position is exophoric at far and the AC/A ratio is normal. The far and near exo deviations are approximately equal in magnitude. An example would be a symptomatic patient who presents with 8Δ exophoria at 6 m and 8Δ exophoria at 40 cm. The basic exophoria patient may experience visual symptoms at both far and near. Much clinical literature indicates that significant exophoria is more prevalent in people experiencing reading difficulties.[78]

Management
The management of basic exophoria is similar to convergence insufficiency, with additional training methods done at farpoint. (See Chapter 14 for a discussion of therapy for exo deviations.) Because fusional convergence can easily be expanded, vision therapy for exophoria (and intermittent exotropia) is effective in these cases. BI prism is also effective in managing basic exophoria if there is little prism adaptation, because it reduces the convergence demand equally at all distances, and the amount of needed prism usually is not excessive.

Divergence Excess
Characteristics
Divergence excess exophoria is indicated when a significantly large exo deviation at far is combined with a high AC/A ratio. If a patient presents with 10Δ exophoria at far and 3Δ exophoria at near then divergence excess is indicated. This condition is often associated with strabismus and a fuller discussion is given in Chapter 7.

Some patients presenting with divergence excess actually have *simulated (pseudo) divergence excess*. For example, with prolonged occlusion, a nearpoint deviation of 3Δ exophoria may increase to 10Δ exophoria. If the far exo deviation is 10Δ, the correct diagnostic category would be basic exophoria. A spasm of fusional convergence at near is one possible explanation for a spurious result

from the initial cover test. Prolonged occlusion is necessary for convergence to decrease sufficiently to reveal the full magnitude of the exo deviation at near. Therefore, these apparent cases of divergence excess are called *simulated divergence excess*, also known as *pseudo-divergence excess*.

Management
In the case of true divergence excess, which indeed has a high AC/A ratio, the patient may experience esophoric problems at very near viewing distances. If fusion is maintained most of the time at far and the AC/A ratio is not extremely high, divergence excess patients often respond well to vision training, but they are not generally as successful as patients with other types of exo deviations. In some cases, a minus add prescribed overall helps the patient to control the far deviation, acting through the high AC/A ratio, but the amount of overminus must be carefully considered so as not to induce an esophoric problem at near. BI prisms, too, may be useful, but there remains the same reservation about inducing an esophoria at near. Many clinicians recommend plus-add bifocals along with vision therapy in the management of divergence excess cases (see Chapter 14 for further discussion of treatment for divergence excess).

Divergence Insufficiency
Characteristics
Divergence insufficiency esophoria is the least prevalent of the esophoria cases. The clinician should be aware that a sudden onset of divergence insufficiency can be associated with a paresis of the 6th cranial nerve and can require referral for scanning and neurological evaluation. It is defined as a significant esophoria (high tonic convergence) at far, combined with a low AC/A ratio. An example would be 12Δ esophoria at far and 3Δ esophoria at near. These patients can lapse into an occasional esotropia at far if fusional divergence is poor. For them, driving a vehicle, particularly at night, can be a serious problem.

Management
Successful management of some cases of divergence insufficiency is difficult. One approach that seems moderately effective is to prescribe BO prism correction in single-vision lenses for general wear. For this example, this may be 8Δ BO if the far esophoria is 12Δ. If there is no prism adaptation, the resulting farpoint esophoria would be 4Δ,

which considerably reduces the fusional divergence demand. However, with these spectacles in place, the near eso deviation would measure 5Δ exophoria instead of 3Δ esophoria. This amount is not excessive by Morgan's norms, but caution is needed in that an induced exo deviation at near is not compatible with the esophoria at far because the patent is experiencing base-out training at near rather than base-in training which is desired at near as well as at distance. A vision training goal to increase divergence ranges would be preferable, but sometimes BO prism can be tried initially to maintain comfortable fusion for sustained viewing at far distances. (Therapy for divergence insufficiency is discussed in Chapter 13.)

Basic Esophoria
Characteristics
Basic esophoria is characterized by a significant eso deviation at far and a moderate AC/A ratio, so that the far and near angles of deviation are approximately equal. An example would be esophoria of 10Δ at all viewing distances. Other associated findings often include reduced NFV, a low PRA, and high NRA.

Management
BO prism is an obvious and safe treatment approach in basic esophoria and usually is effective, because most symptomatic esophores do not adapt to prisms. Vision training is also useful in combination with prism prescription. Without the prism, completion of divergence training often takes several months, and there can be frequent regression of fusional divergence skills. If the basic esophoria patient is symptomatic only at near due to work requirements (e.g., computer or desk work), a reading add (either single-vision lenses or bifocals) may also be considered. (See chapter 13 for a discussion of therapy for basic esophoria.)

Convergence Excess
Characteristics
Convergence excess esophoria is the case that typically presents with little or no esophoria at far but with a high AC/A ratio. An example would be orthophoria at far and 7Δ esophoria at near. Patients with convergence excess often report experiencing nearpoint problems because the esophoria increases dramatically as the viewing distance becomes closer. Eyestrain, blurring, and intermittent diplopia often are reported. These patients

are vulnerable to developing an accommodative esotropia. Associated findings include low NFV, low PRA, high NRA and, possibly, esotropia at very near fixation distances. Latent hyperopia also is frequently associated with convergence excess; therefore, cycloplegic refraction is advisable in many cases of convergence excess.

Management
Usually the full hyperopic refractive error must be corrected if it measures +1.00 D or more. Because of the high AC/A ratio, plus-add bifocals usually are indicated for reading and other nearpoint activities. The amount of the plus-add should be determined empirically by measuring with the cover test and listening to subjective reports of improvement of vision and comfort. BO prism may also be necessary if there is a significant eso deviation at far. Vision therapy is recommended to break any suppression and to expand the range and facility of fusional divergence. Frequent progress checks after therapy usually are indicated, as regression may occur in the absence of an active home maintenance program of vision therapy.

Basic Orthophoria with Restricted Zone
Characteristics
Schapero[72] discussed *restricted zone* cases, which he described as basic ortho cases with restricted fusional vergences and patient-reported visual symptoms. Heterophoria may be present, but its magnitude is insignificant at far and near. The NFV or PFV or both are deficient, as can be the NRA and PRA. Sometimes the entire zone is found to be restricted. These patients often report visual fatigue after prolonged detailed visual activity and intermittent blurring, particularly when changing fixation distance. Reduced accommodative amplitude and facility are often found. The etiology usually is functional in that the patient's visual demands surpass his or her physiologic oculomotor and fusional capabilities. It must be kept in mind that the same clinical findings and visual symptoms can result from drug side effects and general health conditions (similar to those affecting accommodation that were discussed in Chapter 2). Carefully obtaining a patient history is necessary for differential diagnosis. There may also be refractive causes of a restricted zone, such as uncorrected astigmatism, uncorrected anisometropia, and aniseikonia. Optical management is indicated in these cases.

Management

If the condition proves to be caused by accommodative and vergence dysfunctions, then vision training is recommended. This mode of vision therapy is usually successful within a matter of a few weeks. The vision training goal would be to expand the range of the entire ZCSBV and improve the facility of all oculomotor functions.

NORMAL ZONE WITH SYMPTOMS

Schapero[72] also discussed the case of *symptoms but no signs*, in which a patient presents with symptoms that sound uniquely binocular in nature but clinical testing fails to find any component of the ZCSBV that is deficient by clinical standards. Accommodative and fusional amplitudes are normal. No significant heterophoria is measured, and the NPC is within 6 cm of the bridge of the nose. The clinician must search for other possibilities before concluding that the patient has psychogenic problems (e.g., hysteria, malingering, or emotional instability). Some questions and recommendations follow: Is there either latent hyperopia or pseudomyopia? Presence of either condition can be assessed with cycloplegic refraction. Is there a latent phoria? Testing for this condition is by prolonged occlusion. Is there poor accommodation or vergence stamina? Tests of accommodative or vergence facility can be helpful to see if the patients manifests reduced performance over time. The patient can also be tested at the end of the workday.

To determine whether the symptoms are truly of binocular origin, the patient should be instructed to wear a patch over the nondominant eye on alternate days and to keep a log of resulting symptoms. If symptoms decrease, some type of binocular dysfunction is indicated. If symptoms remain the same or increase, then other causes must be identified (e.g., general health problems, drug reactions, or psychological distress). Sometimes diagnostic vision therapy can be undertaken to determine whether symptoms decrease. If the final conclusion is that the symptoms are not of binocular origin, a referral for a medical or psychological evaluation is in the best interest of the patient.

BIOENGINEERING MODEL

Maddox[31] believed that the vergence system could be categorized by four additive components—tonic, accommodative, proximal (psychic), and fusional (disparity) vergence. Graphical analysis based on this concept was developed gradually by several notable individuals such as Percival, Sheard, Morgan, Fry, and Hofstetter and became the scientific foundation for binocular case analysis. We have emphasized the graphical analysis perspective in this chapter and adapted the Duane-White classification scheme to heterophoric as well as heterotropic (strabismic) disorders. We also applied Morgan's normative analysis, which is consistent with classic graphical analysis. In Chapters 2 and 3, the emphasis was on evaluating various oculomotor systems over time, testing the dynamic components of each system. Accuracy, speed, and stamina are distinctive clinical features in that analysis. These two perspectives, graphical analysis and vision efficiency analysis, reinforce one another; however, each delineates visual functions, and disorders thereof, that the other may neglect. For example, disorders of accommodation, other than accommodative insufficiency, are ignored by classic graphical analysis. Vision efficiency analysis of accommodation, however, includes evaluation of lag of accommodation (accuracy), facility (speed), and stamina (sustainability).

Originating in the 1950s, fixation disparity analysis tended to reinforce and supplement the vergence evaluation of graphical analysis. Graphical analysis and fixation disparity analysis emphasized different aspects of vergence and accommodative dynamics, but the systems were intimately related, as they both described the same underlying oculomotor physiology. What has become clear since the time of Maddox is that vergence and accommodative physiology, and disorders thereof, are substantially more complex than Maddox originally formulated. This realization has largely come to light through a bioengineering systems control approach used in basic research.

One of the most useful research tools of bioengineers is to build mathematic control models of biological systems and then to compare them with empiric physiologic evidence. The model is modified until its features accurately simulate physiologic responses and are consistent with what is known about the anatomy of the biological system. Several important insights have evolved from the relation between control systems modeling and physiologic evidence.

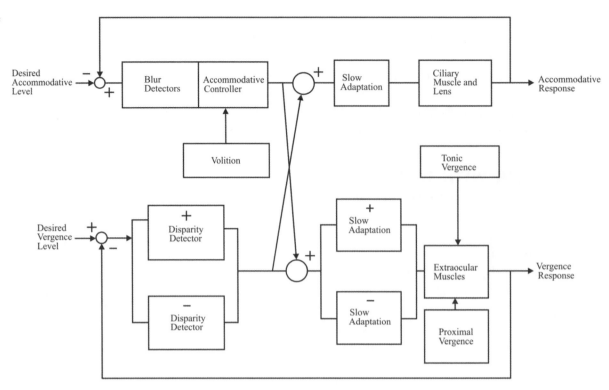

Figure 3-15. Theoretical bioengineering model illustrating interaction between accommodation and vergence in a closed-loop system. (Modified from J J Saladin. Horizontal Prism Prescription. In: Clinical Uses of Prism. SA Cotter, ed. St. Louis: Mosby; 1995:123.)

accommodative system of the eyes and the vergence system are cross-linked and dynamically influence each another. Accommodation drives convergence (AC/A) and convergence drives accommodation (CA/C). When both systems are stimulated simultaneously, the cross-links interact and respond differently from when either system is stimulated in isolation.[79] Classic graphical analysis has not taken into account this dynamic relationship and has largely ignored the influence of the CA/C. Nevertheless, clinicians have long been aware that disorders of accommodation and vergence often are associated.

Stimulation of some adaptive mechanisms for the AC/A, CA/C, and fusional vergence result in tonic changes in both accommodation and vergence. Therefore, there are both momentary and more lasting adaptations to prism and lens stimuli; a particular patient's physiologic responses to added lenses or prisms cannot be accurately predicted in all conditions of clinical management. Schor[80] suggested that the lack of vergence adaptation is an important, if not the most important, characteristic of patients having vergence disorders. Clinical observations that are consistent with this viewpoint include the finding that a steep FDC is one indi-

cator of resistance to "good" vergence adaptation and that good vergence adaptation may increase when vision training is successfully completed.[81] In other words, prism adaptation does increase and the FDC tends to flatten with training.[82] What we mean by "good" vergence adaptation must be distinguished from "bad" prism adaptation, which normally takes place in symptom-free individuals with normal binocularity in which a compensating prism will be "eaten up." For this reason, prisms are considered poison for compensation unless they are absolutely necessary. A prism should not be prescribed in cases of heterophoria unless there are symptoms (associated with vergence dysfunction) that can be relieved by lessening the vergence demand with this optical compensation. *Good vergence adaptation* relates to vision training in which increased prism demand (rather than compensating prism) is introduced for the purpose of increasing fusional vergence ability and, ultimately, favorably affecting tonic vergence.

The influence of proximal vergence on near-point vergence eye position has been largely ignored in classic case analysis, yet in some patients the amount of proximal vergence can significantly influence the associated phoria status, for better or worse.[83] Wick and London[84] proposed a version of the Hung-Semmelow model of interactions between accommodation and vergence that takes into account the influence of proximal convergence. They emphasized that one difficulty with the traditional system of binocular case analysis is that the vergence deviation that exists under binocular (associated) conditions often is not the same as that measured under dissociated viewing conditions (e.g., Maddox rod test). They joined Saladin[85] in a strong appeal for evaluating binocularity under closed-loop (associated) conditions (e.g., fixation disparity testing). Wick and London[84] suggested that an improved graphical analysis approach would result from plotting and evaluating a graph of the *associated* gradient AC/A ratio (derived from FDCs), the proximal vergence ratio, and far and near FDCs. Such an approach may indeed prove to be a significant improvement over traditional methods, but its incorporation into a practical clinical examination probably awaits technologic advances that would allow oculomotor measurements to be easily taken and transcribed directly into a computer program for analysis.

We have drawn our concept of a very simplified hypothetical model (Figure 3-15)—modified from other bioengineering models, particularly that of Saladin[86]—to illustrate the possible interaction between accommodation and vergence and the ways in which responses may be affected by the interaction between accommodative convergence and convergence accommodation as well as feedback information, accommodative and vergence adaptations, and proximal convergence.

We believe it is expedient to evaluate binocular vision using the techniques of classic case analysis and vision efficiency analysis. If clinical findings point to a dysfunction of accommodation, vergence, or their interactions, a complete fixation disparity evaluation is recommended. With this baseline clinical data and the analysis procedures recommended in this chapter, we believe the clinician has sufficient tools for successful and efficient treatment of the vast majority of nonstrabismic binocular anomalies. In patients who do not respond to vision therapy as expected, it is always prudent to retest, re-evaluate, and reconsider other approaches to vision therapy, including referral to other professionals when indicated. Flexibility in the clinical approach is another lesson to be learned from our new appreciation of the complexity of binocular vision interactions, as suggested by bioengineering models.

REFERENCES

1. Rouse M, Borsting E, Mitchell G, Schieman M, Cotter S, Cooper J, Kulp M, London R, Wansveen J, CITT Study Group. Validity and reliability of the revised convergence insufficiency symptom survey. Ophthal and Physiol Opt 2004;24:384-90.

2. Borsting E, Rouse M, Mitchell G, Schieman M, Cotter S, Cooper J, Kulp M, London R, CITT Study Group. Validity and reliability of the revised convergence insufficiency symptom survey in children ages 9-18. Opt Vis Sci 2003;80:832-8.

3. Morgan M. Anomalies of the Visual Neuromuscular System of the Aging Patient and Their Correction. In: Hirsch M, Wick R, eds. Vision of the Aging Patient. Philadelphia: Chilton, 1960.

4. Rainey BB, Schroeder T, Goss DA, Grovesnor TP. Interexaminer repeatability of heterophoria tests. Optom Vis Sci. 1998;75:719-26.

5. Saladin J. Phorometry and Stereopsis. In: Benjamin W, ed. Borish's Clinical Refraction. Philadelphia: WB Saunders, 1998.

6. Flom M. Treatment of Binocular Anomalies of Vision. In: Hirsch M, Wick R, eds. Vision of Children. Philadelphia: Chilton, 1963.

7. Griffin J. Vision Efficiency Therapy, Course 637A, Laboratory Syllabus. Fullerton, Calif.: Southern California College of Optometry, 2001.

8. Hoffman L, Rouse M. Referral recommendations for binocular function and/or developmental perceptual deficiencies. J Am Optom Assoc. 1980;51:119-25.

9. Hayes G, Cohen B, Rouse M, DeLand P. Normative values for the nearpoint of convergence of elementary school children. Optom Vis Sci. 1998;75:506-12.

10. Convergence Insufficiency Treatment Trial (CITT) S. Randomized clinical trial of treatments for symptomatic convergence insufficiency in children. Arch Ophthalmol.;126(10):1336-49.

11. Convergence Insufficiency Treatment Trial (CITT) Study Group. The convergence insufficiency treatment trial: design, methods, baseline data. Ophthalmic Epidemiol 2008;15:24-36.

12. Wick B. Vision Therapy for Preschool Children. In: Rosenbloom A, Morgan M, eds. Pediatric Optometry. Philadelphia: Lippincott, 1990.

13. Rouse M, Borsting E, Deland P, CIRS group. Reliability of binocular vision measurements used in the classification of convergence insufficiency. Opt Vis Sci 2002;79:254-64.

14. Schor C. Visuomotor Development. In: Rosenbloom A, Morgan M, eds. Pediatric Optometry. Philadelphia: Lippincott, 1990.

15. Schor C. Fixation Disparity and Vergence Adaptation. In: Schor C, Ciuffreda K, eds. Vergence Eye Movements. Boston: Butterworth-Heinemann, 1983.

16. Grisham J. Treatment of Binocular Dysfunctions. In: Schor C, Ciuffreda K, eds. Vergence Eye Movements. Boston: Butterworth-Heinemann, 1983.

17. Scheiman M, Herzberg H, Frantz K, Margolin M. A normative study of step vergence testing in elementary school children. J Am Optom Assoc 1989;60:276-80.

18. Antona B, Barra F, Barrio A, Gonzalez E, Sanchez I. Repeatability intraexaminer and agreement in amplitude of accommodation measurements. Graefes Arch Clin Exp Ophthalmol. 2009;247:121-7.

19. Ciuffreda M, Ciuffreda K, Wang B. Repeatability and Variability of Near Vergence Ranges. J Behav Optom. 2006;17(2):39-46.

20. Grisham J. The dynamics of fusional vergence eye movements in binocular dysfunction. Am J Optom Physiol Opt. 1980;57:645-55.

21. Gall R, Wick B. The symptomatic patient with normal phorias at distance and near: what tests detect a binocular vision problem? Optometry 2003;74(5):309-22.

22. Kenyon R, Ciuffreda K, Stark L. *Dynamic vergence eye movements in strabismus and amblyopia: symmetric vergence.* Invest Ophthalmol. 1980;19:60-74.

23. Pierce J. *Lecture. Northern Central States Optometric Conference.* Minneapolis, Minn., 1973.

24. Stuckle L, Rouse M. *Norms for Dynamic Vergences.* On file in the M.B. Ketchum Memorial Library. Fullerton, Calif.: Southern California College of Optometry, 1979.

25. Mitchell R, Stanich R, Rouse M. *Norms for Dynamic Vergences.* On file in the M.B. Ketch um Memorial Library. Fullerton, Calif.: Southern California College of Optometry, 1980.

26. Moser J, Atkinson W. *Vergence Facility in a Young Adult Population.* On file in the M.B. Ketch um Memorial Library. Fullerton, Calif.: Southern California College of Optometry, 1980.

27. Rosner J. *Course 548, Lecture Notes.* Houston: University of Houston, College of Optometry, 1979.

28. Jacobson M, Goldstein A, Griffin J. *The Relationship Between Vergence Range and Vergence Facility.* On file in the M.B. Ketchum Memorial Library. Fullerton, Calif.: Southern California College of Optometry, 1979.

29. Delgadillo H, Griffin J. *Vergence facility and associated symptoms: a comparison of two prism flipper tests.* J Behav Optom. 1992;3:91-4.

30. Donders F. *On the Anomalies of Accommodation and Refraction of the Eye.* In: Moore W, ed. London: The New Sydenham Society, 1864.

31. Maddox E. *The Clinical Use of Prisms and the Decentering of Lenses,* 2nd ed. Bristol, U.K.: John Wright, 1893.

32. Sheard C. *Ocular discomfort and its relief.* EENT 1931;7.

33. Morgan M. *Analysis of clinical data.* Am J Optom Arch Am Acad Optom. 1944;21:477-91.

34. Morgan M. *Accommodation and convergence.* Am J Optom Arch Am Acad Optom. 1968;45:417-91.

35. Scheiman M, Wick B. *Clinical Management of Binocular Vision.* Philadelphia: Lippincott Williams & Wilkins, 2002.

36. Ogle K, Martens T, Dyer J. *Oculomotor Imbalance in Binocular Vision and Fixation Disparity.* In. Philadelphia: Lea & Febiger, 1967.

37. Schor C, Ciuffreda K. *Vergence Eye Movements: Basic and Clinical Aspects.* London: Butterworths, 1983:467.

38. Mallett R. *The investigation of heterophoria at near and a new fixation disparity technique.* Optician 1964;148:547-51.

39. Cole R, Boisvert R. *Effect of fixation disparity on stereo-acuity.* Am J Optom. 1974;51:206-13.

40. Levin M, Sultan B. *Unpublished senior student research study.* On file in the M.B. Ketchurn Memorial Library. Fullerton, Calif.: Southern California College of Optometry, 1972.

41. Dittemore D, Crum J, Kirschen D. *Comparison of fixation disparity measurements obtained with the Wesson Fixation Disparity Card and the Sheedy Disparometer.* Optom Vis Sci. 1993;70:414-20.

42. Ngan J, Goss DA, Despirito J. *Comparison of fixation disparity curve parameters obtained with the Wesson and Saladin fixation disparity cards.* Optom Vis Sci 2005;82:69-74.

43. Cooper J, Feldman J, Horn D, Dibble C. *Reliability of fixation disparity curves.* Am J Optom Physiol Opt. 1981;58:960-4.

44. Kwan L, Lam A, Kwan C, Yeung P. *The characteristics of near prism induced fixation disparity curve in Hong Kong Chinese.* Ophthalmic Physiol Opt. 1999;19:393-400.

45. Wick B. *Forced vergence fixation disparity at distance and near in an asymptomatic young adult population.* Am J Optom Physiol Opt. 1985;62:591-9.

46. Wick B, Joubert C. *Lens-induced fixation disparity curves.* Am J Optom Physiol Opt. 1988;65:606-12.

47. Daum K. *The stability of the fixation disparity curve.* Ophthalmic Physiol Opt. 1983;3:13-9.

48. Rutstein R, Eskridge J. *Studies in vertical fixation disparity.* Am J Optom Physiol Opt. 1986;63:639-44.

49. Garzia R, Dyer G. *Effect of near-point stress on the horizontal forced vergence fixation disparity curve.* Am J Optom Physiol Opt. 1986;63:901-7.

50. Yekta A, Pickwell L, Jenkins T. *Binocular vision, age and symptoms.* Ophthalmic Physiol Opt . 1989;9:115-20.

51. Yekta A, Jenkins T, Pickwell D. *The clinical assessment of binocular vision before and after a working day.* Ophthalmic Physiol Opt. 1987;7:349-52.

52. Karania R, Evans B. *The Mallett Fixation Disparity Test: influence of test instructions and relationship with symptoms.* Ophthal and Physiol Opt 2006;26:507-22.

53. Dowley D. *Fixation disparity.* Optom Vis Sci. 1989;66:98-105.

54. Wildsoet C, Cameron K. *The effect of illumination and foveal fusion lock on clinical fixation disparity measurements with the Sheedy Disparometer.* Ophthalmic Physiol Opt. 1985;5:171-8.

55. Debysingh S, Orzech P, Sheedy J. *Effect of a central fusion stimulus on fixation disparity.* Am J Optom Physiol Opt. 1986;63:277-80.

56. Sheedy J, Saladin J. *Validity of Diagnostic Criteria and Case Analysis in Binocular Vision Disorders.* In: Schor C, Ciuffreda K, eds. Vergence Eye Movements. Boston: Butterworths, 1983.

57. Sheedy J, Saladin J. *Phoria, vergence, and fixation disparity in oculomotor problems.* Am J Optom Physiol Opt. 1977;54(7):474-8.

58. Percival A. *The Prescribing of Spectacles.* Bristol,U.K.: John Wright, 1928.

59. Sheedy J. *Actual measurements of fixation disparity and its use in diagnosis and treatment.* J Am Optom Assoc. 1980;51:1079-84.

60. Worrell B, Hirsch M, Morgan M. *An evaluation of prism prescribed by Sheard's criterion.* Am J Optom Physiol Opt 1971;48:373-6.

61. Payne C, Grisham J, Thomas K. *A clinical evaluation of fixation disparity.* Am J Optom Physiol Opt. 1974;1:88-90.

62. Grisham J. *Treatment of Binocular Dysfunctions.* In: Schor C, Ciuffreda K, eds. Vergence Eye Movements. Boston: Butterworths, 1983.

63. Otto J, Kromeier M, Bach M, Kommerell G. *Do dissociated or associated phoria predict the comfortable prism?* Graefes Arch Clin Exp Ophthalmol. 2008;246:631-9.

64. Scheiman M, Cotter S, Rouse M, Mitchell G, Kulp M, Cooper J, Borsting E, The Convergence Insufficiency Treatment Trial (CITT) Study Group. *Randomized clinical trial of the effectiveness of base-in prism reading glasses versus placebo reading glasses for symptomatic convergence insufficiency in children.* Br J Ophthalmol. 2005;89:1318-23.

65. O'Leary C, Evans B. *Double-masked randomised placebo-controlled trial of the effect of prismatic corrections on rate of reading and the relationship with symptoms.* Opthal Physiol Opt 2006;26:555-65.

66. Stavis M, Murray M, Jenkins P. *Objective improvement from base-in prisms for reading discomfort associated with mini-convergence insufficiency type exophoria in school children.* Binocul Vis Eye Muscle Surg Q 2002;17:135-42.

67. Teitelbaum B, Pang Y, Krall J. *Effectiveness of base-in prism for presbyopes with convergence iInsufficiency.* Optometry and Visual Science 2009;86(2):153-6.

68. Gerling J, de Paz H, Schroth V, Bach M, Kommerell G. *Can fixation disparity be detected reliably by measurement and correctional techniques according to HJ. Haase (MKH)?* Klin Monatsbl Augenheilkd 2000;216:401-11.

69. Kommerell G, Gerling J, Ball M, de Paz H, Bach M. *Heterophoria and fixation disparity: a review.* Strabismus 2000;8:127-34.

70. Jenkins T, Abd-Manan F, Pardhan S. *Fixation disparity and near visual acuity.* Ophthalmic Physiol Opt. 1995;15:53-8.

71. Duane A. *A new classification of the motor anomalies of the eyes based upon physiological principles.* Ann Ophthalmol Otolaryngol. 1897;6:84.

72. Schapero M. The characteristics of ten basic visual training problems. Am J Optom Arch Am Acad Optom. 1955;32:333-42.

73. Grisham J. Visual therapy results for convergence insufficiency: a literature review. Am J Optom Physiol Opt. 1988;65:448-54.

74. Rouse M, Borsting E, Hyman L, Hussein M, Cotter S, Flynn M, Scheiman M, Gallaway M, Deland P, CIRS, group. Frequency of convergence insufficiency among fifth and sixth graders. Optom Vis Sci 1999;76:643-9.

75. Scheiman M, Mitchell L, Cotter S, Cooper J, Kulp M, Rouse M, Borsting E, London R, Wensveen J, The Convergence Insufficiency Treatment Trial (CITT) Study Group. A Randomized Clinical Trial of Treatments for Convergence Insufficiency in Children. Arch Ophthalmol. 2005;123:14-24.

76. Wick B. Vision training for presbyopic nonstrabismic patients. Am J Optom Physiol Opt. 1977;54:244-7.

77. Cohen A, Soden R. Effectiveness of visual therapy for convergence insufficiency for an adult population. J Am Optom Assoc. 1984;55:491-4.

78. Simons H, Grisham J. Binocular anomalies and reading problems. J Am Optom Assoc. 1987;58:578-87.

79. Schor C. Models of mutual interactions between accommodation and convergence. Am J Optom Physiol Opt. 1985;62:369-74.

80. Schor C. Analysis of tonic and accommodative vergence disorders of binocular vision. Am J Optom Physiol Opt. 1983;60:1-14.

81. North R, Henson D. Adaptation to prism-induced heterophoria in subjects with abnormal binocular vision or asthenopia. Am J Optom Physiol Opt. 1981;58:746-52.

82. Luu C, Green J, Abel L. Vertical fixation disparity curve and the effects of vergence training in normal young adult population. Optom Vis Sci. 2000;77:663-9.

83. Wick B. Clinical factors in proximal vergence. Am J Optom Physiol Opt. 1985;62:1-18.

84. Wick B, London R. Analysis of binocular visual function using tests made under binocular conditions. Am J Optom Physiol Opt. 1987;64:227-40.

85. Saladin J. Convergence insufficiency, fixation disparity, and control system analysis. Am J Optom Physiol Opt. 1986;63:645-53.

86. Saladin J. Horizontal Prism Prescription. In: Cotter S, ed. Clinical Uses of Prism. St. Louis: Mosby, 1995.

History	82	Spatial Localization Testing	100
Time of Onset	82	Signs and Symptoms	101
Mode of Onset	83	Diplopia	101
Duration of Strabismus	84	Abnormal Head Posture	101
Previous Treatment	85	Subjective Testing	101
Developmental History	85	Single-Object Method	102
Summary of Clinical Questions	85	Two-Object Method	102
Measurement of Strabismus	85	Frequency of the Deviation	105
Direct Observation	86	Classification	105
Angle Kappa	86	Evaluation	106
Hirschberg Test	86	Patient History	106
Krimsky Test	88	Testing	106
Unilateral Cover Test	88	Direction of the Deviation	107
Alternate Cover Test	89	Classification	107
Four Base-Out Prism Test	90	Objective Testing	107
Bruckner Test	90	Subjective Testing	108
Comitancy	91	Magnitude of the Deviation	109
Causes	91	Classification	109
Criteria and Terminology	91	Testing Procedures	110
Primary and Secondary Deviations	93	Accommodative-Convergence/ Accommodation Ratio	110
Ductions	94	Eye Laterality	111
Versions	95	Eye Dominancy	111
Three-Step Method	95	Variability of the Deviation	112
Recording Incomitant Deviations	97	Cosmesis	112

When the status of a patient's strabismus is evaluated, the first step is to make a diagnosis of the deviation. Much information about the strabismic deviation can be obtained by a careful case history. After that, objective testing can verify nine important diagnostic variables: comitancy, frequency, direction, magnitude, accommodative-convergence/accommodation (AC/A) ratio, eye laterality, eye dominancy, variability, and cosmesis.

HISTORY

Besides giving tentative determination for each of the aforementioned variables, a patient history is needed to assess the time of onset of a manifest deviation, its mode of onset, its duration, previous treatment and results, and pertinent developmental history that may have a bearing on the binocular status of the patient.

Time of Onset

A vital part of any strabismus diagnosis is to ascertain whether the strabismus is congenital. More correctly, congenital strabismus should be referred to as *essential infantile strabismus* because, in many such cases, the manifest eye turn is not present at the time of birth. In cases of essential infantile strabismus, clinical experience has shown that the prognosis for normal binocular vision is very poor unless treatment occurs very early.

We believe that the age of 4 months is the critical cutoff between essential infantile and *early acquired strabismus*, because by that time the accommodation and vergence has developed to a large degree.[1,2] The classification of *late acquired strabismus* pertains to occurrence of strabismus beyond the age of 2 years. For example, an infant with intermittent esotropia at 6 months of age may have an accommodative-convergence component that results in the strabismus. For children 2 years of age and younger, parents should be questioned to determine the specific month of onset. For example, an essential infantile esotropia at birth probably has a poorer prognosis for cure with early treatment (e.g., surgery before age 2 years) than if the onset were at 4 months of age. In the latter case, the infant has presumably experienced 4 months of cortical development for binocular vision.

To ascertain the time of onset, a complete report of previous professional examinations should be obtained. However, this is not always possible and information from parents, relatives, and

Table 4-1. General Guidelines for Characteristics That Might Differentiate between Essential Infantile and Later-Acquired Esotropia

Essential Infantile Esotropia (birth-4 mos)	Acquired Esotropia
Alternating deviation (often a midline switch/cross fixation pattern)	Unilateral deviation (in majority of cases)
Possible lack of any correspondence (often unable to prove any correspondence with testing)	Presence of correspondence (either normal or anomalous)
Often no awareness of diplopia (only alternate perception of images)	Diplopic awareness possible (true simultaneous perception)
Double hyper deviation and often excyclorotation of covered eye (dissociated vertical deviation in majority of cases)	No double hyper deviation (dissociated vertical deviation possible but rare)
Insignificant refractive errors (occurring occasionally but as a separate component of the strabismus)	Significant refractive errors (e.g., hyperopia causing accommodative esotropia)
Normal or low AC/A ratio (may be high, but usually normal)	High AC/A ratio (e.g., high ratio causing nearpoint accommodative esotropia)
Little or no functional amblyopia (alternating fixation preventing unilateral amblyopia)	Unilateral functional amblyopia (constant unilateral strabismus causing amblyopia)

AC/A = accommodative-convergence/accommodation

friends is often erroneous. Pseudostrabismus can be confused with true strabismus; the appearance of esotropia can be simulated by epicanthal folds, negative-angle kappa, narrow interpupillary distance, and other cosmetic factors. Any of these factors can cause parents to believe that their baby has esotropia, when in fact there is only pseudostrabismus. Further confusion as to time of onset is introduced when a pseudostrabismus later becomes an acquired strabismus. A patient history obtained from the parents is not always reliable for accurate timing of the onset. Parents can also be misled by the poorly coordinated eye movements usually present in the early postnatal period, which can cause a report of congenital strabismus when, in fact, the infant's binocular status was normal with respect to age.

The prevalence of infantile esotropia is approximately 10% of all cases of constant esotropia.[3] In the majority of esotropes (whether constant or intermittent), onset is after the age of 4 months and usually before 6 years and has an accommodative component.[3] Because time of onset is important in the prognosis for functional cure, the clinician must differentiate infantile from later-acquired esotropia. When the history fails to pinpoint the onset of esotropia, certain testing may indicate whether the esotropia was essential infantile or acquired: Some possible characteristics of essential infantile esotropia can be compared with those of acquired esotropia (Table 4-1). These findings are useful when the patient history is insufficient. It also may be helpful to have parents bring early childhood photographs for inspection, particularly those taken before the child reached the ages of 1 and 2 years.

The prevalence of essential infantile exotropia is lower than that of infantile esotropia. Onset of acquired exotropia, however, may be early, often before the age of 2 years.

Mode of Onset

It is important to know whether the strabismus was intermittent or constant when it became apparent. An intermittent strabismus is relatively more noticeable than one of equal magnitude that is constant and unchanging. Although an intermittent strabismus may cause cosmetic concern, it has a less deleterious effect on sensory fusion than does constant strabismus. Even if treatment were delayed, it can be assumed that the child with an intermittent manifest deviation did not completely lose central binocular fusion, as would happen in constant strabismus. This is a particularly important point for consideration in cases of small-angle esotropia with a monofixation pattern. Even though the eyes are apparently straight, a small constant esotropia may be present. Only when peripheral fusion breaks down and the larger eso component is manifest will the esotropia be cosmetically noticeable. This seemingly intermittent esotropia is, nevertheless, constant.

Exotropia, on the other hand, tends to be either purely intermittent or constant; the deviating eye is likely to be either all the way out or all the way aligned for bifoveal fixation. Mode of onset reported in the history is usually more reliable in cases of exotropia than in esotropia. Early acquired exo deviations tend to be intermittent as compared with eso deviations, which tend to have a sudden constant mode of onset. Typically, an intermittent exo deviation that begins at approximately 2 years of age continues to be intermittent for many months. Frequently, intermittent exotropia in young children gradually becomes more frequent and may become constant over time, unless treatment is instituted. An eso deviation of comparable magnitude, however, often begins as a constant strabismus.

Whether the deviation was *alternating* or *unilateral* at the time of onset is an important fact to establish, especially in the evaluation of amblyopia. An alternating strabismus is less likely to cause amblyopia than is strabismus that is unilateral. The onset of amblyopia, therefore, cannot be equated with the onset of alternating strabismus; a history of unilateral strabismus is more definitive in regard to time of onset of amblyopia.

Reports of noticeable *variations* of the strabismus angle may be useful. Changes of magnitude in different positions of gaze suggest an acquired paresis as the probable cause of strabismus. If, however, the angle in the primary position is reported to vary from time to time, the deviation may be comitant and due to physical illness, emotional disturbances, or other causes affecting the tonic angle of convergence. For example, psychogenic strabismus (either eso or exo) is a possibility, although psychogenic esotropias are much more frequent than are psychogenic exotropias. The conceivable way that an individual could experience a psychogenic exotropia is by letting go of fusion to allow the latent deviation to lapse into an exotropia. This usually occurs in individuals who use this condition to get their way, to receive sympathy, or for other reasons designed to gain something from others.

In the event that a patient has not been examined previously by another ophthalmologist or optometrist and reports of the patient's refractive, visual acuity, and binocular status are unavailable, the practitioner must depend largely on the patient's or parents' statements for any history. A good line of questioning directed to parents of young patients is the following: "When the turning of the eye was first noticed, did the eye turn out toward the ear or in toward the nose? Was it always the same eye that turned, or did the other eye turn some of the time? Was the turning more noticeable at different times of the day? Was it more noticeable when the child looked up, down, to the left or right?" Answers to these questions may indicate the mode of onset of strabismus.

Duration of Strabismus

The *duration* of time elapsing between the onset of a manifest deviation and therapy is a crucial factor in the re-education and recovery or further development of normal binocular vision. This is particularly so in the child younger than 6 years. The best surgical results in infantile esotropia, as indicated by long-term random-dot stereopsis, occur primarily in those children with a short duration between onset of strabismus and surgical intervention.[4,5] Clinical experience indicates that several months without bifoveal fusion can cause irreparable loss of central fusion to the infant or very young child if treatment is delayed. When the duration is inordinately long and treatment is delayed, peripheral fusion may also be irrecoverable.

The duration time factor is not as critical in the ages beyond the developmental years as it is in the plastic years below the age of 6. Nevertheless, loss of the faculty of bifoveal fixation is not uncommon in adults who have had to give up bifoveal fixation over a long period for one reason or another (e.g., unilateral cataract of long standing, acquired strabismus of many years due to paresis). It is not always possible to regain bifoveal fusion, even though the obstacles may cease to exist (e.g., good visual acuity after a cataract operation).

Total duration (time of onset to patient's current age) and the time elapsing from onset to treatment must be differentiated. Although both time periods are important determinants in prognosis for functional cure, the period between the time of onset and the beginning of treatment is usually more important. If effective therapy is wisely and immediately instituted, the chance for recovery of binocularity is greater than if treatment is delayed. This is not meant to imply that treatment (e.g., surgery) should be performed instantly and with reckless abandon; rather, caution and discretion should be observed in all cases. It is very unwise just to let things be, as valuable time is lost. For instance, a case in which the onset is early and there is constant unilateral esotropia, alternate occlusion might be prescribed as a measure for preventing amblyopia. Also, base-

Table 4-2. Information to Obtain from Patients with a History of Extraocular Muscle Surgery

Age when surgery performed

Eye undergoing operation
  Right
  Left
  Both

Muscle(s) undergoing operation
Technique (e.g. recession, resection)

Cosmetic appearance
  Preoperatively
  Immediately postoperatively
  Later postoperatively

Functional result (much depending on professional reports)
Repeat preceding information for additional surgeries

Table 4-3. Typical Questions in Patient History Regarding Time and Mode of Strabismus Onset

When was the eye turn first noticed?
Was it an inward or outward turning?
Was it just one eye, or did either eye turn?
If either eye turned, what percentage of time did the right eye turn, and what percentage did the left eye turn?
Did the turning take place all the time or just some of the time?
If the turning was just some of the time, how often was it?
Was there any particular time or activity that caused the eye turn?
Has the eye turn gotten worse, more frequent, or larger?
What treatment was given, and what were the results?
What are the cosmetic concerns, symptoms, or other problems?

out (BO) prisms (e.g., Fresnels) should be considered as a holding action, particularly if the patient is below the orthoptic training age (younger than 4 years). In certain cases, the use of BO prisms may be undertaken in conjunction with plus-lens therapy. If good binocularity cannot be recovered after a reasonable period, extraocular muscle surgery may be the recommended treatment.

Previous Treatment

After questioning regarding time, mode, and duration of onset has been completed, another important fact to determine from the patient history is the extent and type of previous treatment that the patient has actually received. However, treatment all too often is recommended but not sufficiently undertaken. Treatment usually takes the form of patching an eye, but in many cases it is found to have been inadequate. The lack of proper occlusion therapy impedes recovery; in addition, a history of a patient's having been patched can lead to erroneous conclusions on the part of a subsequent examining clinician. The second doctor may mistakenly conclude that everything possible was done for the patient and that any existing amblyopia cannot be eliminated by means of patching, as such therapy has been tried without success. To avoid such incorrect assumptions, questions regarding previous treatment must be pursued in depth. This rule applies not only to occlusion therapy but to any of the other various forms of treatment for binocular anomalies. Table 4-2 lists information that should be obtained when a patient has undergone extraocular muscle surgery. It is frequently necessary to acquire records from previous doctors.

Developmental History

The purpose of obtaining a *developmental* history is to determine the important milestones at different ages in a child's life. Of interest are the physical, mental, and emotional development of the child mainly in the plastic years before age 6. A developmental history may explain why a patient has a particular binocular anomaly.

Fisher[6] stated that gross neurologic dysfunction has been found in almost 25% of patients with infantile esotropia. In contrast, the prevalence of such coexisting anomalies is low in cases of acquired esotropia. Hence, a history of neurologic signs may indicate infantile strabismus. A mild lag in neurologic development may produce detrimental factors in the development of good binocularity. A developmental history can be important in many cases of strabismus.

SUMMARY OF CLINICAL QUESTIONS

Table 4-3 outlines sample questions on a typical clinical form for the purpose of strabismus diagnosis. Each of these questions can be explored in depth, but the basic format is similar in most cases when strabismus testing is begun.

MEASUREMENT OF STRABISMUS

Several methods may be used for detection of strabismus. Some are more sensitive than others, meaning that detection is more likely using those methods. For example, the unilateral cover test is more likely to detect strabismus than is direct observation. Objective methods are listed in Table 4-4, and the relative sensitivity for detection of each is shown.

Table 4-4. Objective Testing Procedures for Detection of Strabismus in Ascending Order of Sensitivity

Direct observation
Hirschberg test
Krimsky test
Four base-out prism test
Unilateral cover test
Brückner test

Direct Observation

Horizontal manifest deviations greater than 20Δ can often be detected by observation alone, because they are cosmetically noticeable in most cases. Deviations of less than 10Δ usually are not detectable by direct observation alone. Moderately sized angles may or may not be noticeable, depending on other factors such as angle kappa and epicanthal folds. A great problem with reliance on direct observation is that pseudostrabismus often is confused with true strabismus by this method. More sensitive testing is required, such as the Hirschberg test, which involves evaluation of angle kappa.

Angle Kappa

Angle kappa is the angle between the visual axis and the pupillary axis. It is practically the same as angle alpha, which is the angle formed at the first nodal point by the intersection of the optic axis and the visual axis. Because angle alpha cannot be measured by clinical means, angle kappa is the traditionally designated clinical term, although technically the clinician is measuring angle lambda (the angle subtended at the *center of the entrance pupil* of the eye by the intersection of the pupillary axis and the visual axis).

The magnitude of angle kappa (actually lambda) customarily is referred to in terms of millimeters rather than prism diopters (Δ) or degrees. Although the normally expected magnitude is from 0.25 mm positive (nasalward) to 0.5 mm positive, there is nothing abnormal about a larger or smaller angle kappa (even a negative, or temporalward, angle) provided the magnitude is the same for each eye. The distance in millimeters between the corneal reflection of the fixated penlight and the center of the pupil determines the magnitude (Figure 4-1).

Testing is performed monocularly under dim room illumination. The patient fixates a penlight at a distance of approximately 50 cm. The examiner's sighting eye must be directly behind the light

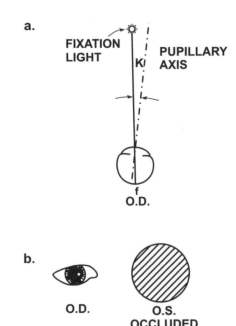

Figure 4.1. Illustrations of angle kappa (K). a. Top view of right eye, illustrating a positive angle kappa, b. Front view of right eye, illustrating a positive angle kappa. The light reflection is displaced nasally by approximately 1 mm. (f = fovea).

source. The position of the corneal light reflection in relation to the center of the pupil is observed and estimated. For example, a finding of 1 mm nasal is expressed as 1 mm positive angle kappa for the eye (+1 mm). The same procedure is repeated for the other eye. The usual causes of an observable difference in angle kappa between the two eyes are (1) large eccentric fixation of an eye; (2) a displaced pupil (corectopia); and (3) a displaced fovea (macular ectopia).

Hirschberg Test

In the latter part of the nineteenth century, Julius Hirschberg[7] introduced a quick and practical test for measuring the angle of strabismus. The procedure has remained the same over the years, although interpretation has varied. The Hirschberg test is performed by directing a small light source, such as a penlight (Hirschberg used a candle flame), onto the patient's eyes. From behind the light, the examiner sights the eyes while the patient is fixating the light. The examiner's dominant eye for sighting is directly behind the light, preferably less than 10 cm from the light source. Hirschberg recommended approximately a 30-cm distance between the light and the patient, although this may be increased to 1 m and still maintain accuracy. We recommend a range between 0.5 and 1.0 m for clinically measuring an angle of strabismus.

Hirschberg attempted to quantify the strabismic angle by comparing the first Purkinje image (clinically referred to as the corneal reflex), located in the entrance pupil of the fixating eye, with the apparent location of the corneal reflex on the deviating eye. Because the cornea acts as a small convex mirror, a virtual image of the bulb of the penlight is formed. The reference points for judging the position of the reflection on the strabismic eye include the center of the pupil, the pupillary margin, and the limbus. In the past, guidelines for quantification were used: For example, a reflex appearing to be on the temporal limbus of the deviating eye was estimated to represent 100Δ of esotropia. This method is not reliable, because factors of corneal size, corneal steepness, and angle kappa must be taken into account for accurate measurement.

Various clinicians have proposed simple ratios for measuring the magnitude of strabismic deviations. In the past, the commonly accepted ratio was 12Δ per 1 mm displacement of the reflex of the deviating eye, relative to its location on the fixating eye. A much higher ratio of 22Δ/mm was proposed by Jones and Eskridge.[8] Griffin and Boyer[9] used photographic means to study subjects with known magnitudes of strabismus. The position of each corneal reflex in the photographs was determined by microscopical analysis. Their results concurred closely with those of Jones and Eskridge.[8,10,11] Studies in children indicate that the ratio of 20-22 mm is essentially stable throughout development, except at ages younger than 5 months.[10,11] For clinical purposes, the same ratio can be used for children and adults.

Interpretation of the Hirschberg test is illustrated in Figure 4-2 in which a 22/1 ratio is assumed and the pupil size is 4 mm. In Figure 4-2a and 4-2b, angle kappa (more correctly, angle lambda) is zero. In Figure 4-2c and 4-2d angle kappa is +1 mm, and in Figure 4-2e angle kappa is -1 mm. The importance of accounting for angle kappa for Hirschberg testing is evident in these illustrations. Angle kappa is normally between +0.5 and +1.0 mm, and a zero angle kappa is the exception. Therefore, the center of the pupil and the corneal light reflection usually are not in conjunction; rather, the reflex usually is displaced nasalward from the center of the pupil.

The sensitivity of the Hirschberg test is limited to approximately 5Δ for horizontal deviations.[12] A convenient clinical ratio is 20Δ/mm, which

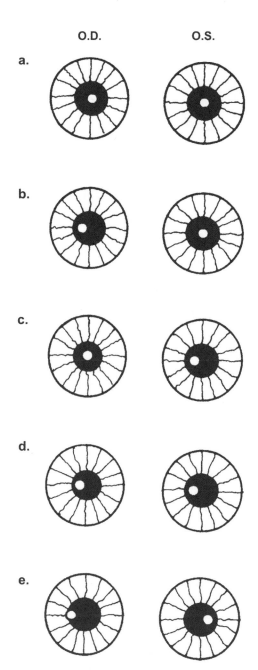

O.D.   O.S.

a.

b.

c.

d.

e.

Figure 4-2—Interpretation of the Hirschberg test in five examples, a. Bifoveal fixation, 0 angle kappa, b. O.S. fixating, 0 angle kappa, and 22Δ esotropia of O.D. c. OS fixating, +1 -mm angle kappa, and 22Δ esotropia of OD. d. OS fixating, +1 -mm angle kappa, and 44Δ esotropia of OD. e. OS fixating, -1 -mm angle kappa, and 22Δ esotropia of OD.

means that a relative displacement of 0.25 mm of the corneal reflex on the deviating eye represents 5Δ. This is the best a clinician can expect, because a displacement of less than 0.25 mm is almost impossible to discern.

The accuracy of a Hirschberg estimate tends to decrease with the size of the strabismic deviation, even among experienced clinicians. The amplitude of large esotropias and exotropias are most often underestimated by the Hirschberg test as

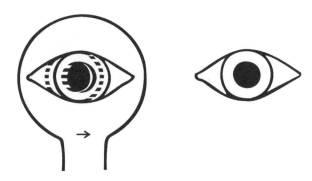

Figure 4-3. Unilateral cover test in an example of esophoria. A translucent cover paddle (as depicted here) may be used for observation of the eye behind the occluder; if an opaque occluder is used, the examiner can look around the paddle to observe the occluded eye.

compared with results by the alternate cover test.[13] Hirschberg test accuracy and reliability can be improved by video enhancement of the image of the eyes with a millimeter scale in the field, so that direct measurements can be made.[14] This method may be applicable in infants and small children in whom other methods are not providing consistent results.

Krimsky Test

The Krimsky test has slightly more sensitivity than the Hirschberg test, yet it is similar, with one exception: Prisms are used to reposition the corneal light reflex of the deviating eye to the same relative location as the reflex on the fixating eye. The magnitude of the prism necessary to accomplish this is the measurement of the angle of strabismus. A confounding factor in the Krimsky test is the possibility of prism adaptation. Therefore, the testing time must be brief, 2-3 seconds at most. For this reason and because the Krimsky test is more complicated and less natural for the patient, we routinely use the Hirschberg test rather than the Krimsky test.

Unilateral Cover Test

The *unilateral cover test* is also known as the *cover-uncover test*. Its main purpose is to detect strabismus by distinguishing it from heterophoria. For example, assume a patient has an esophoria, and the cover is placed before the patient's right eye. The left eye would continue to fixate, but the right eye would move in a nasal direction behind the occluder (Figure 4-3). When the occluder is removed from the right eye, the eye would move in a temporal direction for resumption of bifixation. Similarly, when the occluder is placed before the

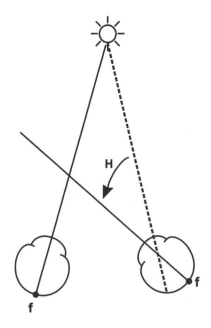

Figure 4-4. Esotropia of the right eye. (f = fovea; H = magnitude of the horizontal angle of strabismus.)

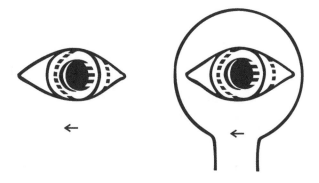

Figure 4-5. Examiner's view of eye movements on the unilateral cover test when the occluder is placed before the fixating left eye. If an opaque occluder is used, the examiner must look behind the occluder to see the movement of the covered eye.

left eye, that eye would move inward behind the cover and, when the cover is removed, the left eye would move outwardly in the case of esophoria.

An esotropia of the right eye is illustrated in Figure 4-4. If the cover is placed before the right eye, there will be no movement of either eye because only the left eye is fixating. When the cover is placed before the left eye, however, the right eye will have to move outwardly to fixate the target. Also, the left eye will make an inward movement and be in an eso posture behind the occluder (Figure 4-5). The movement of the uncovered eye is the distinguishing feature of strabismus on the unilateral cover test.

Alternate Cover Test

The alternate cover test is also referred to as the Duane cover test. It may be used with prisms to measure the angle of deviation of either a strabismus or phoria. Although it is a very sensitive method for detecting a deviation of the visual axes, a limitation of the alternate cover test is that it cannot differentiate between heterotropia and heterophoria (i.e., strabismus versus phoria) as can the unilateral cover test. This is because, during the procedure, only one eye is fixating at any given moment; the eyes are in a state of dissociation, making fusion impossible. The alternate cover test cannot determine whether a deviation is concealed by fusion.

The test is performed by alternately occluding one eye and then the other while watching for any conjugate movement of the eyes, which would indicate a deviation. The greater the conjugate movement, the greater is the deviation (either strabismic or phoric). An exo deviation will result in conjugate movement in the same direction as the movement of the occluder ("with" motion), whereas an eso deviation causes an "against" motion during the alternate cover test.

The testing procedure is best explained by using an example. Assume that the patient in this example has an esotropia of the right eye of 25Δ. The first step is to occlude the eyes alternately at a rate of 1-2 seconds per occlusion to determine whether there is an eso, exo, or hyper deviation. The direction and magnitude of the conjugate movement of the eyes indicate the direction and magnitude of the deviation.

Assuming the unilateral cover test was done previously, certain information about the deviation of the visual axes is already known (i.e., whether the deviation is strabismic or phoric, the dominant eye preferred for fixation, the direction and estimated magnitude of the deviation). Bearing in mind the knowledge gained from the unilateral cover test, the examiner's next step is to occlude the nondominant deviating eye. In this example, the right eye is occluded and no movement of either eye is expected, because the left eye remains the fixating eye and is motionless. When, however, the occluder is switched to the left eye, the right

Table 4-5. Effects of Eccentric Fixation on Measurement Results of the Cover Test

Direction of Deviation	Nasal Eccentric Fixation	Temporal Eccentric Fixation
Eso	Smaller measurement	Larger measurement
Exo	Larger measurement	Smaller measurement

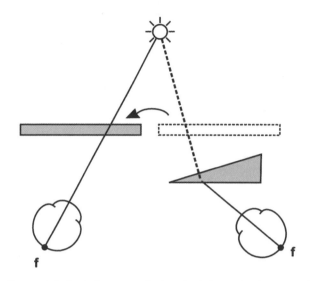

Figure 4-6. Occluder is switched to the left eye. In this example, no eye movement is seen because the base-out prismatic power is equal to the magnitude of the strabismic deviation (i.e., neutralization of the conjugate movement on the alternate cover test), (f = fovea.)

eye takes up fixation, which causes a conjugate eye movement to the patient's right-hand side.

The next step is to switch the occluder to the right eye and place a prism between the eye and the occluder. Then the occluder is switched to the left eye, and any conjugate movement is noted; if there is no movement, the prismatic power represents the magnitude of the deviation (Figure 4-6). If there is an "against" motion, the BO neutralizing prismatic power is insufficient, with a residual eso deviation. If there is a "with" motion, the prismatic power is overcorrecting the eso deviation (as though the patient has an exo deviation).

A pitfall of the cover test is that its validity is vitiated if there is eccentric fixation. (Refer to the discussion on eccentric fixation in Chapter 5.) For example, suppose the patient has nasal eccentric fixation of 5Δ of the right eye and has an esotropia of the right eye of 5Δ. The *measured* magnitude on the cover test would be zero. If, in another case, the *true* angle of esotropia is 8Δ, the cover test would yield a magnitude of 3Δ of eso deviation. Eskridge[12] proposed rules to differentiate between

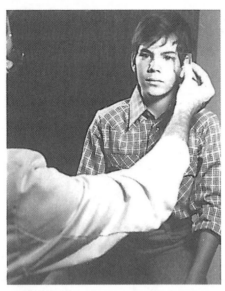

Figure 4-7. Preparing for the four base-out prism test in the case of a small esotropia of the right eye.

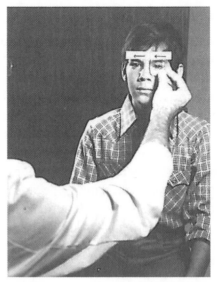

Figure 4-8. When the 4Δ base-out prism is placed before the fixating left eye, it adducts (toward the apex of the prism), and the esotropic right eye abducts. This is dextroversion, but no convergence is seen in this case of strabismus. If the patient were heterophoric rather than strabismic, a convergence would follow the initial dextroversion.

the measured and true deviation. Nasal eccentric fixation causes the measured angle H to be smaller than the true angle H in esotropia but larger than the true angle H in exotropia. In contrast, temporal eccentric fixation causes the measured angle H to be larger in esotropia but smaller in exotropia (Table 4-5).

When evaluating the angle of deviation the practitioner can expect some variation when measuring at different times. The reliability of the alternate cover test with prism neutralization in esotropia was recently investigated by the Pediatric Eye Disease Investigative Group.[15] Children with esotropia younger than five years of age were evaluated at two different times. If the angle of deviation was larger than 20Δ, then the 95% limits of agreement were approximately +/- 10Δ . If the angle of deviation was between 10 to 20Δ, then the 95% limits of agreement were approximately +/- 5Δ.

Four Base-Out Prism Test

When an esotropic angle is small (10Δ or less), the four BO prism test may be helpful in detecting a microstrabismus. Assume a patient has a small, unnoticeable esotropia of the right eye and the 4Δ prism is placed in a BO orientation before the fixating left eye. The right eye will abduct; it will move approximately 4Δ (Figures 4-7 and 4-8). Conversely, if the BO prism is placed before the strabismic right eye, no movement of either eye is expected, presumably because of suppression of the deviating eye. Exceptions to this result may occur in very small esotropic angles, less than 4Δ,

because the prism power is larger than the angle of deviation. This is because peripheral (extramacular) fusion may allow a convergence response to the prism, although usually not the full 4Δ of convergence.

If the deviation were esophoric rather than esotropic, the left eye, and later the right eye, would be expected to adduct. Clinical results from this test and the unilateral cover test provide information on tropia versus phoria, assessment of suppression in an objective manner, and information about which eye tends to be strabismic. In both tests, analysis of the patient's eye movements requires keen observation. These tests appear to be very simple, but they probably require more clinical acumen than other tests for assessing binocular vision.

Brückner Test

An extremely sensitive, although not always reliable, method for detecting strabismus is the Brückner test.[16, 17] It is performed by using an ordinary direct ophthalmoscope held at approximately 75 cm from the patient's eyes with the beam of the ophthalmoscope directed to the bridge of the nose and equidistant from each eye. The examiner observes the fundus (red) reflex and compares the brightness between the two eyes. The strabismic eye, as a rule, will appear brighter (Figure 4-9), although there are frequent exceptions to this rule. Pigmentary difference, unequal pupil size,

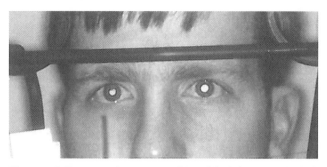

Figure 4-9. Patient with esotropia of 3Δ of the left eye in which the fundus reflex is brighter on the Brückner test.

and anisometropia invalidate the Brückner test: That is, the fixating eye may appear brighter than the deviating eye in such cases. Nevertheless, the Brückner test is a good adjunct method for detecting microstrabismus.

COMITANCY

All deviations are classified as being either *comitant* or *noncomitant*. (The correct etymological terms are *concomitant* and *nonconcomitant* but the shortened words generally are preferred for ease in clinical usage.) *Comitancy* (or *comitance*) means that the angle of deviation of the visual axes remains the same throughout all positions of gaze. This implies that there are neither abnormal underactions nor overactions of any of the 12 extraocular muscles controlling eye movements. In contrast, *noncomitancy* (or *noncomitance*) means that the magnitude of the deviation changes when the eyes move from one position of gaze to another. Thus, there is either abnormal restriction to movement or overaction of one or more of the extraocular muscles.

Causes

Underactions are the result of one of three basic malfunctions. First, the extraocular muscles themselves may be paretic, as in cases of direct traumatic injury. Second, and more frequently, mechanical reasons such as faulty muscle insertion and ligament abnormalities may restrict ocular motility. Third, and most frequently, the extraocular muscle paresis responsible for underactions is caused by innervational deficiencies due to impairment of the cranial nerves (III, IV, and VI) that innervate the muscles. Nerve impairment is commonly attributable to vascular problems, such as hemorrhages, aneurysms, and embolisms in older patients. Infectious diseases that affect the central nervous system also are frequent causes and should be suspected, particularly in young patients.

Table 4-6. Yoked Muscles

Right lateral rectus (RLR) and left medial rectus (LMR)
Right medial rectus (RMR) and left lateral rectus (LLR)
Right superior rectus (RSR) and left inferior oblique (LIO)
Right inferior rectus (RIR) and left superior oblique (LSO)
Right superior oblique (RSO) and left inferior rectus (LIR)
Right inferior oblique (RIO) and left superior rectus (LSR)

Overactions may be due to mechanical anomalies, such as a faulty muscle insertion giving mechanical advantage to the particular muscle. More often, however, the overaction can be explained by Hering's law of equal innervation to two yoked muscles. This law states that the contralateral synergists are equally innervated when a movement is executed by both eyes. If, for example, the right lateral rectus muscle is paretic and requires an abnormally high level of innervation to abduct the right eye, the equally high level of innervation is sent to the medial rectus of the left eye (the yoke muscle of the lateral rectus of the right eye) (Table 4-6). This results in an overaction of the left medial rectus, which further increases an eso deviation due to the paretic right lateral rectus. If this overaction continues for several months, a permanent state of contracture may result, whereby the tissues of the left medial rectus eventually become fibrotic and nonelastic. This worsens the prognosis for cure of an eso deviation. In this example of a paretic right lateral rectus muscle, the right medial rectus (homolateral antagonist) can also become spastic and, eventually, fibrotic. Precautions and appropriate therapy in such cases are discussed in Chapter 15.

Criteria and Terminology

Few individuals have perfect comitancy in the strictest sense, if the term is used to mean that the angle of deviation remains exactly the same throughout all positions of gaze. The frequent lack of perfect comitancy occurs because the basic deviation of most individuals varies slightly from one direction of gaze to another. Therefore, some allowance must be made so that the term noncomitance is not misleadingly overused. For clinical purposes, the allowable amount of change of deviation is 5Δ, thus providing for the deviation to be classified as comitant. If the change in deviation in any of the various positions of gaze is greater than 5Δ, the deviation is considered to be noncomitant.

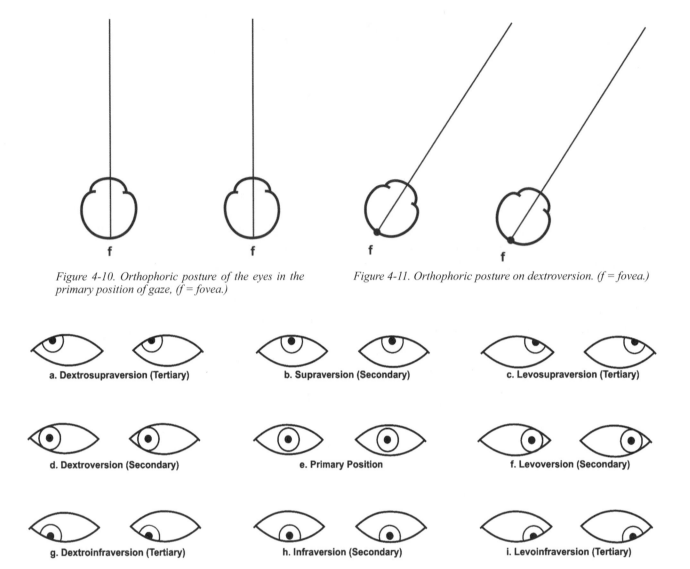

Figure 4-10. Orthophoric posture of the eyes in the primary position of gaze, (f = fovea.)

Figure 4-11. Orthophoric posture on dextroversion. (f = fovea.)

a. Dextrosupraversion (Tertiary)　　b. Supraversion (Secondary)　　c. Levosupraversion (Tertiary)

d. Dextroversion (Secondary)　　e. Primary Position　　f. Levoversion (Secondary)

g. Dextroinfraversion (Tertiary)　　h. Infraversion (Secondary)　　i. Levoinfraversion (Tertiary)

Figure 4-12. The nine diagnostic positions (a-i) of gaze for conjugate eye movements, with secondary and tertiary positions indicated.

The severity of noncomitancy can be evaluated by applying the following qualifications:

Mild: 6-10Δ change in deviation

Moderate: 11-15Δ change in deviation

Marked: 16Δ or larger change in deviation

A noncomitant deviation of the visual axes may or may not be paretic. *Paresis* is an etiologic term, whereas *noncomitancy* is a descriptive term. Unless the etiology is known with absolute certainty, it is wise to avoid using the word *paresis* or similar terms such as *palsy* or *paralysis*, because noncomitancy can also be due to a mechanical problem, such as restriction due to faulty muscle insertion. When the etiology is uncertain, it is best to describe the condition as noncomitant or to use a synonymous term (e.g., *incomitant*) until the exact cause is established.

The term paresis is used in this text rather than *paralysis*. Although these words are used synonymously in the literature, *paralysis* seemingly denotes total loss of function, although loss of function may not always be complete. If there is total loss of muscle function due to nerve lesions, *paralysis* would be an appropriate term; this condition may also be called *complete paresis*. As a rule, when the totality of loss of function is in doubt, paresis is probably the preferred term.

In testing for noncomitancy, it is important to know the relationship of the visual axis of one eye to that of the other. If the axes (lines of sight) are parallel, the eyes are postured in the ortho position. Figure 4-10 illustrates parallelism with the eyes in the primary position of gaze. Similarly, Figure 4-11 shows the eyes in the orthophoric posture in the secondary position of gaze of dextroversion,

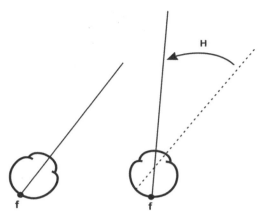

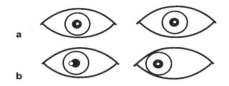

Figure 4-15. Hirschberg test in primary gaze and dextroversion, a. Ortho posture in the primary position of gaze. b. Esotropia of the right eye in right gaze.

Figure 4-13. Esotropia of the right eye on dextroversion (right gaze), (f = fovea; H = magnitude of the horizontal angle of strabismus.)

Figure 4-14. Direct observation of esotropia of the right eye on dextroversion due to insufficient abduction; the left eye is fixating.

in which each eye made an equal movement to the right so that the orthophoric posture was maintained. Another helpful way of illustrating eye posture is by showing a confrontation view. Nine diagnostic positions of gaze are demonstrated in Figure 4-12. These illustrations depict a patient's eyes in the orthophoric posture as seen by the examiner.

To illustrate a noncomitant deviation, Figure 4-13 shows the eyes in a nonorthophoric posture with dextroversion: The left eye made a nasal movement (adduction) larger than the temporal movement (abduction) of the right eye. Assuming that the left eye is the fixating eye, this results in an esotropic deviation of the right eye in rightward gaze. This same deviation is clinically depicted in Figure 4-14. This indication of noncomitancy is even more evident when Hirschberg testing is used (Figure 4-15).

Primary and Secondary Deviations

Measurements of the primary and secondary deviations are customarily made in the straight-ahead gaze (primary position) using the alternate cover test with prisms, usually at far (6 m), although the test may also be conducted at near (e.g., 40 cm). The magnitude of one angle is compared with the magnitude of the other. If a patient has a paretic muscle in only one eye, the primary angle of devi-

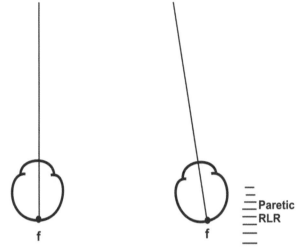

Figure 4-16. Esotropia of the right eye in a case of paresis of the right lateral rectus muscle (RLR). The nonparetic eye is fixating a distant target, revealing the primary angle of deviation, (f = fovea.)

ation is the angle measured when the nonparetic eye fixates, whereas the secondary angle is the angle measured when the paretic eye fixates.

The literature too often obfuscates the true meaning of the secondary angle by implying that it is the angle measured when the nondominant eye (or the deviating eye in strabismus) is fixating. This can be misleading, as the nondominant eye may possibly be the nonparetic eye and the dominant eye the paretic one. Under such circumstances, the primary angle of deviation would be the one measured when the nondominant eye is used for fixation. For this reason, we prefer to restrict the use of the terms *primary* and *secondary deviations* to the question of comitancy rather than commingling the issue of dominancy (as discussed later in this chapter).

The secondary angle of deviation is almost always significantly larger than the primary angle, according to Hering's law of equal innervation. Figures 4-16 and 4-17 are examples of paresis of the right lateral rectus muscle. The excessive innervation involved in contracting the right lateral rectus is carried over to the yoke muscle, the left

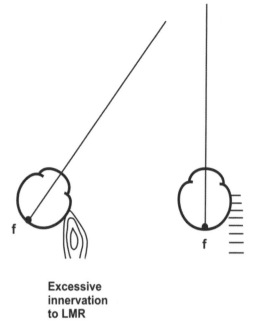

**Excessive
innervation
to LMR**

Figure 4-17. Esotropia of the left eye is illustrated in a case of paresis of the right lateral rectus muscle when the right eye is fixating. This is the secondary angle of deviation, which is much larger than the primary angle, (f = fovea; LMR = left medial rectus muscle.)

Table 4-7. Classification of Ductions and Vergences

Classification	Ductions	Vergences
Horizontal	Adduction (nasal)	Convergence
	Abduction (temporal)	Divergence
Vertical*	Supraduction (elevation)	Positive
	Infraduction (depression)	Negative
Torsional	Incycloduction (intorsion)	Incyclovergence
	Excycloduction (extorsion)	Excyclovergence
Tertiary positions	Dextrosupraduction	--
	Levosupraduction	
	Dextroinfraduction	
	Levoinfraduction	

*Vertical vergence is also known as vertical divergence. It is positive if the right eye elevates and negative if the left eye elevates.

medial rectus. The left eye is turned inward to an excessive degree, thus causing the eso deviation to be larger when the paretic eye is fixating.

Differences between the primary and secondary deviations may be due to noncomitancies caused by circumstances other than paresis. A faulty muscle insertion may test positive in this regard. However, the difference between primary and secondary angles usually is less remarkable than when a paretic muscle is involved. The disparity is usually greater in the case of a newly acquired paresis than in one of long duration. (There is a tendency for a noncomitant deviation of very long duration to evolve toward comitancy, but not to become completely comitant, in almost all cases.) If there is a difference greater than 5Δ between the primary and secondary angles, noncomitancy should be suspected. Although a lack of difference would indicate comitancy, there may be exceptions. Mild noncomitancies not caused by nerve impairment are often overlooked, as they may not produce a significant difference in the deviations. Even some paretic muscles with nerve impairment etiology may show a false-negative finding (i.e., appear normal) when they are of long duration. Conversely, a false-positive finding of noncomitancy (the appearance of abnormality when, in fact, none exists) sometimes occurs in cases of uncorrected refractive errors. For example, a

patient fixating with the right eye that is plano may be orthophoric, but the patient may have an eso deviation when fixating with the left eye that is 2 D hyperopic. In general, however, positive findings tend to be true indications of noncomitancy.

Ductions

The words *duction* and *vergence* have caused confusion in clinical usage. Technically, *ductions* are monocular eye movements (Table 4-7). The common interchanging of the two terms probably arose from clinicians' misuse of the word *ductions* when *vergences* was meant.

Duction testing is useful when evaluating noncomitancy. It is not as sensitive, however, as version testing, but ductions can be very informative if the extraocular muscles are tested in their diagnostic action fields (DAFs) (Table 4-8). Each DAF is evaluated by having the patient look in the appropriate direction, which may be either a voluntary saccadic eye movement or a following pursuit to the gaze testing point. To test the integrity of the right lateral rectus muscle, for example, the left eye is occluded while the patient fixates a target with the right eye in right gaze. To test the right superior oblique muscle in its DAF, the patient's right eye fixates a target that is to the left and down. Any underaction indicates a restriction, possibly due to paresis.

Distinguishing between a true paresis and a mechanical, or anatomic, problem is often difficult. In many cases, this distinction can be ascertained by a good patient history in combination with results obtained from the various methods of testing and careful observation during duction evaluation. The *saccadic velocities* test can help to make this distinction. The clinician observes the saccadic speed of the strabismic eye as it moves

Table 4-8. Diagnostic Action Field of Each Extraocular Muscle

Right Eye Muscle	Gaze	Left Eye Muscle	Gaze
Right lateral rectus	Right	Left lateral rectus	Left
Right medial rectus	Left	Left medial rectus	Right
Right superior rectus	Right and up	Left superior rectus	Left and up
Right inferior rectus	Right and down	Left inferior rectus	Left and down
Right superior oblique	Left and down	Left superior oblique	Right and down
Right inferior oblique	Left and up	Left inferior oblique	Right and up

toward and away from the restricted field. If the saccadic speed is approximately equal in both directions before the eye enters the restricted field, a mechanical etiology is suggested. However, if saccades are slower when moving toward the restricted field, a paresis can be suspected.

Another useful differential diagnostic procedure is the *forced duction test*. This procedure requires local anesthesia of the bulbar conjunctiva and a sterile forceps. A cotton-tipped applicator stick is soaked in a local anesthetic such as proparacaine hydrochloride (Ophthaine) 0.5% and then is pressed firmly to the bulbar conjunctiva at the limbus in the direction of the observed restriction. The conjunctiva is gripped with the forceps at the point of anesthesia, and the eye is slowly moved in the direction of gaze limitation. Mechanical restrictions such as contracture or space-taking lesions can be detected by the sensation of physical resistance. In cases of extraocular muscle (EOM) paresis, the eye will move to the extreme position. To help verify a paresis, the doctor holds the patient's eye in the primary position as the patient is asked to make a voluntary saccadic movement in the DAF (right gaze in the example given earlier of right lateral rectus paresis). If no pulling (tugging) is felt by the doctor, paresis is assumed. However, if a tugging is felt and the forced duction is restricted on passive rotation, a mechanical restriction is indicated.

Versions

Versions are conjugate movements of both eyes. Testing for noncomitancy is more sensitive with versions than with ductions, because a change in the deviation of the visual axes from one position of gaze to another can be measured fairly

precisely in version testing, in contrast to duction testing, in which only one eye is being examined and a restriction or overaction must be relatively large to be observed. Detecting a change in deviation under binocular seeing conditions during versions is relatively easy. For example, assume the patient has a mild paresis of the right lateral rectus muscle. On duction testing, the patient may be able to abduct the right eye with a large excursion, complicating the diagnosis of noncomitancy. Dextroversion testing, however, would probably detect the restriction in the DAF of the right lateral rectus in this case, because an eso deviation would increase dramatically on rightward gaze.

The three objective methods of version testing, ranging from least to most sensitive, are (1) direct observation, (2) Hirschberg testing, and (3) the alternate cover test with prism. Each method may be used in the nine DAFs illustrated in Figure 4-12. For example, with dextroversion, the DAFs are for the right lateral rectus and the left medial rectus. If the right lateral rectus muscle is paretic, esotropia is likely on rightward gaze, whereas if instead the left medial rectus is paretic, exotropia is likely on rightward gaze.

Three-Step Method

Ordinarily, analyzing the eight cyclovertical muscles is more difficult than analyzing the four horizontally acting recti. A useful paradigm for identifying an isolated paretic cyclovertical muscle, taking into account a vertical deviation, was introduced by Parks.[18] The three basic steps of this method are shown in Table 4-9 for each cyclovertical muscle.

The three-step method is best explained by using as an example of a known paretic muscle and then proceeding to the three differentially diagnostic steps. Suppose the patient has a paretic right superior oblique muscle. This muscle's main action is infra-duction and, secondarily, intorsion. In the primary position, the superior oblique has a slight action of abduction, but this can be considered negligible for purposes of our discussion. When the patient fixates in the primary position of gaze, the right eye is likely to have a small degree of hyper deviation. This could be either hypertropia or hyperphoria, depending on the results of the unilateral cover test. The likelihood that a right hyper deviation will be present is attributable to

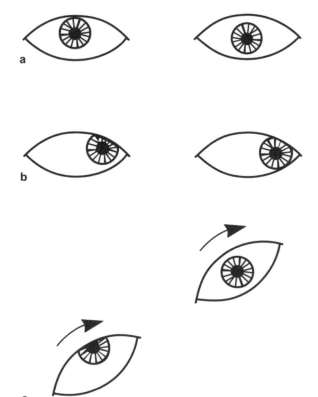

Figure 4-18. The three-step method for diagnosing an isolated paretic cyclovertical muscle. The right superior oblique muscle is affected in this example, a. Right hypertropia in the primary position, b. Hypertropia increases in left gaze. c. Further increase of the hypertropia when head is tilted toward patient's right shoulder. Arrows indicate direction of compensatory torsional movements.

Table 4-9. The Three-Step Method for Identifying a Paretic Cyclovertical Muscle

Right or Left Hyper Deviated Eye in Primary Position	Hyper Deviation Greater on Either Right or Left Gaze	Hyper Deviation Greatest on Either Right or Left Tilt	Paretic Muscle
R	R	R	Left inferior oblique
R	R	L	Right inferior rectus
R	L	R	Right superior oblique
R	L	L	Left superior rectus
L	R	R	Right superior rectus
L	R	L	Left superior oblique
L	L	R	Left inferior rectus
L	L	L	Right inferior oblique

L = left; R = right.

weakened depressing (infraduction) action of the paretic superior oblique muscle. The magnitude of the right hyper deviation may be estimated objectively, either by direct observation or with the unilateral cover test. For the exact measure of magnitude, the alternate cover test with a base-down (BD) prism placed in front of the right eye is used.

The first column of Table 4-9 lists hyper deviations of either the right or left eye. The fourth column lists the affected muscles from among the eight cyclovertical muscles. When there is a right hyper deviation in the case of an isolated paretic muscle, any of three muscles besides the right superior oblique may be the cause. They are the left inferior oblique, the right inferior rectus, and the left superior rectus. A paretic left inferior oblique could cause a hyper deviation (of the right eye) because its yoke muscle, the right superior rectus, receives excessive innervation (Hering's law). In addition, the left inferior oblique is an elevator, and the weakened muscle would cause the left eye to have a hypo deviation (relative right hyper deviation).

The same reasoning applies to a paretic left superior rectus, as its yoke muscle, the right inferior oblique, would receive excessive innervation to cause a right hyper deviation. Similar explanations can be supplied for each muscle when using the three-step method.

The number of possibilities can be narrowed from four to two by having the patient fixate in two lateral positions of gaze approximately 30 degrees each way. In right gaze, the amount of the hyper deviation is measured with the alternate cover test and BD prism. The same procedure is performed in left gaze. If the hyper deviation of the right eye increases in left gaze, the paretic muscles are narrowed to two possibilities, right superior oblique and left superior rectus, because both of these muscles have an isolated vertical action in left gaze.

Theoretically, the right superior oblique becomes a pure depressor only when the right eye is adducted 51 degrees, and the left superior rectus a pure elevator only when the left eye is abducted 23 degrees (see Chapter 1). For clinical purposes, however, 30 degrees for each lateral gaze is a satisfactory and workable compromise. When the possibilities are narrowed to two muscles, the Bielschowsky head-tilt test is necessary (Figure 4-18). The patient is instructed to tilt the head approximately 40 degrees toward the right shoulder. The same instructions then are given for head tilt to the left shoulder. An *increase* in an existing hyper deviation is the important observation. Usually, the up-shooting of the hyper deviated eye is obvious on right head tilt in this example of right superior oblique paresis. If fusion is strong and the vertical deviation remains latent, the alternate cover test must be used to dissociate the eyes and assess the hyper deviation. A subjective measurement of the hyper deviation can be misleading, because the tilting itself produces a "hyper" eye, which should not be confused with a true hyper deviation that can be seen objectively. Because of this artifact, subjective testing is unreliable; the examiner must make such an assessment by objective means. Objective assessment is best accomplished by both the examiner and the patient tilting their heads in the same direction (e.g., simultaneously toward patient's right shoulder and toward doctor's left shoulder). In this orientation, the alternate cover test with prisms can be performed as though both the doctor and patient were facing each other with their heads in the upright position. A small fixation light (if testing is done at near) may be held by either the patient or an assistant, as the doctor may require both hands to hold the occluder and loose prisms. The tip of the doctor's nose is also a convenient and satisfactory target for this purpose.

In the case of a right superior oblique paresis, the hyper deviation increases with a right head tilt, because postural reflexes cause compensatory torsional eye movements. (With a right head tilt, the right eye must make an incycloduction movement; that is, the top of the eyeball must move nasally around its anteroposterior axis.) At the same time, the left eye must make an excycloduction movement. The impulse to keep the visual fields upright is compelling, which explains why the head tilt test is definitive in so many cases. In the case of a right superior oblique paresis, the other intorsion muscle—the right superior rectus—is engaged to help incycloduct the eye. The action of this elevating muscle is the principal reason for the increased right hyper deviation with a right head tilt. Another reason involves the fellow eye: The left inferior rectus is the yoke muscle of the right superior oblique. Because of Hering's law, a hypo deviation of the left eye is produced, making the right eye relatively more hyper deviated.

The responses of the other cyclovertical muscles on the Bielschowsky head-tilt test can be analyzed similarly by accounting for the torsional action of each muscle. The rule to remember is that a superior muscle rotates the eye inwardly (intorsion), and an inferior one rotates the eye outwardly (extorsion). The mnemonic expression "inferior people extort" may help one to remember the torsional actions

of the eight cyclovertical muscles. For clinical purposes, the four lateral recti have no significant torsional action.

The chief advantage of the three-step method is that it is an objective means of testing that requires little participation by the patient, other than fixating a target and tilting the head. If the patient has a hypertropia large enough to be noticeable, direct observation (with or without Hirschberg testing) may be all that is required. If either the deviation is latent (phoric) or the hypertropia is too small to discern, the alternate cover test is used.

A convenient analysis system for the three-step method is illustrated in Figures 4-19 through 4-22. This visual portrayal conforms to the flowchart in Table 4-9.

Bajandas[19] suggested adding a fourth procedure to the three-step method, which involves having the patient look in upward and downward positions of gaze. If there are questionable results and a clear differential diagnosis cannot be made between, for example, a right superior oblique and a left superior rectus muscle, the downward gaze will tend to increase the right hyper deviation and, thus, implicate the right superior oblique. Conversely, an increasing vertical deviation on upward gaze would implicate the left superior rectus. Similar reasoning applies for the other cyclovertical muscles when applying this fourth step.

Because many cases of noncomitancy tend to evolve toward comitancy (often referred to clinically as *spread of comitancy*), the three-step method may give nebulous results. Therefore, this method is most useful when there is a newly acquired paresis of a cyclovertical muscle, whereas it may not be differentiating in cases of long duration. Also, mechanical problems do not always provide a clear-cut diagnosis, as in cases of newly acquired paresis. Furthermore, if more than one cyclovertical muscle is involved, the three-step method will not be valid.

Recording Noncomitant Deviations

Jampolsky[20] recommended a direct and efficient system of evaluating and recording the motoric aspects of a strabismus. The objective testing and recording procedure can be divided into four parts. The evaluation is done with the patient wearing the habitual refractive correction to ascertain the current oculomotor status. If the examination indi-

Primary Position: RE Hyper

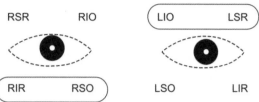

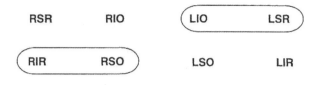

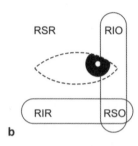

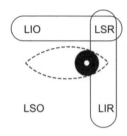

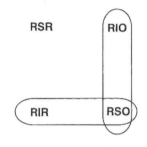

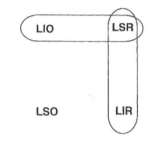

a

Lateral Gazes: Hyper increases on left gaze

Hyper increases on left gaze

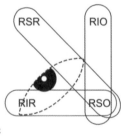

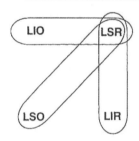

b

Head Tilt: Hyper Increases on Right Tilt

Hyper Increases on Left Tilt

c

Figure 4-19. A convenient analysis system for identifying an isolated paretic muscle using the three-step method. In step 1 (a), assuming a right-eye hyper deviation (RE hyper) in the primary position of gaze, the paretic muscle would be one of four possibilities, including the right inferior rectus (RIR), right superior oblique (RSO), left inferior oblique (LIO), and left superior rectus (LSR). These four muscles are shown in the horizontal oval-like demarcations in step 1. In step 2 (b), assuming an increased right hyper deviation (hyper) in left gaze, the possibilities are reduced to two: RSO and LSR muscles. This is shown by the two ovallike demarcations intersecting with the previously drawn horizontal demarcations, the RSO and LSR muscles being common to both horizontal and vertical demarcations. In step 3 (c), assuming a further increase of right hyper deviation on right head tilt, the corresponding tilted, oval-like demarcation shows an intersection with the horizontal and vertical demarcations in which the RSO is common to all three. Hence, the diagnosis is RSO paresis. (LIR = left inferior rectus; LSO = left superior oblique; RIO = right inferior oblique; RSR = left superior rectus.)

Figure 4-20. Analysis of an isolated left superior rectus (LSR) paresis using oval-like demarcations. (LIO = left inferior oblique; LIR = left inferior rectus; LSO - left superior oblique; RE hyper = right-eye hyper deviation; RIO = right inferior oblique; RIR = right inferior rectus; RSO = right superior oblique; RSR = right superior rectus.)

cates a significant change in refractive error, spectacles are prescribed, and the patient is scheduled for an additional examination after she or he has adapted to the lenses.

- *Step 1*: Without correcting for head posture, the presenting deviations at far and near are meas-

ured with a prism bar or loose prisms and are recorded.

- *Step 2*: While the patient holds fixation with the dominant eye on a distant target (e.g., 6 m), the patient's head is rotated by the examiner so the eyes move to the extreme position in up, down, left, and right fields of gaze. The deviation at each horizontal or vertical position is neutralized with prisms and recorded on a diagram, as illustrated in Figure 4-23. If necessary, the primary deviation is measured again and recorded on the diagram, without allowing the patient to assume the habitual head posture.

- Step 3; The patient's head is rotated to extreme tilted positions, right and left, and any resulting

Primary Position: LE Hyper

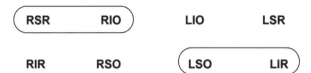

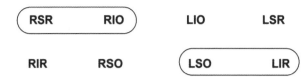

Primary Position: LE Hyper

Hyper increases on right gaze

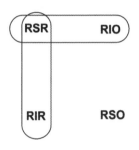
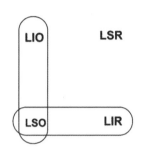

Hyper increases on right gaze

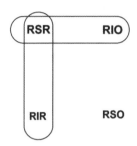
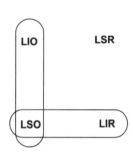

Hyper Increases on Left Tilt

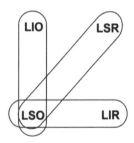

Hyper Increases on Right Tilt

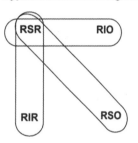

Figure 4-21. Analysis of an isolated left superior oblique (LSO) paresis using oval-like demarcations. (LE hyper = left-eye hyper deviation; LIO = left inferior oblique; LIR = left inferior rectus; LSR = left superior rectus; RIO = right inferior oblique; RIR = right inferior rectus; RSO = right superior oblique; RSR = right superior rectus.)

Figure 4-22. Analysis of an isolated right superior rectus (RSR) paresis using oval-like demarcations. (LE hyper - left-eye hyper deviation; LIO = left inferior oblique; LIR = left inferior rectus; LSO = left superior oblique; LSR = left superior rectus; RIO = right inferior oblique; RIR = right inferior rectus; RSO = right superior oblique.)

hyper deviation is measured. The results of the head-tilt test are simply recorded close to the diagram.

- *Step 4*: The patient is instructed to follow a penlight, or a toy target, as it is moved into eight extreme DAFs. The examiner qualitatively grades on a ranking scale any observed overaction or restriction in each field of gaze, as illustrated in Figure 4-24. Restrictions are graded and recorded on the diagram in the affected field of gaze. An advantage of this method of recording (as compared with the Hess-Lancaster test, for example) is the direct and easy visualization of the affected fields of gaze and comitancy

pattern. A similar method for grading overactions is illustrated in Figure 4-25 in an example of an overacting right inferior oblique muscle. In cases of paretic strabismus, overaction of the yoked muscle (contralateral synergist) usually is seen. However, in cases of developmental comitant strabismus of long standing, particularly esotropia, overactions of the oblique muscles often occur also. Overactions can present either unilaterally or bilaterally. Thorough diagnosis requires the grading of overactions on a 4-point scale. The clinician moves the fixation target, often a penlight, to direct the patient's fixation into an extreme field of gaze. For example, when checking for an overac-

2 eso	5 eso	20 eso
2 eso	5 eso	20 eso
2 eso	5 eso	20 eso

5 eso	15 eso	35 eso
5 eso	15 eso	35 eso
5 eso	15 eso	35 eso

Figure 4-23. Recordings in a case of left lateral rectus paresis (examiner's view).

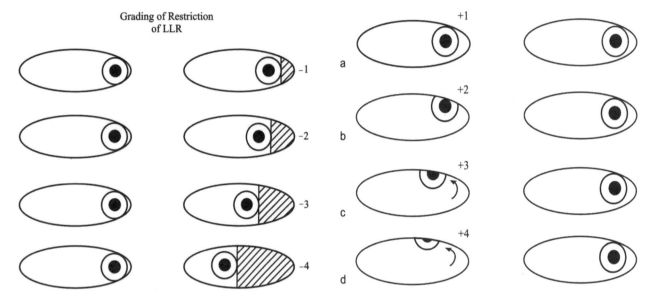

Grading of Restriction
of LLR

Figure 4-24. Grading of ocular motility—in this case, restriction of the left lateral rectus muscle (LLR)—on a ranking scale similar to that of Jampolsky, with -1 being the most mild and -4 being the most marked in severity. The right eye in this diagram is fixating a target in extreme left gaze.

Figure 4-25. Example of grading of overaction of the right inferior oblique muscle. In this example, the left eye is fixating a target in extreme left gaze. a. Right eye is approximately 1 mm higher than left eye. b. Right eye is approximately 2 mm higher than left eye. c. Right eye is approximately 3 mm higher than left eye, part of pupil is obscured by upper eyelid, and right eye is slightly diverging (arrow represents upward and outward movement of the eye, as well as extorsion). d. Right eye is nearly 4 mm higher than left eye, most of pupil is obscured by the upper eyelid, and right eye may be markedly diverging.

tion of the right inferior oblique muscle, the clinician should direct the patient to fixate with the left eye in extreme left gaze (see Figure 4-25). Also, testing should be performed with the patient's left eye in extreme upper left gaze. (Likewise, to check for overaction of the right superior oblique muscle, the fixating left eye would be directed to the extreme lower left field.) Then the vertical alignment of the two eyes should be compared for differences. We recommend the following convention: If the nonfixating eye is 1 mm higher than the fixating eye in up-gaze or 1 mm lower than the fixating eye in down-gaze, the overaction is graded as +1; if the difference is 2 mm, then the grade is +2; if a 3-mm difference, then +3; and if a 4-mm or greater difference, then +4. Divergence often accompanies overactions of the oblique muscles in grades +3 and +4, as is indicated in Figure 4-25. In the primary position of gaze, the oblique muscles

have the tertiary action of abduction. On extreme adduction, the eye does not move to 51 degrees, where there would be purely vertical action, but falls short, allowing for some abduction. In extreme overactions of the oblique muscles, the abduction becomes apparent.

Spatial Localization Testing

Patients who have a newly acquired paresis usually have spatial localization errors, as evidenced by pointing beyond the target's DAF location (clinically referred to as *past pointing*). For example, assume that the right superior oblique muscle is paretic. This muscle should be tested in its DAF (levoinfraduction). For such testing, the left eye is occluded. Then, with the right eye fixating, the patient is instructed to look at a penlight (or any suitable target) located in the DAF position (to the patient's left and down) and to touch it with an index finger (i.e., pointing). Although testing distance is not critical, approximately 40 cm is recommended. The patient is told to move a hand quickly from behind the shoulder (out of view) to touch the light. This must be done rapidly; otherwise, judgment corrections may be made and the patient will touch the target accurately (although slowly). Unless the procedure is performed correctly, localization may falsely appear to be normal. Correctional judgments of localization are learned over time, which explains why sensitivity of this test diminishes in cases of paresis of long duration.

If testing is conducted correctly in a newly acquired case of a paretic right superior oblique muscle, the patient will likely miss the target by pointing to the left of the target (i.e., patient's left) and below it. All 12 extraocular muscles can be tested in this manner, in the DAF of each. Clear-cut evidence of spatial localization error implicates a newly acquired paresis as the cause of noncomitancy.

SIGNS & SYMPTOMS

Noncomitancy may or may not cause noticeable problems or be reported. For many young children, the deviations must be obvious before their parents are prompted to pursue examination of such children by an eye care professional. Subjective complaints arising from noncomitancy are relatively infrequent in children younger than 7 years. The situation is most often that of the parent noticing signs of intermittent deviation rather than the child reporting diplopia. Likewise, other subjectively reported symptoms, such as nausea and vertigo, are believed to be more frequent in adults.

Diplopia

Young children infrequently report diplopia. We have seen many children who, when examined and asked, replied, "I thought everybody sees double." Their lack of life experience and difficulty in articulating what is and what should be may explain in part why reports of diplopia may not be heard from many young children who are strabismic. Another reason is that young children can usually suppress the aggravating image caused by the deviating eye.

Suppression is more difficult to achieve with maturity. Most adults have trouble coping with diplopia that results from a manifest deviation of sudden onset, such as from a newly acquired paretic muscle. In such cases, diplopia is the main reason for an office visit. If, however, a patient has always had poor binocular vision with deep suppression, diplopia may not be noticed and would not be a warning of a newly acquired paresis.

Abnormal Head Posture

An affected extraocular muscle can often be identified merely by observation of the head posture of the patient. Interpretation of abnormal posture is facilitated by the knowledge that the patient's face points in the same direction as the DAF of the affected muscle (Tables 4-8 and 4-10). For example, a paretic right superior oblique muscle causes a patient to turn the head abnormally to the left and to lower the chin. (The right superior oblique muscle is in its DAF when the right eye is turned to the left and downward.)

Another similar rule explains the presence of an abnormal head tilt. A paretic right superior oblique muscle, for example, causes the head to be tilted toward the left shoulder in habitual natural seeing conditions. Because the right superior oblique muscle is an intorter, it moves the top of the eye in a leftward direction and, because the muscle is weak, the patient's head tilts in a leftward direction as compensation. The rule to remember is that the compensatory abnormal head tilt is in the same direction as the torsional movement of the eyeball that would result from the muscle's contraction.

Diagnosis is complicated when more than one muscle is affected. Nevertheless, the patient is likely to have an abnormal head posture and one that tends to be biased toward the DAF of the most severely affected muscle. Multiple pareses require careful analysis, as with the Hess-Lancaster method (discussed later in this chapter). Unlike past pointing, the mere passage of time does not tend to compensate for head posture abnormalities when the muscle or muscles remain paretic. Consequently, it is likely that a noncomitancy of long duration can be detected by means of head posture observation.

SUBJECTIVE TESTING

Subjective comitancy testing, when feasible, is usually more precise than are objective testing

Table 4-10. Abnormal Head Posture (Position of Face) Related to Affected Extraocular Muscles

Muscle	Turn	Elevation	Tilt
Right lateral rectus	R	--	--
Right medial rectus	L	--	--
Right superior rectus	R	Up	L
Right inferior rectus	R	Down	R
Right superior oblique	L	Down	L
Right inferior oblique	L	Up	R
Left lateral rectus	L	--	--
Left medial rectus	R	--	--
Left superior rectus	L	Up	R
Left inferior rectus	L	Down	L
Left superior oblique	R	Down	R
Left inferior oblique	R	Up	L

L = left; R = right.

methods. The patient may be able to notice a very small displacement of two images resulting from misalignment of the visual axes. Observations of small deviations sometimes is difficult for the examiner, making objective testing less sensitive. This is particularly true for cyclo deviations, for which subjective testing must often be relied on for accurate diagnosis.

There are, however, disadvantages to subjective testing. This type of examination is greatly dependent on the cooperation of a capable and aware patient. An uncooperative or unperceptive patient can give either invalid or no results. Objective testing must be relied on in such cases. The presence of anomalous retinal correspondence (ARC) also may invalidate subjective findings, because the objective and subjective angles are different. Moreover, the subjective angle itself is often variable when this condition is present. (ARC is discussed in Chapter 5.)

Single-Object Method

The traditional way to make a patient aware of pathologic diplopia is by using a single target (see Chapter 1). If a patient has an exotropic deviation, a bright penlight in a darkened room should be perceived by that patient as a double image. A deviating right eye sees the image of a light to the left of the fixated light seen by the left eye. This is *heteronymous (crossed) diplopia* and the type normally expected with exo deviations. In contrast, *homonymous (uncrossed) diplopia* is normally expected with eso deviations.

Two rules apply when testing for noncomitancy using the single-object method. First, the patient should perceive the target seen by the deviating eye in an opposite direction from that in which the eye is deviating. Hence, an exotropic right eye sees the image to the left, whereas an esotropic right eye sees the image to the right. Second, the distance between the diplopic images becomes greater when there is an increase in either an underaction or an overaction during versions. Neutralization with loose prisms, however, can determine the direction and magnitude of the subjective angle of directionality, which is the same as the objective angle of deviation of the visual axes if there is normal retinal correspondence.

The subjective angle of directionality (angle S) can also be measured by using a black tangent screen and can be performed in all nine diagnostic positions of gaze. The examiner marks on the screen the separation of the diplopic images reported by the patient. If a 1 m test distance is used, each centimeter displacement of the images represents 1Δ. Nevertheless, many practitioners find the single-object method confusing, because they have to think in reverse as to direction of the deviating eye and the diplopic image. This confusion is eliminated by employment of the two-object method.

Two-Object Method

Two fixation targets are required for the two-object method. Special filters, usually red and green, are used. The right eye sees only one target (customarily through a red filter), and the left eye sees the other target (customarily through a green filter). The Hess-Lancaster test may be custom-made by drawing red lines on a white board to form a grid, a rectangular coordinate tangent screen with a white background and red lines and red fixation spots (Figure 4-26). The red lines and spots are invisible to the eye wearing the red filter. This is because the white background is more intense than the red lines and spots; they are, consequently, washed out. They are visible, however, to the eye wearing the green filter. The lines and spots appear as dark gray, because the red hue is not transmitted by the green filter, but the white background is. A convenience when interpreting the results is that the directions in which the flashlights are pointed correspond to those of the visual axes.

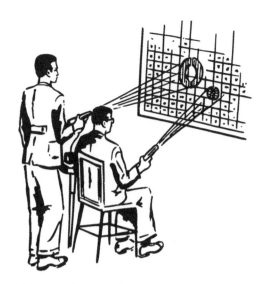

Figure 4-26. Procedure for Hess-Lancaster testing. The patient (wearing green and red glasses) is given hand projector and instructed to place the projected green spot (seen by the left eye) on the projected red spot (seen by the right eye). Relationship of dot to circle makes diagnosis possible.

Figure 4-27 illustrates a recording chart for the Hess-Lancaster test. The separation between the lines represents approximately 7Δ. The fixation spots are five squares from the center; therefore, they are 35Δ (almost 20 degrees) laterally displaced. The spots are placed 28Δ vertically above and below the level of the central fixation spot. Because of changing tangent values, the magnitude represented by each separation of lines is variable. The prism diopter value diminishes as fixation changes from the primary position to the periphery. Despite this mathematic variable, it is generally unnecessary to compensate for these changes for clinical purposes. The mathematic error amounts to only 1Δ or 2Δ within the range of the test. Fixations would have to be much greater than 35Δ away from the primary position before tangent values would create a significantly invalidating factor. The chart also includes the names of the 12 extraocular muscles. The location of each represents the DAF for those particular muscles.

The following procedure is recommended for performing the Hess-Lancaster test. To evaluate the right field (i.e., to test the muscles of the right eye), the patient puts on red-green spectacles with the red filter over the right eye. The spectacles stay in place throughout testing for both the right and left fields. The room is dimly illuminated. While the examiner holds the green projecting flashlight, the patient holds the red one. Test distance from the patient to the center of the screen is 1 m. The deviation in the primary position is measured first. The examiner projects the green light onto the central spot, and the patient attempts to superimpose the projected red spot of light (being seen only by the right eye) with the green spot, which is seen and fixated only by the left eye. An exotropic or exophoric patient with a deviating right eye will point the red flashlight to the right of the central target to achieve the perception of superimposition of the red and green images (Figure 4-28). Note that a vertical streak projected by each flashlight would be preferable to a spot, because a cyclo deviation can be revealed at each testing position.

If the patient is either esotropic or esophoric, the red spot should be projected to the left of the fixated green spot. The rule is that the patient projects the light in the same direction as that of the deviating eye. This is direct foveal projection; interpretation is facilitated by not having to think in reverse, as in the single-object method.

If the patient does not understand this testing procedure, which often is true of young children, it is instructive to remove the colored spectacles and to ask the patient to superimpose the projected

Left Field

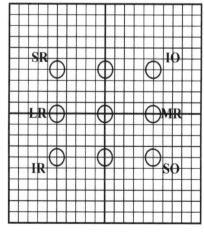

Right Field

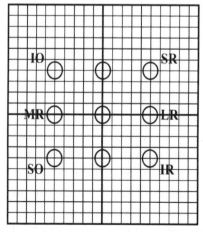

Figure 4-27. Form used for charting results of the Hess-Lancaster test. (IO = inferior oblique; IR = inferior rectus; LR = lateral rectus; MR = medial rectus; SO = superior oblique; SR = superior rectus.)

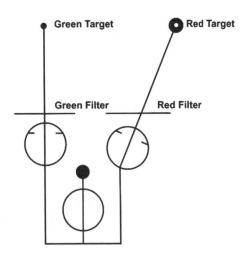

Figure 4-28. Diagram showing patient's perception of superimposition on the Hess-Lancaster test in an example of an exo deviation of the right eye. This could be either an exotropia of the right eye or an exophoria that is decompensated by the dissociating red and green filters, and one in which the left eye is the dominant eye.

spots. Because there is no binocular demand, this latter task should be accomplished easily. It is wise to allow the parent of a young child to watch this procedure. When the child feels confident about superimposing the spots, the red-green spectacles are put on. Because fusion is broken and the eyes are now dissociated, the visual axes must be in ortho alignment for superimposition to occur. When a deviation is present, the child will have the perception that the spots are superimposed on the screen, but the parent can see that they actually are separated. This observation is helpful in explaining the nature of a deviation to the parent of a young patient.

After measuring the subjective angle in the primary position of gaze, the other eight positions should be tested in a similar manner. For right-eye field testing, the left eye remains the fixating eye. For left-eye field testing, however, the examiner exchanges flashlights with the patient. The examiner directs the red spot to the central fixation circle, and the patient fixates with the right eye and tries to superimpose the green spot with the red. All nine positions of gaze are measured for the left field, following the same procedure as is used in testing the right field. It is important that the red filter remain over the right eye and the green over the left eye, so that this method can be followed consistently; otherwise, interpretation of results may be confusing, particularly true when two or more affected muscles are involved.

Examples are provided to explain interpretation of the measured deviations. Figure 4-29 shows the charting of a paretic right lateral rectus muscle. In right gaze, the paretic right lateral rectus is in its DAF and is underacting. The left medial rectus is in its DAF and is overacting (Hering's law). The Xs represent the positions of the spots seen by the deviating eye, whereas the circles represent the fixation spots for the fixating eye. An outline of the eight outside Xs is made by connecting them to form an enclosure. The area of the enclosure of each field is compared. In this example, the right enclosure is smaller than the left, which means that the paresis causing the underaction is in the right eye. The left enclosure is larger, indicating overaction by the left eye, thus graphically illustrating the effect of Hering's law. For clarification with a contrasting example, an exotropic deviation due to paresis of the right medial rectus is shown in Figure 4-30. The area of the enclosure for the right field is much smaller than for the left. Hence, the overaction of the left lateral rectus muscle is large when the paretic right medial rectus muscle is in its DAF.

This method of charting is very useful when two or more muscles are affected. Figure 4-31 illustrates an example of paresis of both the right lateral rectus and the right superior oblique muscles. Besides the similar effect of the paretic lateral rectus, there is also an underaction in the DAF of the right superior oblique, which results in an overaction of its yoke muscle, the left inferior rectus. The two underacting muscles of the right eye cause the enclosure of the right field to be much smaller than that of the left field. Visual inspection of muscle field charting facilitates diagnosis of the affected muscles.

The Hess-Lancaster test is the most sensitive of all clinical tests for noncomitancy. There are, however, some pitfalls, including ARC, deep suppression, and poor cooperation by the patient. If any of these exists, testing may have to be performed entirely by objective means. Furthermore, results of one test should confirm the results of another; therefore, it is wise to perform different types of tests on a patient when noncomitancy is suspected. Management of cases of noncomitancy is discussed in subsequent chapters, particularly Chapters 8 and 15.

FREQUENCY OF THE DEVIATION

Next in importance to comitancy evaluation is determination of the frequency of a manifest deviation. This knowledge helps the practitioner to assess the status of a patient's binocularity. For example, a patient who is strabismic 95% of the time has poorer control on bifoveal fusion than does a patient who is strabismic only 5% of the time.

Classification

Frequency refers to the amount of time a deviation is manifest, which may range from 1% to 100%. If a strabismus is not present any of the time under natural habitual seeing conditions, the patient is necessarily classified as either orthophoric or heterophoric (if there is a latent deviation of the visual axes). More patients are heterophoric than orthophoric because there is usually at least some deviation present, even though it may be small. Any latent deviation (1Δ or greater) is classified as heterophoria. As in strabismus, the heterophoric deviation may be horizontal, vertical, or torsional.

Strabismus is classified as intermittent if it is present from 1% to 99% of the time. A synonymous term for *intermittent* is *occasional*. The latter term is used by some clinicians, but we believe it implies a state of infrequency: The semantic connotation to

Left Field   **Right Field**

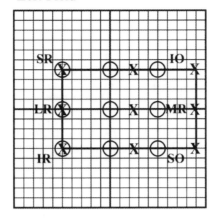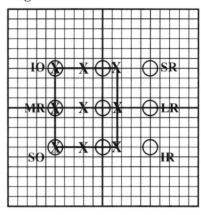

Figure 4-29. Chart of the results of the Hess-Lancaster test in the case of a paretic right lateral rectus muscle. (IO = inferior oblique; IR = inferior rectus; LR - lateral rectus; MR = medial rectus; SO = superior oblique; SR = superior rectus.)

Left Field   **Right Field**

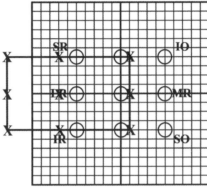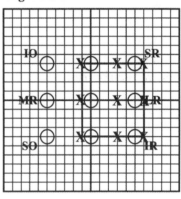

Figure 4-30. Chart of the results in the case of a paretic right medial rectus muscle. (IO = inferior oblique; IR = inferior rectus; LR = lateral rectus; MR = medial rectus; SO = superior oblique; SR = superior rectus.)

LEFT FIELD   **RIGHT FIELD**

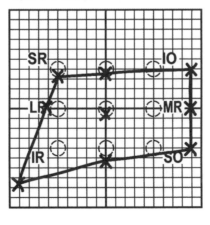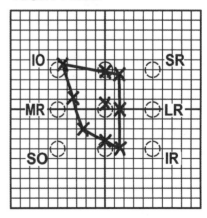

Figure 4-31. Chart of the results of paresis of both the right lateral rectus and the right superior oblique. (IO = inferior oblique; IR = inferior rectus; LR = lateral rectus; MR = medial rectus; SO = superior oblique; SR = superior rectus.)

most practitioners is that the deviation is manifest only once in a while, which may not state the true situation. It would be misleading, for example, to a strabismus that is present 95% of the time as *occasional*. We believe the term *intermittent* is more neutral as to frequency, and we recommend it along with including the estimated percentage of time a strabismus is present at far and at near.

Table 4-11 classifies frequency of strabismus based on the percentage of time (during normal waking hours) that there is a manifest deviation of the visual axes. Strabismus is constant when it is present 100% of the time. Synonymous terms include *continuous strabismus*, *permanent strabismus*, and *absolute strabismus*. We prefer the term *constant*.

An intermittent strabismus may be either periodic or nonperiodic, although in most cases it is the latter. If a strabismus is to be called *periodic*, its occurrence must be predictable and regular. A periodic intermittent strabismus may be either direct or indirect. *Direct* means that the strabismus occurs regularly only at near, under specified conditions. Typically, this is the patient with intermittent esotropia at near caused by the combination of esophoria at far, uncorrected hyperopic refractive error, and a high AC/A ratio. Accommodation brought into play for nearpoint demands can precipitate a manifest deviation.

An intermittent strabismus that is periodic and indirect occurs only at far. This is typified by the patient who has intermittent exotropia at far but who is exophoric at near. Such a patient usually has a high AC/A ratio that allows the deviation to be less at near. At far, however, the individual may regularly lapse into an exotropia unless there is strong compensational fusional ability.

Another cause for periodicity may be noncomitancy. For example, a patient with complete paresis of the right lateral rectus muscle has a marked noncomitancy, which would likely result in the patient always having esotropia in right gaze.

In the majority of cases, however, the intermittent regularity of strabismus is uncertain and cannot be absolutely predicted. Hence, most cases of intermittent strabismus are *nonperiodic*.

Evaluation

There are two principal ways to evaluate the percentage of time that there is a manifest devia-

TABLE 4-11. Classification of Frequency of the Deviation

Type of Strabismus	Percentage of Time Deviation Is Manifest
Constant strabismus	100
Intermittent strabismus	1-99
Periodic	
Direct (strabismus at near)	
Indirect (strabismus at far)	
Certain cases of noncomitancy	
Nonperiodic (unpredictable intermittence)	
Nonstrabismus	0
Heterophoria (deviation always latent under normal seeing conditions)	
Otrhophoria	

tion of the visual axes: patient history and results of testing procedures.

Patient History

Patient history information can come from reports of how others see the patient. Parents of young children may report that a child is "cross-eyed about half the time, especially when he is tired" or "walleyed when he looks out the window or daydreaming." This information is important, because young patients seldom report experiencing diplopia.

Older children and adults may give an index to the frequency of strabismus by reporting the amount of time that diplopia is noticed. This, however, is not always highly correlated with the frequency of strabismus, because the individual may use the antidiplopia mechanisms of suppression and ARC. Questioning of the patient's self-perceived appearance of the eyes and that observed by family and friends must, therefore, be pursued.

Testing

Estimation of the frequency of strabismus is not made by a rigid system of testing. Rather, it is done by using professional judgment based on impressions from the patient history and results of various testing procedures. Some guidelines for testing are given here.

It is better to observe the patient before rather than after dissociative testing is begun. The eyes are not dissociated when making direct observation, either with or without the Hirschberg test.

The cover test, however, fully dissociates the eyes. When the cover is removed, any refusion movements should be noted and evaluated. A slow rather than a quick recovery indicates that the frequency of strabismus is relatively high.

Diplopia testing reveals the patient's ability to notice pathologic diplopia. If this condition is

Table 4-12. Classification of Direction of Deviation

Deviation	Direction of Deviating Eye When Fixating Eye Is In Primary Position
Horizontal	
Eso	Inward rotation of eye
Exo	Outward rotation of eye
Vertical	
Hyper	Upward rotation of eye
Hypo	Downward rotation of eye
Torsional	
Incyclo	Inward rotation of top of eye
Excyclo	Outward rotation of top of eye

TABLE 4-13. Examples of Testing Procedures to Determine the Direction of Deviation of the Visual Axes

Objective procedures
  Direct observation
  Hirschberg test
  Krimsky test
  Unilateral cover test
  Alternate cover test
Subjective procedures
  von Graefe (vertical prism dissociation)
  Colored filters
  Maddox rod
  Apparent motion

easily noticed when the patient becomes strabismic, the frequency of strabismus is relatively low. In contrast, if diplopia seldom is perceived when the deviation is manifest, the frequency is relatively high. This is because compensatory fusional vergence tends to be better when suppression is less. In other words, diplopia is not likely to be noticed in most cases of constant strabismus (because of suppression and ARC).

Many other sensory and motor fusion tests (see Chapters 2, 5, and 6) can contribute to the overall estimation of frequency of a manifest deviation. This estimation should be determined for far and near fixation distances.

DIRECTION OF THE DEVIATION

The direction of a deviating eye may be horizontal, vertical, or torsional, or a combination of these. Table 4-12 lists the directions in which an eye may deviate.

Classification

Horizontal deviations in the majority of cases are isolated, without a vertical or torsional component, when all strabismus and phoria cases are considered. In contrast, vertical deviations are different in that they often have a horizontal component (e.g., esotropia with hypertropia). Torsional deviations (cyclo deviations) almost always have both vertical and horizontal components.

Some clinicians speak only of hyper deviations, thus avoiding use of *hypo deviations*. We believe that this is misleading. For example, it is preferable to call a constant unilateral downward deviation of a nonfixating right eye a *right hypotropia* rather than a *left hypertropia*. In this case, the left eye is the fixating eye and is not deviating upward, which invalidates the diagnosis of left hypertropia.

Testing procedures to determine the direction of deviation may be either objective or subjective (Table 4-13).

Objective Testing

When there is a manifest deviation, direct observation, the Hirschberg test, or the Krimsky test is useful if the strabismus is large enough to be noticeable. If, however, the manifest deviation is either small or latent, the cover test is necessary for diagnostic purposes. Unilateral occlusion is good for detecting the direction of deviation for lateral and vertical components. It has limitations, however, for determining cyclo deviations. (Subjective methods are more sensitive.)

For example, in the case of a right exotropia combined with right hypertropia and right excyclotropia, covering the left eye would result in the following movements: The right eye would be seen to move inward and downward, with the top of the eye (the 12-o'clock position on the limbus) moving inward. This is the required movement that the right eye must make to go from the deviated position to the position of fixation. Unilaterally covering the strabismic right eye would result in no movement. If, however, there is an exophoria combined with a right hyperphoria and an excyclophoria, occlusion of the right eye would cause the anterior segment of the right eye to drift outwardly and upwardly, and the top of the eye would rotate outwardly.

The alternate cover test is another good method for determining the direction of the deviation. Neutralizing prisms will provide the desired information. When the lateral (horizontal) component is neutralized, either with BO or BI (base-in) prism, the vertical component is much easier to observe. If the vertical component also is neutralized with either BU (base-up) or BD prism, it may be possible to isolate and observe cyclo deviations as small as 3 degrees. Smaller cyclo deviations usually must be detected and measured by subjective means.

Subjective Testing

The subjective angle of directionalization may be determined with two targets (e.g., Hess-Lancaster test) or, more commonly, with a single target, using any of several methods for either phorias or tropias. The horizontal subjective angle is easily determined with the von Graefe method using vertical prism dissociation. This is performed routinely to measure phorias in primary eye care examinations. As the patient sees the diplopic images of the single target (e.g., penlight), the examiner introduces a sufficient horizontally oriented prism, either BI or BO, to create vertical alignment of the two images. This is the subjective angle of directionalization.

Colored filters can be used in conjunction with the von Graefe method, or they can be used without the vertical dissociation. If, for example, a red lens is placed before a right esotropic eye that is being suppressed, the filter creating a color difference between the eyes may serve to break the suppression. In some cases in which suppression is very deep in the deviating eye, the red filter should be switched to the fixating eye. This reduces the intensity of the light entering the eye and acts as a mild occluder, giving an advantage to the deviating eye. In any event, assuming normal retinal correspondence, the patient should perceive homonymous (uncrossed) diplopia when there is an eso deviation. If the patient has an exo deviation, the perception should be heteronymous (crossed) diplopia.

The Maddox rod can also be used to determine both the direction of the subjective angle and the magnitude. Although the original design by Maddox was a single, elongated, cylindric lens, most clinicians prefer multiple rods for dissociative testing. Nonetheless, this method that uses multiple rods is known as the *Maddox rod* (singular). If the Maddox rod is placed with its axis at 180 degrees (rod horizontal) before the right eye, the eye should see a vertical streak. If, for example, the patient is exotropic (or if exophoric), the vertical streak should be seen to the left of the fixation light. If the patient has an esotropia (or esophoria), the vertical streak should be seen to the right of the fixation light.

The Maddox rod measurement of the far deviation appears to have good test-retest repeatability.[21]

Cyclo deviations require the use of a Maddox rod for each eye. If a Maddox rod is placed before the right eye with its axis at 180 degrees and another Maddox rod with its axis at 180 degrees is placed before the left eye, two vertical streaks may be seen (assuming a horizontal deviation is also present to prevent the superimposition of the two vertical streaks). If a cyclo deviation is not present, the streaks appear parallel. If, however, the right eye is exotropic and excyclotropic, the top of the leftward streak (seen by the right eye in this example) will appear inclined away from the vertical streak seen by the fixating left eye. In regard to the direction of the perceived slant, the rule is that the patient perceives the streak as slanting in the direction opposite the cyclo deviation of that eye, as illustrated and clarified in Figure 4-32.

Another subjective method for determining the direction of the deviation, when there is normal retinal correspondence, is the use of the apparent motion, which is a patient's perception of movement of a stationary single target during rapid alternate occlusion. The apparent movement is perceived when a deviation of the visual axes is present. The apparent motion is based on the stimulation of disparate retinal points and not on eye movements. For illustration of this point, refer to Figure 4-4, in which the right eye is shown to be esotropic. On rapid alternate occlusion, the right eye can be briefly exposed while an occluder is shifted from the right to the left eye. The fixated target will appear to move to the right (opposite movement from that of the occluder). When the occluder is shifted back to the right eye, the target will appear to move to the left (opposite direction).

In cases of exo deviations, the shift of the apparent movement is the same as the motion of the occluder. In vertical deviations, when the hyper deviated eye is exposed, the apparent movement is downward. If the patient has a torsional deviation, a vertical line is used for fixation, and a shift in the inclination during alternate occlusion reveals a cyclo deviation. If, for example, a patient has an excyclotropic eye, the top of the line will appear to move in the same direction as the occluder. If the eye has an incyclo deviation, the top of the line will appear to move in the opposite direction.

If there is no deviation of the visual axes, the apparent movement should not be perceived. There may also be no perception of the movement if the alternate occlusion is too rapid so that the patient is allowed to see as though looking through the blades of a fan. We recommend switching the occluder approximately every 0.5 second to achieve the most reliable results for the apparent motion.

MAGNITUDE OF THE DEVIATION

Unless otherwise specified, the *magnitude of the deviation* customarily refers to the angle of deviation of the visual axes when fixation is in the primary position. This parameter should be measured for both the farpoint (optical infinity) and the nearpoint. The most frequently used fixation distances are 6 m (20 ft) for far and 40 cm (16 in.) for near. Accommodation must be carefully controlled, particularly at near, if measurement of horizontal deviations is to be valid (because of effects of accommodative convergence). The best objective test for measuring the magnitude of deviations for far or near is the alternate cover test combined with loose prisms. There is an advantage of using loose prisms rather than prism racks, because both the horizontal and vertical components of a deviation can be conveniently measured simultaneously. In addition, the prism rack is bulky, making measurement of more than one component awkward. For example, to use the prisms in measuring an esotropia of the right eye that also has a hypertropia, two loose prisms, one BO, the

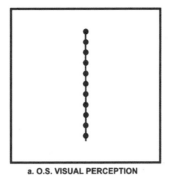

a. O.S. VISUAL PERCEPTION

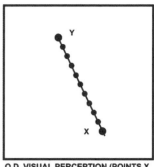

O.D. VISUAL PERCEPTION (POINTS X AND Y ARE NOT SEEN, BUT ARE ONLY FOR EXPLANATION PURPOSES)

b. IMAGE OF MADDOX ROD

POSTERIOR VIEW OF RETINAS

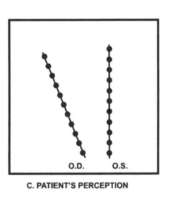

C. PATIENT'S PERCEPTION

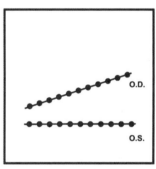

D. PATIENT'S PERCEPTION

Figure 4-32. Explanation of cyclo deviation testing using Maddox rods, a. The patient perceives the imaged line as being vertically oriented for the fixating left eye. However, the line seen by the right eye appears to be slanting, with the top oriented in a leftward position, b. Posterior view of the eyeballs, illustrating the excyclo deviation of the right eye. The analogy of visual fields and retinal projection is used here for clarification. Point x stimulates the superior nasal retina and is therefore projected into the inferior temporal field. Likewise, point y on the inferior temporal retina is projected into the superior nasal field, c. The slanted line seen by the right eye is seen to the left of the vertical line because of a horizontal exo deviation of the right eye. d. Many practitioners prefer to place the axis of the rods at 90 degrees so the patient sees horizontal streaks (in this example, by the left eye). If a vertical prism is placed base-down before the right eye, the excyclo deviation causes the perceived streak for the right eye to slant upward in the temporal field and downward in the nasal visual field. The vertical prism is necessary to create the doubling so that one line is above the other. This may be unnecessary if the patient has an existing vertical deviation.

other BD, are simply placed together between the occluder and the right eye.

Classification

Classification of the magnitude of heterophoric deviations is somewhat nebulous in that the deviation is latent and, thus, not cosmetically noticeable. Although cosmesis is not of concern, binocular function may sometimes be related to magnitude. In general, a very large deviation tends to cause symptoms and may affect performance in school, work, and play. There are many exceptions, however. For example, a small esophoria may play havoc with an individual's comfort and performance when reading, if fusional divergence is inadequate and there is an eso fixation disparity. On the other hand, we have seen patients with relatively large esophoria who are comfortable and perform well at school, work, or play, possibly because of excellent fusional divergence and the absence of fixation disparity. The factors discussed in Chapters 2 and 3 relating to visual skills efficiency must be taken into account when correlating magnitude of heterophoria with comfort and performance. Nevertheless, the magnitude classifications that follow for strabismus may also be useful as guidelines in heterophoria.

The question of what constitutes small and large strabismus needs answering. The classification of von Noorden (as cited by Press[22]) states that an acceptable surgical result in infantile strabismus is less than 20Δ, which is classified as small; an unacceptable result exceeds 20Δ, which is classified as large-angle strabismus. This classification is based mainly on cosmetic evaluation, and we concur with the determination that a 20Δ finding should be considered large, as the deviation is usually noticeable and may be a cosmetic problem. This is somewhat in accord with our recommendations. Classification of strabismus magnitude based on cosmetic acceptability is given in Table 4-14. Horizontal strabismic deviations greater than 20Δ and vertical strabismic deviations greater than 15Δ are often unacceptable cosmetically.

Another aspect of magnitude classification is the functional cure approach (Table 4-15). This classification determinant involves the predicted outcome if nonsurgical means (i.e., prism compensation, vision training techniques, or both) are used to cure the strabismus. An esotropia greater than 20Δ may require surgical reduction, because excessive prismatic power is needed to compensate for the deviation. Comfort and cosmetic acceptance may be problems, as may limitations of fusional divergence training, which often does not produce the desired result in large strabismic deviations. A greater magnitude is allowed in exotropia because fusional convergence is more robust than is fusional divergence in most cases, and it can

TABLE 4-14. Classification of Magnitude of Strabismic Deviation on Basis of Cosmesis

Cosmetic Effect	Esotropia & Exotropia (Δ)	Hyper-tropia (Δ)
Small (usually acceptable)	1-15	1-10
Moderate (sometimes unacceptable)	16-30	11-20
Large (usually unacceptable)	>30	20

usually be increased sufficiently with functional training techniques. However, patients with an exo deviation greater than 25Δ should be considered as possible candidates for surgery. Vertical deviations cannot be improved greatly with training in most cases, and they may require prismatic compensation. Hypertropia greater than 10Δ is, therefore, considered large. These are only general guidelines for a functional description; there are many exceptions in clinical practice. Decisions, as to the extraocular muscle surgery are discussed in subsequent chapters.

Testing Procedures

Testing for magnitude can be undertaken with the procedures listed in Table 4-13, which determine the direction of a deviation of the visual axes. Although the magnitude may be measured by subjective and objective methods, there are times when measurement by subjective means is preferable. This is because objective testing may lack necessary precision, as in cyclo deviation. Subjective testing, however, is not always reliable, especially when there is deep suppression or ARC or the patient is a poor observer.

Subjective methods designed for the determination of the magnitude of deviation are variations of either the single-object or the two-object method. The measuring tools are either prisms or calibrated scales. The scales may be in true space. For example, in the Hess-Lancaster test, the patient directly views the test targets, and their separation can be converted into prism diopters by using the measurement lines on the screen. In contrast, when haploscopes such as the major amblyoscope (discussed in subsequent chapters) are used, the deviation is measured from scales on the instrument.

ACCOMMODATIVE-CONVERGENCE/ ACCOMMODATION RATIO

The AC/A ratio means that for every diopter of accommodative response, a certain amount of

TABLE 4-15. Classification of Magnitude of Strabismic Deviation on Basis of Prognosis for Functional Cure (with Prism Compensation and/or Training Techniques)

Magnitude	Esotropia (Δ)	Exotropia (Δ)	Hypertropia (Δ)
Small	1-10	1-15	1-5
Moderate	11-20	16-25	6-10
Large	>20	>25	>10

Table 4-16. Classification of Alternation of Strabismus at Far and Near

Unilateral	Strabismic right eye
	Strabismic left eye
Alternating	Habitual alternation
	Right eye preferred for fixation
	Left eye preferred for fixation
	Forced alternation

accommodative convergence is brought into play, depending on the value of the ratio. For example, if the AC/A is 6Δ per 1.00 D of accommodative response, a patient who accommodates 2.50 D will have an increased convergence of 15Δ. In strabismus cases, the *calculated* AC/A is determined in the same manner as was described in Chapter 3. However, a *gradient* AC/A in strabismic patients usually is not defined using phoropter measurements, although it may be determined by finding the effect of spherical lenses (from a trial lens set) on convergence (with the alternate cover test). At the farpoint, minus lenses are used for this purpose. At the nearpoint, either plus or minus lenses will give the value. Regardless of the testing distance, the AC/A ratio should be determined with the patient wearing full-plus farpoint refractive correction (i.e., corrected ametropia most plus [CAMP] lenses) (see Chapter 2).

The following is an example of the gradient method. Assume that the patient has an exotropia of 15Δ at far. A spherical lens of -2.50 D is placed before each eye in free space, and the patient is instructed to focus and clear the fixation target while looking through the lenses. When the target is reported to be clear, another measurement of the angle of deviation is made (e.g., alternate cover test). If the lenses cause the angle to change from 15Δ exo to ortho, the AC/A ratio is 6 to 1, determined by dividing the change in magnitude of the deviation by the change of accommodative stimulus.

EYE LATERALITY

In cases of strabismus, *eye laterality* refers to whether only one eye or either eye is able to maintain fixation. This determination should be made at far and near fixation distances. If only one eye is able to fixate, the strabismus is classified as *unilateral*, whereas if either eye can fixate, it is an *alternating* strabismus (Table 4-16). Alternation should be classified as either habitual or forced. *Habitual alternation* means the patient switches fixation naturally, without being aware of doing so. *In*

forced alternation, the patient must be made aware of the need or instructed to alternate. The degree of forcing indicates the patient's tendency to alternate or not alternate. This important information should be included in the evaluation of eye laterality.

Evaluation is made by such means as the Hirschberg test, unilateral cover test, patient history, and direct observation of the patient. A judgment is made regarding whether a patient fixates with either eye (and the frequency of fixation with each) or whether fixation is confined to one eye. An interesting characteristic of many strabismics is alternation of fixation on lateral versions. The clinician can observe whether a patient switches fixation at the midline with lateral pursuits to the right and left. For example, in left gaze, an esotropic patient may prefer the right eye for fixation, whereas in right gaze, the left eye may be preferred. The presence of such a midline switch should be recorded. This often is associated with infantile esotropia or ARC (or both). The midline switch also is referred to as a *cross-fixation pattern*: Although each eye is used at various times, this is not truly an alternating strabismus as regards switching fixation in the primary position of gaze.

EYE DOMINANCY

Eye dominancy refers to the superiority of one eye over the other, in either the motor or sensory realm. Sighting tests that determine the eye preferred for fixation are examples in the motor realm. In strabismus, the terms *eye preference* and *eye dominancy* are used synonymously. The unilateral cover test can be used to determine the fixating eye in strabismus. If the deviation is large enough to be observed, the Hirschberg test is a practical means for such evaluation.

In heterophoria, in which the deviation is latent and not observable except on dissociation, sighting tests such as the hole-in-the-card test should be used. With both hands, a patient holds, at arm's length, a card having a small hole in the center and sights a distant fixation target. The clinician alternately occludes each of the patient's eyes to determine which eye the patient is using to sight the target.

The nearpoint of convergence is another means of determining which eye is superior in motoric functioning. The eye that stops first in following the advancing target is considered to be nondominant, at least for very near fixation distances. Testing of accommodative facility (monocularly) and fixation disparity are other indices of motor dominance (see Chapters 2 and 3).

Dominancy testing in the sensory realm includes retinal rivalry, color fusion, and suppression and applies particularly to cases of heterophoria. (In strabismus evaluation, eye dominancy generally is based on the finding of which eye is preferred for fixation.) Dominancy should be determined at far and near, as there may be a difference when fixation distance is changed. The latter situation is an example of *mixed dominancy* meaning that one eye is preferred for some functions but not for others.

In evaluation of heterophoria, eye dominancy is determined by testing for both sensorial and motoric superiority between the two eyes. In the past, great interest was shown in crossed dominancy (i.e., the dominant eye and the dominant hand being on opposite sides of the body). The relation between crossed dominancy and learning disabilities was once considered by some to be significant, although modern thinking tends to disregard this association.

VARIABILITY OF THE DEVIATION

There are many influences on tonic convergence which, in turn, affect the magnitude of a deviation. According to Maddox (see Chapter 1), tonic convergence is one of the four components of convergence, the other three being accommodative, fusional (reflex), and proximal (psychic).

In cases of heterophoria, changes in tonic convergence are not obvious, unless dissociative testing is performed and each day's findings are compared with those obtained on other days. However, significant changes in cases of strabismus may be observable and can have a striking effect on the patient's appearance if the deviation changes from being just noticeable to being highly noticeable. Cosmetic appearance of a strabismus is often a patient's greatest concern. It is important for the

Table 4-17. Anatomic Factors in Strabismic Cosmesis

Favorable for Esotropia, Unfavorable for Exotropia	Favorable for Exotropia, Unfavorable for Esotropia
Positive angle kappa	Negative angle kappa
Narrow bridge of nose	Wide bridge of nose
Absence of epicanthus	Presence of epicanthus
Large interpupillary distance	Small interpupillary distance
Narrow face	Wide face

clinician to understand this and to have empathy for a patient's feelings in this regard.

Changes in the magnitude of deviation may occur for various reasons. Fatigue, emotional stress, medication, illness, and other factors may be involved. Variation in the magnitude of the angle of deviation may cause a latent deviation to become manifest. A case of intermittent strabismus is usually more noticeable than a case of constant strabismus. It should be noted, however, that intermittence is not usually the result of a change in tonic convergence. In most cases, intermittence probably involves the power of compensatory fusion, whereby a deviation may or may not be held latent.

COSMESIS

In addition to magnitude, its variability, and strabismic intermittence, certain anatomic factors affect cosmesis. The list of such factors presented in Table 4-17 indicates whether each is favorable or unfavorable to the appearance of patients with esotropia or exotropia.

Clinicians should not judge cosmesis exclusively on the basis of the magnitude of the deviation. Rather, all factors must be considered. For example, the recommendation to undergo surgery for cosmetic reasons may be given to a patient having an esotropia of 20Δ. However, surgery for cosmetic reasons alone may not be necessary for such a patient if he or she has a large positive angle kappa, a narrow bridge, no epicanthal folds, a large interpupillary distance, and a narrow face. Under these conditions, the eyes are likely to appear cosmetically straight. It is possible that the eyes would appear exotropic if the eso deviation were significantly reduced by means of surgery. Consequently, it is always wise to observe the patient carefully and weigh the various factors influencing appearance before reaching any conclusion regarding extraocular muscle surgery.

The effect of eyewear on cosmesis should also be taken into account. A certain spectacle frame may either help or hinder the strabismic individual's appearance. Trial of different sizes and patterns and keen observation of the patient's appearance are the rules to follow.

REFERENCES

1. Aslin R. Development of binocular fixation in human infants. J Exp Child Psycho 1977;123:133-50.

2. Aslin R. Motor aspects of visual development in infancy. In: Salapatek P CL, ed. Handbook of infant perception, vol 1: From sensation to perception. New York: Academic Press, Inc, 1978.

3. Greenberg A, Mohney B, Diehl N, Burke J. Incidence and Types of Childhood Esotropia. Ophthalmology 2007;114:170-4.

4. Wong A. Timing of survery for infantile esotropia: sensory and motor outcomes. Can J Ophthalmol. 2008;43:43-51.

5. Birch E, Stager S. Long-term motor and sensory outcome after early surgery for infantile esotropia. J AAPOS 2006;10:409-13.

6. Fisher N. General principles of esotropia. Audio Digest Ophthalmol. 1972;10(18):side B.

7. Hirschberg J. Ober die Messung des Schielgrades und Dosierung der Schieloperation. Centralbl Prakt Augen-keilkd 1885;9:325-7.

8. Jones R, Eskridge J. The Hirschberg test: a re-evaluation. Am J Optom Arch Am Acad Optom. 1970;47:105-14.

9. Griffin J, Boyer F. Strabismus: measurement with the Hirschberg test. Optom Wkly 1974;75:863-6.

10. Riddell P, Heinline L, Abramov I. Calibration of the Hirschberg test in human infants. Invest Ophthalmol Vis Sci. 1994;35:538-43.

11. Hasebe S, Ohtsuki H, Kono R, Nakahira Y. Biometric confirmation of the Hirschberg ratio in strabismus children. Invest Ophthalmol Vis Sci. 1998;39:2782-5.

12. Eskridge J. The complete cover test. J Am Optom Assoc. 1973;44:601-9.

13. Choi R, Kishner B. The accuracy of experienced strabismologists using the Hirschberg and Krimsky tests. Ophthalmology 1998;105:1301-6.

14. Hasebe S, Ohtsuki H, Tadokoro Y, et al. The reliability of a video-enhanced Hirschberg test under clinical conditions. Invest Ophthalmol Vis Sci. 1995;36:2678-85.

15. Pediatric Eye Disease Investigator Group. Interobserver reliability of the prism and alternative cover test in children with esotropia. Arch Ophthalmol. 2009;127:59-65.

16. Griffin J, McLin L, Schor C. Photographic method for Bruckner and Hirschberg testing. Optom Vis Sci. 1989;66:474-9.

17. Griffin J, Cotter S. The Bruckner test: evaluation of clinical usefulness. Am J Optom Physiol Opt. 1986;63:957-61.

18. Parks M. Isolated cyclovertical muscle palsy. Arch Ophthalmol. 1958;60:1027-35.

19. Bajandas F, Kline L. Neuro-Ophthalmology Review Manual. In. Thorofare, NJ: Slack Inc., 1987.

20. Jampolsky A. A Simplified Approach to Strabismus Diagnosis. In: Symptoms on Strabismus, Transaction of the New Orleans Academy of Ophthalmology. St. Louis: C.V. Mosby, 1971.

21. Howarth P, Herm G. Repeated measures of horizontal heterophoria. Optom Vis Sci. 2000;77:616-9.

22. Press L. Topical review: strabismus. J Optom Vision Dev. 1991;22:5-20.

Chapter 5 / Sensory Fusion and Sensory Adaptations to Strabismus

Sensory Fusion	114	Visually Evoked Potentials	138
Simultaneous Perception	115	Interferometry	139
Superimposition	115	Fixation Evaluation	140
Flat Fusion	115	Description of Eccentric Fixation	140
Stereopsis	115	Visuoscopy	141
Vectographic Methods	116	Haidinger Brush Testing	141
Percentage of Stereopsis	117	Refraction Procedures	143
Stereopsis and Binocular Vision	117	Eye Disease Evaluation	144
Norms for Stereoacuity	119	Ophthalmoscopy	144
Sensory Adaptation to Strabismus	119	Visual Fields	144
Suppression	119	Neutral-Density Filters	145
Characteristics of Suppression	120	Tests of Retinal Function	145
Testing for Suppression	123	Screening for Amblyopia	146
History	123	Anomalous Correspondence	146
Red Lens Test	123	Classification	146
Worth Dot Test	123	Characteristics	149
Amblyoscope Workup	124	Horopter in Anomalous Retinal Correspondence	149
Amblyopia	126	Horror Fusionis	152
Classification	127	Etiology of Anomalous Retinal Correspondence	152
Strabismic Amblyopia	127	Depth of Anomalous Retinal Correspondence	153
Anisometropic Amblyopia	127	Prevalence of Anomalous Retinal Correspondence	154
Isoametropic Amblyopia	128		
Image Degradation Amblyopia	128	Testing	154
Amblyopia as a Developmental Disorder	129	Dissociated Red Lens Test	154
Case History	131	Afterimages	155
Visual Acuity Testing	132	Bifoveal Test of Cüppers	156
Snellen Charts	132	Major Amblyoscope	158
Psychometric Charts	133	Bagolini Striated Lenses	161
Amblyopia Treatment Study (ATS) Visual Acuity Protocol	134	Color Fusion	162
HOTV and Lea Charts	134		
Infant Visual Acuity Assessment	136		

SENSORY FUSION

From a clinical perspective, the measurement of the strabismus discussed in Chapter 4 is principally motoric. However, there must be sensory (and usually perceptual and often cognitive) input so that visual functioning can occur. Clinical testing of sensory fusion also involves a motoric component. Nevertheless, for instructional purposes, it is convenient to deal with motor fusion and sensory fusion as though they were separate, keeping in mind that this distinction is artificial and that they are really indissoluble.

On a clinical basis, motor fusion can be considered basically to involve the amplitude and speed of various ranges of vergences. In contrast, the basic clinical concern in sensory fusion is suppression. Sensory fusion is classified according to the Worth taxonomy into three categories: first-, second-, and third-degree fusion. (Refer to Chapter 1 for theoretical discussions of these degrees of sensory fusion.)

In clinical diagnosis, sensory fusion of form can be classified into four levels, a modification of the categories of fusion recommended by Worth (as cited by Revel[1]): Simultaneous perception (diplopia) Superimposition (first-degree fusion) Flat fusion (second-degree fusion) and Stereopsis (third-degree fusion)

These categories of binocular sensory status can be conveniently tested by using vectographic techniques, colored filters, and the numerous stereoscopic methods employing septum arrangements. Many methods and instruments are presented in this chapter and in this book, particularly in case examples.

Simultaneous Perception

Although simultaneous perception is classified as one of the levels of sensory fusion, there is actually no real fusion with this particular binocular demand. Simultaneous perception is determined to be present merely by the patient's awareness of binocular images at the same time. In clinical usage, simultaneous perception refers to the stimulation of non-corresponding retinal points that give rise to diplopia. An example is shown in Figure 1-11, in which the fixated light is seen diplopically because the dioptric image is on a noncorresponding point of the deviated right eye.

The usual test applied in determining whether a patient can appreciate simultaneous perception is to elicit a diplopic response when one object (e.g., a penlight) is fixated. When deep suppression interferes with diplopia testing, stimulating a noncorresponding point somewhere outside the suppression zone may be desirable. This is conveniently accomplished by placing a vertically oriented loose prism in front of the deviating eye to elicit a diplopic response. If a sufficiently large base-down prism is placed before the right eye, the dioptric image of the light is located below the suppression zone (inferior retina) and will be perceived (in the visual field) above the fixated one. When suppression is very deep, this technique is useful in determining the horizontal subjective angle of deviation.

Superimposition

The superimposition of two dissimilar targets is known as first-degree fusion. However, when this occurs, confusion rather than true sensory fusion exists, because similar targets are not being integrated; they merely have common oculocentric directions. Because two dissimilar objects stimulate corresponding retinal points and are perceived as superimposed, the definition of superimposition is satisfied.

With the exception of the Maddox rod test, superimposition testing usually requires more instrumentation than a penlight in free space. Stereoscopes containing a different target for each eye (e.g., a fish seen only by the left eye and a tank seen by the right eye) are usually necessary (see Figure 5-14).

Flat Fusion

Flat fusion is true sensory fusion and is the integration of two similar ocular images into a single percept. There may be one target in free space, such as a page of print, or there may be two identical targets in a stereoscope. In any event, to be classified as a flat-fusion stimulus, this type of target must be two-dimensional and identical in form for each eye.

Such targets are the most frequently employed in testing and evaluating motor fusion (fusional divergence and convergence). Usually Snellen letters or printed words are used as targets, to be fused with the incorporation of unfused suppression clues in the test design. (An example of a flat fusion target with a test design for extrafoveal suppression is shown in Figure 5-15.) If the angular separation from the center of the target to a suppression clue is greater than 5 degrees, testing for peripheral suppression is being accomplished. Testing for foveal suppression requires that a suppression clue be located in or near the center of the target. Therefore, the location of the clues that are suppressed determines the size of the suppression. These specifications regarding targets for determination of suppression size are listed in Table 5-6.

In cases of heterophoria, however, foveal suppression, rather than larger suppression zones occurring in strabismus, is usually the concern. Similarly, depth of suppression is necessarily evaluated in cases of strabismus but rarely is evaluated in heterophoria.

Stereopsis

Stereopsis is the perception of three-dimensional visual space due to binocular disparity clues. Test targets for stereopsis are similar to those for flat fusion with one exception; in the former, there is lateral displacement in certain portions of the target. The displacement of a set of paired points (referred to as homologous points) is relative to the position of other pairs of homologous points on the stereogram. For example, in Figure 1-14, consider the star as the figure that is fixated and fused. The small vertical lines are displaced inwardly (BO, or crossed disparity effect) relative to the fused star. Assume that the patient is concentrating on the fused star. The vertical lines are imaged on each retina temporally in relation to the star, which causes the fused image of the lines to appear closer than the star. The opposite would be true if the lines were disparately nasalward on each retina. The rule to remember is that if the retinal disparity is temporalward ("templeward") from the center of each fovea, the stereoscopic image will appear closer, whereas if the retinal disparity is nasalward, the image will appear farther.

If the disparities become too far separated, the lines can no longer be fused (by remaining within Panum's areas) and are seen diplopically. Because they fall on points too disparate, they cause diplopia in the same manner as in simultaneous perception testing. However, if the disparities are not very great, the targets are fusible even though they do not fall exactly on corresponding retinal points. This is due to the allowance in disparity afforded by Panum's area. It is this small fused disparity that is responsible for stereopsis.

As in flat-fusion testing, there are suppression clues in stereopsis testing, which are those portions of the stereogram that are supposed to be seen in depth, relative to a fixated point. In the preceding example, the clues are the fused lines. The lack of depth may be an indication of suppression.

Vectographic Methods

Most clinical tests of stereopsis use vectographic targets. Applying the principle of polarization to the testing of vision allows the use of suppression clues during fairly natural conditions of binocular viewing. For vectographic testing, the patient wears polarizing filters in the form of spectacles. The polarizing filter for one eye must be rotated to an angle 90 degrees different from the filter for the other eye, thereby achieving mutual exclusion of light coming to each eye. Thus, when the test targets are also polarized, one eye cannot see certain portions of the test target that are visible to the other eye. In the United States, the filters in commercially available polarizing spectacles usually are oriented at 45 and 135 degrees; those manufactured in some other countries are often set at 90 and 180 degrees.

Several frequently used vectographic tests for stereoacuity are listed in Table 5-1. Examples of vectographic tests are depicted in Figures 5-1 through 5-5. Other nonvectographic tests (e.g., Frisby & Lang) are illustrated in Figures 5-6 through 5-8. Most clinical tests of stereopsis are administered at 40 cm but in some cases of strabismus (such as: intermittent exotropia) distance testing is desirable. The recent development of the Distance Stereo test (see Figure 5-2) and the Frisby-Davis Distance test address this need (Figure 5-8).

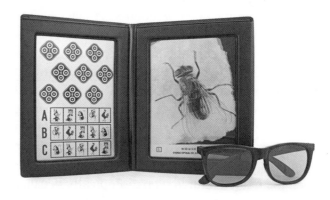

Figure 5-1. The "Fly" stereopsis test contoured targets. (Courtesy Stereo Optical Co.)

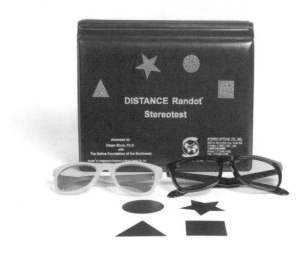

Figure 5-2. The distance randot steretest. (Courtesy Stereo Optical Co.)

Table 5-1. Frequently Used Vectographic Tests of Stereoacuity

Stereotest (Fly) (nearpoint testing)
Distance Randot Test (farpoint testing)
Vectographic Slide (farpoint testing)
Pre-school Stereoacuity test (global stereopsis)
Randot stereotest (nearpoint testing)
Random dot E stereotest (near to far testing)

Stereoacuity may also be evaluated by comparing the relative distance of two objects in free space, such as in the traditional Howard-Dolman peg test, which is designed for farpoint measurements. The test consists of two black, movable vertical rods viewed through an aperture against a white background. The patient is seated at a distance of 6 m from the rods and is instructed not to move his or her head. Otherwise, lateral parallax will be induced, thereby invalidating testing procedures. The rods are moved by the patient, either nearer

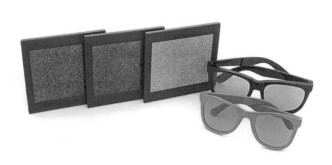

Figure 5-3. Random dot E stereopsis test noncontoured targets. (Courtesy Stereo Optical Co.)

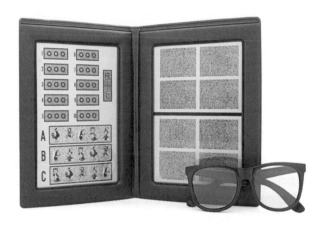

Figure 5-4. Randot stereopsis test noncontoured and semicontoured targets. (Courtesy Stereo Optical Co.)

or farther from each other, by means of strings, until they appear to be equidistant (i.e., in the same plane). The distance error is determined from an average of several trials and is converted from millimeters into seconds of arc; this value represents stereoacuity (Table 5-2). For example, if the error (the distance the patient misaligns the two pegs) is 60 mm, the stereoacuity is 20 seconds of arc. Because there may be a constant error due to a skewed or tilted horopter, however, testing results may be invalid. The standard deviation of the mean would represent a truer index of stereoacuity, but acquiring this information would require completion of approximately 15 trials; hence, it seldom is done on a routine clinical basis. An apparatus of the Howard-Dolman type may be custom-made or obtained through commercial sources.

For similar nearpoint testing, the Verhoeff Stereoptor (formerly made by the American Optical

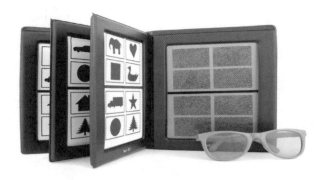

Figure 5-5. Randot Preschool Stereoacuity Test, for 800-40 seconds of arc to test to ages as young as 2 years, a. Three books of the set. b. Book 2, in which the top portion is 60 seconds of arc and the bottom 40 seconds of arc. For book 1, the values are 200 and 100 seconds of arc for the top and bottom, respectively; for book 3, 800 and 400 seconds of arc for the top and bottom, respectively. (Courtesy of Stereo Optical Co.)

Corporation but no longer manufactured; see Appendix J) has been widely used by many government agencies (e.g., military). It has an illuminated white window in which three vertically placed black strips are centered. One of the strips is displaced from the plane of the other two, either forward or backward, and the patient is asked to tell for which strip the distance differs from the other two. The instrument can be adjusted to form eight different strip arrangements (i.e., eight different targets). A patient with a stereoacuity of 31 seconds of arc or better should be able to report all eight targets correctly at a testing (Table 5-3).

Percentage of Stereopsis

Occasionally, practitioners are asked to report percentage values of stereopsis rather than values recorded in seconds of arc. Percentage scales were empirically determined by Dr. Carl F. Shepard for such purposes, and calculations and information pertaining to this method were presented by Fry. Table 5-4 gives percentage values corresponding to stereoacuity in seconds of arc.

Stereopsis and Binocular Vision

The level of stereopsis determines the level of binocular status in most cases: Stereopsis is the "barometer" of binocularity. If stereopsis is good, the binocular status is good, but the opposite cannot always be said with certainty. That is, a patient may be found to have no stereopsis but have normal sensory and motor fusion in all other respects. This is particularly so in small-angle strabismics, who can develop good fusional amplitudes but yet may have a poor prognosis for developing bifixation (with central, fine stereopsis).

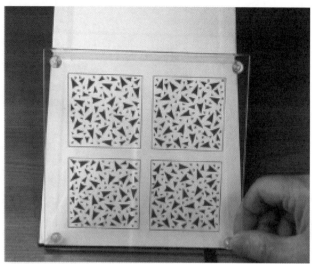

Figure 5-6. Frisby test. Random patterns are printed on each side of a transparent plate. The patient is instructed to locate in which of the four squares is the stereoscopically perceived circular target. (Courtesy of Dr. John Frisby.)

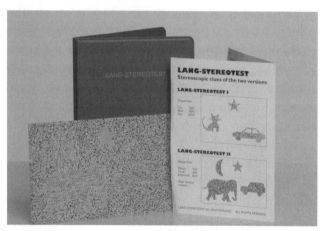

Figure 5-7. Lang test. Images for the eyes are separated by the fine parallel cylindrical strips to create perception of stereopsis by way of lateral displacement of images seen by each eye. Note that this is Lang test 1; another version, Lang test 2, is also available.

In light of this discussion, one may wonder why random-dot stereo tests, even gross ones, apparently seem to be effective in detecting sensory binocular anomalies of suppression, anomalous correspondence, and amblyopia. Conversely, the stereo tests with contoured patterns must be within relatively sensitive criteria to be effective in this regard. The difference in criteria between the two types of stereopsis tests may have something to do with "local" versus "global" stereopsis. Hofstetter et al[2] defined local stereopsis as a "very simple disparity stimulus pattern such as, for example, a stereogram with two parallel vertical line segments seen by each eye with slightly differing lateral separations." This same group defined global stereopsis as that "elicited by the disparity of portions and/or clusters within relatively large stereogram patterns,

Table 5-2. Howard-Dolman Test for Stereopsis, Performed at 6 m

Alignment Error (mm)	Stereoacuity (seconds of arc)
5	2
10	3
20	7
30	10
40	13
50	16
60	20
80	26
100	33
200	66
300	99
400	132
500	165

Note: An interpupillary distance of 60 mm is assumed. Stereoacuities were determined by the following formula: $\eta = \text{IPD} (x)/d^2 \times 206,000$, where η (eta) is the symbol for stereoacuity in seconds of arc; IPD is the interpupillary distance in millimeters; x is the alignment error in millimeters; and d is the testing distance from patient to rods in millimeters.

involving complex textured surfaces and repetitive elements for which many disparately paired details might provide ambiguous or even conflicting stereopsis clues without destroying the overlying percept of depth, believed by Julesz to represent a perceptual interpretation process differentiated from local stereopsis."

In a study investigating the angle of horizontal strabismus and level of stereopsis, Leske and Holmes used both random dot and contour stereo tests to measure stereopsis in 186 strabismic patients.[3] The following tests of stereopsis were used; the Titmus Fly, Titmus Animals, Titmus Circles, Frisby, and Randot Preschool Stereo Tests. Two important results were reported. First, the contour stereo tests have monocular cues to depth and can lead to false positives. The authors found that at stereo acuity levels better than 140 seconds of arc few monocular cues were present. Second, they found that no strabismus patients with an angle of deviation greater than 4 diopters were able to achieve appreciation of random dot stereopsis or have a positive response to contour stereo targets of better than 140 seconds of arc. Thus, in patients who perceive random dot stereopsis or have good stereoacuity the presence of a large angle constant strabismus is unlikely.

TABLE 5-3. Verhoeff Stereopter and Corresponding Stereoacuities

Test Distance (cm)	Stereoacuity (seconds of arc)
10	3,090
20	772
30	343
50	124
60	86
80	48
100	31
110	26
130	18
150	14
200	8
300	3

Note: Response to all eight targets must be correct. The stereo-threshold values in this table are calculated for an interpupillary distance of 60 mm. The η value (stereoacuity) is calculated using an x value of 2.5 mm, which is the displacement of one strip from the plane of the other two strips. Verhoeff stereoacuities are calculated according to the same formula used for the Howard-Dolman test (see footnotes to Table 5-2).

Table 5-4. Approximate Corresponding Values for Stereoacuity in Seconds of Arc and Shepard Percentages

Stereoacuity in Seconds of Arc	Stereoacuity in Shepard Percentages
1,000	4
400	16
200	31
100	51
50	72
40	78
20	95
15	100
10	106

Note: Shepard percentages are calculated using the following formula of Fry (Fry G. Measurement of the threshold of stereopsis. Optom Wkly 1942;33:1032)
Percentage stereopsis = $[10,100/(\eta+81)] - 5$
where η is the symbol for stereoacuity.

TABLE 5-5. Ranking of Results of Stereopsis Testing (Seconds of Arc)

Rank	Description	Contoured	Noncontoured
5	Very strong	≤20	≤30
4	Strong	20-30	31-50
3	Adequate	31-60	51-100
2	Weak	61-100	101-600
1	Very weak	≥100	≥600

Norms for Stereoacuity

Rankings of stereoacuity scores are clinically practical for possible referrals and for assessment of stereopsis before and after vision therapy. These rankings are listed in Table 5-5 for contoured (local) and noncontoured (global) stereopsis.

Note that leniency is given for global stereopsis. These rankings apply to patients at least 7 years old. Professional judgment is required when evaluating test results of children younger than age 7. Because it is an overall indicator of the patency of binocular vision, stereoacuity has been used as part of a vision screening test battery. A preschool test that has good inter-rater test-retest reliability is the Randot Preschool Stereoacuity Test.[4] This test can be used for children as young as 2 years and samples stereoacuity from 800 to 40 seconds of arc (see Figure 5-5).

Sensory Adaptations to Strabismus

Several anomalous sensory conditions can develop secondary to the onset of a developmental strabismus, particularly of early origin. These include suppression, amblyopia, and anomalous correspondence. These conditions and the appropriate testing methods for them are discussed in this chapter. Although it is customary to think in terms of the deviation causing these adaptive conditions, it is also possible that the process may work in reverse. In other words, the strabismus may be the end result rather than the cause of the anomalous sensory conditions.

SUPPRESSION

When a strabismus occurs, the affected individual may experience pathologic diplopia or confusion (or both). Suppression is the defense mechanism that is usually attempted first by an individual to eliminate these perceptual annoyances. *Suppression* is the lack of perception of normally visible objects in all or part of the field of vision of one eye, occurring only under binocular viewing conditions and attributed to cortical inhibition.[5] In normal binocular vision, *physiologic suppression* naturally occurs, particularly, for all objects falling outside the singleness horopter. The suppressed image can usually be brought to consciousness by directing attention to it. On the other hand, *pathologic suppression* is a binocular anomaly. In the presence of strabismus, for example, a suppressed image is not easily perceived by merely directing one's attention to it. There is, apparently, active cortical inhibition of the suppressed eye's image that is not as subject to volitional control; von Noorden[6] noted that even retinal rivalry disappears in some strabismic patients. Retinal rivalry (see Chapter 1) and suppression both occur in the

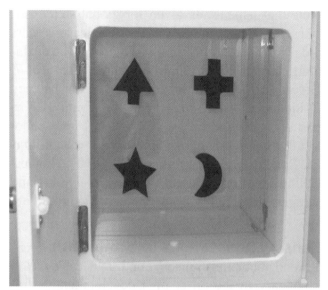

Figure 5-8. The Frisby Davis (FD2) Stereotest can be done between 3 and 6 meters. (Courtesy of Dr. John Frisby)

visual cortex, although they may be mediated by different neural processes.[7]

Suppression that occurs during infancy and early childhood can have a profound effect on the development of the full visual acuity potential of the affected eye and development of stereopsis. When the images of each eye are discordant due to strabismus or uncorrected anisometropia, there is active cortical inhibition in V1 related to the affected eye that slows or halts further sensory development.[8] Stereopsis (binocular depth disparity detection) starts to develop in normal infants at approximately 2.5-4.0 months of age and progresses rapidly.[9] The onset of strabismus at this early time has the most disruptive effect.[10] Amblyopia can quickly develop in the turned eye if the child fails to develop an alternate fixation pattern. Stereopsis, however, can continue to develop in the presence of a constant strabismus, although not to the same degree as when the eyes are straight. In the case of anisometropia, suppression is directly related to the degree of the refractive difference between the eyes, and the development of stereopsis is affected accordingly.[11] Early identification of disorders of binocular vision that cause suppression and result in amblyopia and reduced stereoacuity is a desirable public health goal, as it makes the successful management of such conditions much easier.

In cases of excessive heterophoria and intermittent strabismus (particularly intermittent exotropia), testing for suppression usually requires very sensitive suppression controls, such as the alternate polarized letter test found on the Vectographic Slide (see Figure 3-11) the Mentor B-VAT Binocular Vision Testing System, or newer computerized visual acuity charts.[12]

Characteristics of Suppression

The precise neurologic mechanism for suppression is not thoroughly known, but the phenomenon can be easily demonstrated by diagram. Figure 5-9 illustrates the concept of diplopia and confusion and the resulting zone of suppression. The fixation target is imaged on the fixating left eye. An esotropia of the right eye causes the target's image to fall on the nasal retina. Cyclopean projection shows the patient perceiving two images. When the diplopic image is seen on the same side as the eye that deviates (e.g., right eye seeing the diplopic image in the right field), the diplopia is called *homonymous*, or *uncrossed*. If, however, the diplopic image were to fall on the temporal retina of the deviating eye, *heteronymous (crossed) diplopia* would occur. For the redundant ocular image to be eliminated, the target point on the nasal retina of the right eye must be suppressed. Jampolsky[13] referred to this location as the "zero measure" point (*point zero*). This point and its adjacent area must be suppressed to avoid diplopia. Peripheral diplopia may occur if the deviation is larger than Panum's fusional areas in the peripheral binocular field, but the combined influence of low resolution, suppression, and selective attention to the fixated target usually prevents the perception of double images in these distant locations.

Whereas point zero (the target point, sometimes designated as *T*) usually is suppressed, the fovea in the deviating eye is suppressed even more intensely. If this were not the case, then two dissimilar images would be superimposed, as each fovea is pointing to a different location within the binocular visual field. This intolerable situation is called *confusion*. Suppression of the fovea of the deviated eye occurs more quickly and deeply than at point zero because foveal vision is usually the location of attention. Clinically, strabismic individuals typically do not report confusion, but some do have symptoms of diplopia.

It is probable that suppression begins first at the fovea when a horizontal deviation of the visual axes becomes manifest, as in Figure 5-9; later, point zero is also suppressed. Afterward, a pathologic zone of suppression encompasses the area

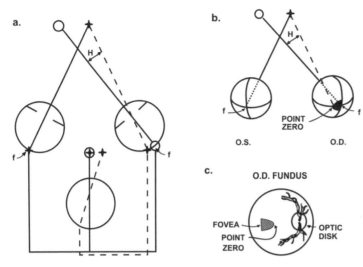

Figure 5-9. Confusion and diplopia in an example of esotropia of the right eye and the resulting pathologic suppression, a. Cyclopean perception of confusion and pathologic homonymous diplopia. The fixation starlike object is seen diplopically. The nonfixated circle falling on the fovea of the deviating right eye causes confusion. Although the circle could possibly be seen diplopically, it is not usually noticed, as the patient is not paying it any attention, b. Theoretical posterior view of the eyes showing the suppression zone that could result from the esotropic right eye. c. Theoretical ophthalmoscopic view of the right fundus, illustrating the shape and location of the suppression zone, (f = fovea; H = horizontal angle of deviation; O.D. = oculus dexter; O.S. = oculus sinister.)

between the fovea and point zero of the deviating eye. The vertical dimension of this zone is usually smaller than the horizontal dimension. The shape of the zone resembles the letter *D*, according to Jampolsky,[13] and the vertical demarcation at the fovea resembles a hemianoptic visual field defect. Although this is a theoretical model of the suppression zone, clinical findings suggest that these demarcations are not always so clear-cut. Pratt-Johnson and MacDonald[14] showed that suppression does not exclusively involve the nasal retina in esotropes and the temporal retina in exotropes, but it may extend in both directions regardless of the direction of the deviation. The shape and size of the suppression zone depends on the targets used and the way the test is performed. The suppression "scotoma" is, therefore, considered *relative* rather than absolute, appearing more extensive and deep in the hemiretina toward point zero. In some cases, however (e.g., a large-angle strabismus with amblyopia of long standing), it appears that most or all of the binocular visual field of the deviating eye is pathologically suppressed.

How does the suppressing strabismic patient perceive visual objects in space? Such a patient does experience continuity of visual space across the visual field, similar to the individual having normal binocular vision (Figure 5-10a). However,

there may be a slight decrease or increase in the horizontal size of the visual field, depending on whether the deviation is esotropic (see Figure 5-10b) or exotropic (see Figure 5-10c), respectively. Fortunately, a strabismic patient who is free of ocular pathology perceives no gaps (missing portions) in the visual field. Suppression of the turned eye occurs only within the binocular overlap area. Suppression is not obvious to the individual except indirectly, possibly because of deficient stereopsis; a vivid spatial sense of three-dimensionality often is missing, depending on the extent and depth of the suppression zone. The extreme peripheral lateral fields of each eye are, however, normal. These temporal crescents, approximately 30 degrees on each side, cannot be suppressed. The crescents are neurally subserved only by monocular fibers from the nasal retina of each eye. The suppressed eye is unresponsive to binocular stimulation but is responsive to the "monocular" stimulation of the peripheral nasal retina.

Foveal suppression may also be found in nonstrabismic patients. Anisometropia may cause image size difference on the retina of each eye (aniseikonia) and also a difference in clarity. Suppression is, therefore, necessary to eliminate the confusion arising from the resulting superimposition of dissimilar ocular images (i.e., one image being larger than the other). The suppression zone in such cases is relatively small and encircles only the fovea, as there is no extrafoveal point zero. Therefore, confusion, and not diplopia, is the problem. Foveal suppression is found also in patients with large heterophoria if fusional vergence compensation is poor. The mechanism is not fully understood, but it is likely that vergence stress or fixation disparity can initiate a suppression response.

Suppression may be classified by size and intensity. In regard to size, suppression is classified as being either *central* or *peripheral*. If a patient has central suppression, the edge of the suppression zone can extend to 5 degrees from the center of the fovea. Beyond this limit, suppression is considered to be peripheral (Table 5-6). It must be remembered that the limits of the suppression zone depend on the testing conditions and the size of the targets used.

Intensity of suppression varies on a continuous scale from *shallow* to *deep* (Table 5-7). This is necessarily a qualitative determination. It is made by finding the ease with which suppression can be broken by using various testing procedures. The more unnatural the environment (laboratory type of testing conditions), the less likely is suppression. For example, the Worth dot test using red-green filters in a dark room is relatively unnatural and serves as a strong stimulus to break through suppression. Conversely, in more natural seeing conditions (e.g., Pola-Mirror), the patient will more likely suppress an eye. Illuminated targets, such as a penlight or Worth lights, become less natural by lowering room illumination.

In effect, intensity is described in terms of the testing procedure that is required to break (eliminate) the suppression response. Some of the methods commonly used to test the intensity of suppression are listed in Table 5-7. The more natural tests appear at the top of the list, with the less natural following in descending order. Using this as a guide, it is reasonable to assume, for example, that a strabismic patient who notices pathologic diplopia when viewing a penlight in an illuminated room has shallow suppression. In contrast, if the room must be darkened and the patient must wear red-green filters to perceive diplopia, then the suppression would be deep.

Several attributes of the strabismic deviation affect the suppression response. Magnitude of the deviation is one: Generally, the larger the deviation, the larger is the suppression zone. The intensity of suppression, however, is not necessarily correlated with the magnitude. It may be that a patient with a constant, small-angle esotropia will have a small suppression zone but one that is suppressed very

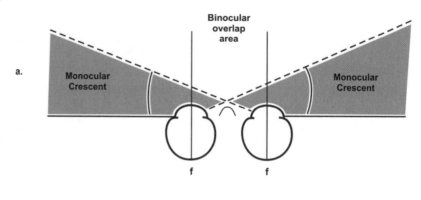

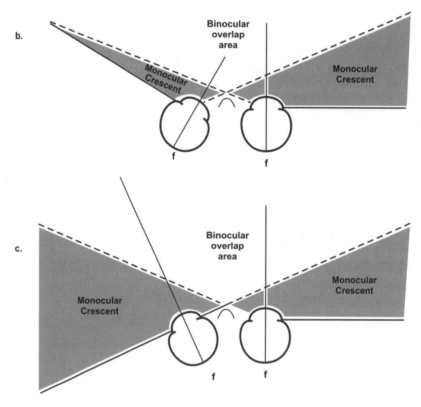

Figure 5-10. Horizontal visual field limits, a. Orthophoria, b. Esotropia of the left eye. c. Exotropia of the left eye. (f = fovea.)

deeply. Another factor is eye laterality. If the strabismus is alternating, the suppression is also likely to alternate from eye to eye. If the strabismus is unilateral, suppression is confined to the deviating eye. Frequency of the strabismus is another important variable. The more frequent the strabismus, the more likely is it that deep suppression will be found. If anomalous retinal correspondence (ARC) is present, these relations do not necessarily apply, because ARC is also an antidiplopia mechanism that partially obviates the need for suppression.

Suppression is usually shallow in noncomitant strabismic patients. Intensity is less because the magnitude of the deviation is continuously changing as

Table 5-6. Size of Suppression Zone in Either Superimposition or Fused Targets

Classification	Separation from Target Center to Suppression Clue
Central	≤5 degrees
Foveal	≤1 degree
Parafoveal	≤3 degrees (but >1 degree)
Paramacular	≤5 degrees (but >1 degree)
Peripheral	>5 degrees

Table 5-7. Tests for Intensity of Suppression

Naturalness of Testing	Method of Testing	Instrumentation	Intensity of Suppression
Natural	Diplopia in space	Ordinary objects Penlight	Shallow
---	Vectographic methods	Pola-Mirror Vis-à-vis (Griffin) test Vectograms	---
---	Septums	Turville test Bar reading	---
	Septums with optical systems	Brewster stereoscope Wheatstone stereoscope	
---	Colored filters	Red lens test	---
Unnatural		Worth four-dot test	Deep

fixation shifts from one field of gaze to another. This means that point zero (the target point) is not at a fixed site on the retina; thus, diplopia is more likely to be perceived. Fortunately, the accompanying diplopia with noncomitant deviations can warn individuals of possible neurologic problems that require immediate health care attention.

Testing for Suppression

The number of tests for suppression is legion. Only some of the basic methods are presented here for assessing suppression associated with strabismus. All of these, except the major amblyoscope, are readily available to the primary eye care practitioner. The patient should be wearing appropriate optical correction (corrected ametropia with most plus [CAMP] lenses for best visual acuity) if needed. For screening purposes, a simple test for suppression can be used effectively for 5-year-old children.[15] We recommend the Pola-Mirror test (i.e., crossed-polarizing filters and a mirror) as a simple, easy, inexpensive, and sensitive screening test for suppression associated with amblyopia, strabismus, and uncorrected anisometropia. The vis-a-vis test, introduced by Griffin, is similar to the Pola-Mirror test except that there is no mirror; rather, the patient and doctor face each other from a distance of approximately 50 cm, with both wearing crossed-polarizing filters. Suppression is

indicated if one of the doctor's eyes appears darkened. (Refer to Chapter 12.)

History

Strabismic patients should be questioned if they notice diplopia under natural viewing conditions: Are the double images only at a particular distance or in a certain field of gaze? Are the double images present at all times or just occasionally? Is diplopia noticed only when the patient is thinking about it and ignored at other times?

Red Lens Test

For the red lens test, the patient, wearing a red filter over one eye, views a fixation light in a normally illuminated testing room at a distance at which the strabismus is manifest. The patient is asked whether one or two lights are visible. Seeing two lights under these conditions indicates that the suppression is either relatively shallow or is absent. If one light is reported, a red lens or filter should be inserted before the fixating eye, and the patient should be asked whether he or she sees one light that is either red or white (a suppression response), one pink light (a fusion response), or both a red and a white light (indicating diplopia). Strabismic individuals having harmonious ARC may report seeing some variation of a pink light, simulating a normal fusion response. Patients who suppress and have alternating strabismus will report seeing the light change from red to white. If only one red light is seen, the depth of suppression can be assessed by sequentially adding neutral-density (gray) lenses to the dominant eye until diplopia can be noticed. When multiple filters are necessary to elicit diplopia, deep suppression is indicated. Another method for assessing the intensity of suppression is to dim the room light until diplopia of the penlight image is noticed. If no diplopia is seen in a dark room, the suppression can be considered to be deep.

Worth Dot Test

The Worth dot (four-dot) test is similar to the red lens test, but it is more popular. Red-green filters are worn by the patient over any needed spectacles. By convention, the red filter is placed before the right eye and the green before the left. The test is administered under two lighting conditions, full room illumination and dark. A Worth flashlight is held with the white dot (of the four dots) oriented on the top (Figure 5-11). The examiner stands across the room from the patient and asks how many lights are perceived. A report of two red dots indicates suppression of the green-filtered eye. A report of three green dots means suppression of the red-filtered eye. A four-dot response suggests second-degree sensory fusion at that testing distance and under those particular test conditions. Alternate suppression is indicated if the patient reports switching between two and three lights. A report of five dots (two red and three green) indicates diplopia. The examiner notes the response at far and then slowly moves toward the patient. The patient reports any changes in the perception of the dots as the examiner advances the Worth flashlight to 10 cm from the patient. It is customary to record the patient's responses at least at far (6 m) and at near (40 cm). If the initial test was done with the room lights on, it is repeated with the lights off.

The interpretation of test results can be complex. The Worth dot test at far assesses central sensory fusion if the angle subtends the dots at less than 10 degrees. As the flashlight is advanced toward the patient, peripheral fusion can be assessed. Also as the flashlight is moved closer, the intensity of the lights on the retina increases, which tends to overcome suppression. For these reasons, the Worth dot test at near, particularly in a dark room, is a strong stimulus to break suppression. The clinician must also take into consideration any change in the patient's strabismic deviation from far to near that has previously been measured on the cover test. Another problem in interpretation is that a light is not a good stimulus for accommodation, and therefore an accommodative response may be inadequate, thereby affecting the magnitude of strabismic deviation. It must also be recognized that red-green filters tend to dissociate the eyes and may cause a latent deviation to become manifest. The dark room conditions exaggerate this tendency, because the only effective fusion stimulus is the small, single, white dot.

Despite these complications, an experienced clinician can obtain much information about a patient's suppression and sensory fusion. For example, suppose that a patient has a comitant, intermittent exotropia of 15Δ at far and 18Δ at near. In a lighted room, the Worth dot responses of this patient are three dots at far and four dots at near. These responses indicate that the patient is suppressing the red-filtered eye at far but has

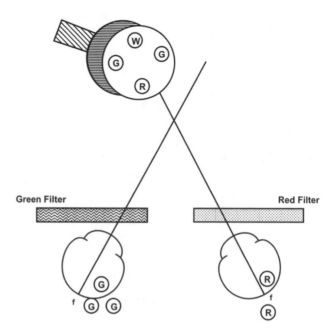

Figure 5-11. Worth four-dot test in a case of esotropia of the left eye. (f = fovea; G = green; R = red; W = white.)

sensory fusion at near. In the dark room, assume that the patient reports five dots at far and at near. The patient is showing a relatively shallow central suppression indicated by suppression at far in the lighted room, with a small retinal image and diplopia in the darkened room. Inadequate fusional convergence also is indicated if a fusion response occurred at near in a lighted room yet fusion was broken in a darkened room.

Preschool children often have difficulty counting accurately, so results of the Worth dot test for these children may have questionable validity. A less ambiguous test is Bernell's three-figure test, which also requires the use of red-green anaglyphic glasses. Three relatively large figures are presented on the face of a flashlight; a red little girl, a green elephant, and a white ball. This presentation seems to communicate well with most children older than 2 years, but because the suppression controls are larger and brighter than the standard Worth dot test, evidence of mild suppression may be missed.

Amblyoscope Workup

The major amblyoscope (e.g., Clement Clarke Synoptophore; see Appendix J for location of supplier) has the advantage that various targets can be placed precisely at the strabismic angle of deviation. Superimposition, flat fusion, and stereofusion targets (i.e., first-degree, second-degree, and third-degree, respectively) are used to assess the patient's sensory fusion ability. If the patient

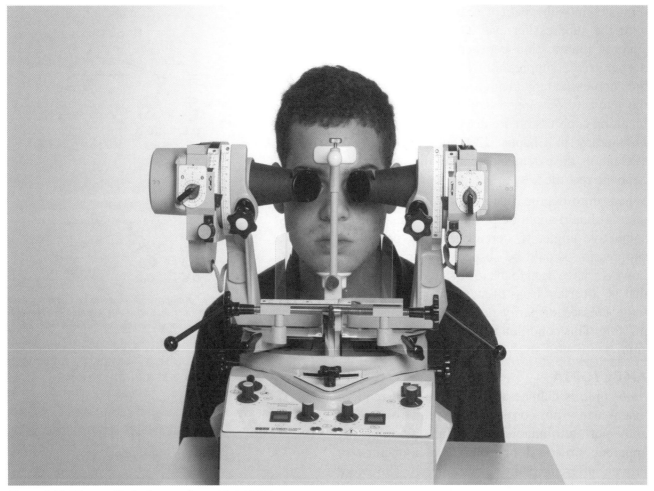

Figure 5-12. Clement Clarke Synoptophore, Model 2001.

has second-degree fusion, vergence ranges can be measured relative to the strabismic angle. In addition, the extent and intensity of suppression can be easily evaluated.

The Synoptophore is one of the most popular major amblyoscopes (Figure 5-12). Each tube of the Synoptophore includes a mirror placed at 45 degrees and a +7-diopter (+7-D) eyepiece lens. Test targets are placed at optical infinity. Figure 5-13 shows the direction of movement of a carriage arm to create base-in and base-out prism demands. Typical first-degree (superimposition) and second-degree targets for sensory fusion assessment are shown in Figures 5-14 and 5-15, respectively. The carriage arms are aligned to the patient's measured, subjective angle of directionality (discussed later in this chapter).

Initially, superimposition targets are placed in the amblyoscope, and equal illumination is used for the two eyes. If one of the targets is not seen, suppression is indicated. Regarding suppression zone size, slide G48 (the fish tank) subtends angular dimen-

sions of 1.5 degrees vertical and 2 degrees horizontal and are useful for foveal and parafoveal suppression testing (see Figure 5-14). The G2 slide (sentry box) subtends angles of 15 degrees vertical and 9.5 degrees horizontal. The soldier and the house slides, therefore, are useful for testing peripheral suppression. The other superimposition targets in these examples, X and square, test for foveal suppression.

An excellent example of second-degree targets containing both peripheral and central suppression clues are those illustrated in Figure 5-15. Again, the targets are placed in the amblyoscope at the subjective angle with equal illumination for the two eyes. A normal fusion response would be the report of seeing a single bug having four wings and three dots on its body. Any missing dots would indicate central suppression, whereas missing wings would indicate peripheral suppression. If suppression is noted, intensity can be assessed by simply changing the relative illumination of the targets. The target of the dominant eye can be dimmed until the patient sees the missing clues with the suppressing eye. The larger the difference in illumination between the two eyes, the deeper is the suppression. Flashing and moving the suppressed target can also provide an index to the intensity of suppression. (These methods for breaking suppression are discussed in the sections on therapy in Chapter 12.) Subsequent to this evaluation, the extent and depth of the suppression zone are recorded.

When third-degree fusion slides are used, the targets should again be positioned at the patient's subjective angle. If stereopsis is not perceived, suppression should be suspected. Some patients, however, have been found to be stereoanomalous— that is, a certain class of stereodisparity detectors (e.g., crossed disparity detectors) is congenitally missing. This condition is independent of suppression.

AMBLYOPIA

Amblyopia is defined as the condition of reduced visual acuity not correctable by refractive means and not attributable to ophthalmoscopically apparent structural or pathologic anomalies or proven afferent pathway disorders.[5] The word *amblyopia* literally means "dullness of vision." Best correctable visual acuity worse than 20/30 (6/9) is considered to meet a descriptive criterion for amblyopia. Generally speaking, amblyopia of 20/30-20/70 is mild (shallow), 20/80-20/120 is moderate, and worse than 20/120 is marked or deep.

Amblyopia also is defined by a difference in visual acuity between the two eyes. For clinical purposes, if the acuity difference is two lines of letters on the Snellen chart, amblyopia of the poorer eye may be present. For example, if the better eye is 20/15 (6/4.5) and the poorer eye is 20/25 (6/7.5), this aspect of the definition is met. Ciuffreda et al.[16] made the important point that amblyopia is not merely any reduction of visual acuity but that the etiology of the acuity loss must be some recognized amblyogenic factor (e.g., constant unilateral strabismus, anisometropia, or high refractive error bilaterally [isoametropia]). Amblyopia refers to a developmental loss of acuity during early childhood due to one or more of the preceding etiologic factors. For consistency with health science clas-

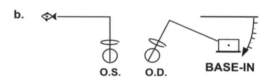

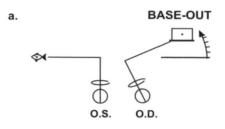

Figure 5-13. Schematic of a major amblyoscope. a. Carriage arm moved toward examiner results in a base-out demand, b. Carriage arm moved away from the examiner results in a base-in demand.

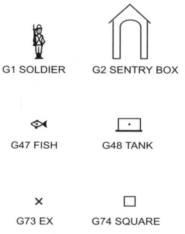

Figure 5-14. Superimposition (first-degree fusion) slides used in the Synoptophore. Gl and G2 test for peripheral suppression. G47 and G48 test for parafoveal suppression. G73 and G74 test for foveal suppression.

sification, amblyopia must be described by the associated etiologic factors.

The prevalence of any condition depends on how the condition is defined and the sampling characteristics of the surveyed population. For these reasons, there is considerable variation in the prevalence of amblyopia reported in the professional literature. In a major review of the topic by Ciuffreda et al.[17], their most accurate estimates were 1.6% for military personnel, 1.8% for preschool and school-aged children, and 2.3% for clinical patients seeking vision care. Premature infants are particularly vulnerable to developing amblyopia

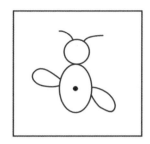

Figure 5-15. Target designed to test second-degree fusion while monitoring peripheral suppression (wings) and central suppression (dots).

(21 %) or strabismus (28%) in the first three years of life, according to Schalij-Delfos et al.[18]

Classification

Amblyopia usually is considered to arise from a deprivation of form vision, abnormal binocular interaction (i.e., suppression), or both during early development, probably before 7 years of age. The form deprivation can be either unilateral or bilateral but most often occurs unilaterally. Those patients in whom visual acuity is reduced significantly due to obvious ocular disease or in whom there is proven pathology in the visual pathways are classified as having *low vision*, in contradistinction to amblyopia. *Organic amblyopia*, however, is the term sometimes used (rather than *low vision*) in certain cases of reduced vision in which ocular pathology is not obvious (even though there may be a small central scotoma in some cases). Examples include a reduction of acuity from nutritional factors, tobacco, alcohol, salicylates, and other toxic agents. Another type of reduced visual acuity that often is labeled as *psychogenic amblyopia* is due to causes such as hysteria or malingering. It is fairly common in children and adolescents and occurs sometimes in adults who are in stressful situations. Perimetric studies usually reveal tubular fields. In this book, however, we discuss developmental amblyopia due to form deprivation and suppression rather than organic and other causes of reduced visual acuity.

A current classification system for amblyopia is based on the specific etiology of the condition: strabismic amblyopia, anisometropic amblyopia, isoametropic amblyopia, and image degradation amblyopia.

Strabismic Amblyopia

Amblyopia may occur as a result of long-standing suppression when there is constant unilateral strabismus at all viewing distances during early child-hood. The foveal area is suppressed to prevent confusion. Subsequently, there is active cortical inhibition of point zero in the deviating eye and often of the entire binocular overlap area in the amblyopic eye. Stereopsis is usually severely reduced or absent in strabismic amblyopia. The suppression mechanism may be similar in strabismic and anisometropic amblyopia, but it may be more intense in strabismic amblyopia. The acuity loss in strabismic amblyopia tends to be worse than in anisometropic amblyopia, but the severity of amblyopia is not consistently correlated with the size of the strabismic deviation.[19] When both strabismus and anisometropia coexist, the amblyopia tends to be deeper than in the presence of only one of the conditions.

Because constant unilateral esotropia is much more prevalent than constant unilateral exotropia, amblyopia is more frequently associated with esotropia. Most esotropic patients have constant strabismus, whereas most exotropes exhibit intermittent strabismus. Helveston[20] found amblyopia in 80% of his sample of esotropes but in only 17% of the exotropes. If reduced unilateral acuity is associated with intermittent strabismus in the absence of anisometropia, the clinician should suspect an organic cause.

Strabismic amblyopia is often associated with eccentric fixation (EF). When the amblyopic eye is forced to pick up fixation, the time-averaged position of fixation is not the fovea but an extrafoveal point. The patient's sense of straight-ahead or oculocentric direction has also shifted to the extrafoveal point or area used for fixation, which may explain why EF develops initially (see subsequent section for a comprehensive explanation of EF).

Anisometropic Amblyopia

Some clinical studies indicate that anisometropia is the most common cause of amblyopia.[20-22] However, in a retrospective study of 544 amblyopes in whom microtropia was assessed, Flynn and Cassady[23] found pure anisometropic amblyopia to be the least prevalent type. They reported 20% of the cases of amblyopia were due solely to anisometropia, 48% were purely strabismic, and 32% were both anisometropic and strabismic. Anisometropia deforms foveal images in a different way than strabismus does. In strabismus, the two foveas are presented with two different images (confusion), a disparity of form perception, thus strongly stimulating suppression. In anisometropia, the suppression is less intense; the dissimilarities of the foveal images are in relative clarity, size (aniseikonia), and contrast.

The amount of anisometropia presuming no treatment (i.e., optical correction or vision training) is given directly influences the depth of amblyopia and its prevalence.[24, 25] A 1-D difference in refractive error is considered to define anisometropia, but this amount does not usually cause amblyopia to develop. However, Tanlamai and Goss[26] found an amblyopia incidence of 50% for hyperopic anisometropes of 2 D and of 100% incidence for 3.5 D or greater. Most investigators have found a strong correlation between the amount of hyperopic anisometropia and severity of amblyopia;[13,27,28] however, it is possible for a patient with only a small amount of anisometropia and no strabismus to have deep amblyopia.[16] Generally speaking, binocular fusion becomes weak and stereoacuity decreases in proportion to the depth of anisometropic amblyopia, according to Tomac and Birdal.[29]

Myopic anisometropia does not generally result in deep (or as prevalent) amblyopia as does the hyperopic variety unless the amount of anisometropia is very high. The uncorrected hyperopic anisometrope typically focuses to the level of the least hyperopic eye, leaving the more hyperopic eye permanently deprived of a clear image. The uncorrected myopic anisometrope, on the other hand, often alternates fixation, because each eye is independently in focus at a different near distance. Tanlamai and Goss[26] reported an amblyopia incidence of 50% among myopic anisometropes of 5 D and of 100% for 6.5 D and greater. If reduced unilateral visual acuity is found associated with a small degree of myopic anisometropia (e.g., OD, -2.00 20/60; OS, plano 20/20) and strabismus is absent, then the clinician should suspect an organic or other cause of reduced acuity until proven otherwise.

Generally, anisometropic amblyopia is not highly associated with EF, although there are many exceptions. In most cases, the fixation is central but unsteady. There appears to be increased spatial uncertainty regarding visual direction, but the time-averaged position of fixation usually is not shifted away from the fovea.

Uncorrected astigmatic anisometropia of 1.50-D cylinder or greater early in life can also result in amblyopia for sharp contours in the deprived meridional orientation. *Meridional amblyopia* is usually not severe. Patients frequently show significant improvement after a few weeks or months of wearing the appropriate spectacle or contact lens correction. Part-time occlusion of the dominant eye also promotes rapid progress in these cases, unless the ametropia is of long duration since early childhood.

Isoametropic Amblyopia

Isoametropic amblyopia is relatively rare. Agatston[30] reported this condition in approximately 0.03% of Army draftees. It is secondary to high symmetric refractive error (hyperopia, myopia, or astigmatism) that remained uncorrected during early childhood (before age 7 years). These patients typically have a mild impairment of acuity, 20/30-20/70, in each eye when the ametropia is first optically corrected.[16] Due to the bilateral nature of this type of amblyopia, it usually is detected earlier than is anisometropic amblyopia, because the child cannot see clearly with either eye. Because the images are equally blurred, there is little or no suppression.[31] This may explain, in part, why the effects of a bilateral loss of acuity are less severe than with anisometropia and, consequently, why the condition usually responds well to vision therapy. Fortunately, visual acuity often improves after spectacles or contact lenses are worn for a few weeks or months, however, optimal visual acuity may not be obtained until 1 year after optical correction.[32,33] Vision training sometimes proves useful too and, frequently, normal or nearly normal visual acuities are achieved.

Image Degradation Amblyopia

Reduced visual acuity caused by a physical obstruction to clear vision during early childhood that results in severe light and form stimulus deprivation is sometimes called *image degradation amblyopia*. The most common causes of this type of amblyopia are congenital cataracts that are removed much later in life (Table 5-8). Because of abnormal binocular interactions, unilateral light or form deprivation results in deeper amblyopia than would binocular deprivation for the same period.[34] Stimulus deprivation of one or both eyes before age 1 year can lead to profound and permanent visual acuity loss as well as nystagmus. Early and effective treatment is absolutely critical for remediation of acuity.

AMBLYOPIA AS A DEVELOPMENTAL DISORDER

Amblyopia may be considered to be a developmental disorder of spatial vision caused by some type of visual form deprivation during early childhood.[16] If anisometropia, strabismus, or other causes of form deprivation occur relatively late in life, amblyopia does not develop. If there is no impedance to clear retinal imagery or binocular coordination of the eyes, visual acuity develops fairly rapidly from the time of birth. There is a rapid increase of visually evoked potential acuity to near-adult levels within 8 months of age, which actually reaches an adult level by 13 months.[35] The receptive field organization of foveal vision (retinal, lateral geniculate nucleus, and cortical) undergoes a poorly understood process of neural tuning to higher spatial frequencies of contours at all orientations in the environment. However, the consolidation of these neural processes takes considerable time, probably 5-7 years. A clinical study by Keech and Kutschke[36] concluded that the upper age limit for the development of amblyopia is 73 months (approximately 6 years). Anisometropia, constant unilateral strabismus, high refractive error, and visual form deprivation can all interrupt the normal process of acuity development and consolidation within this time period.

About a century ago, Worth[37] referred to the acuity loss due to lack of development as *amblyopia of arrest* and the acuity loss due to interference with consolidation as *amblyopia of extinction*. He believed the former to be irrecoverable by patching or other therapy and the latter to be reversible through proper treatment. This view of amblyopia still strongly influences many clinicians and scientists alike, although aspects of it do not appear to be supported by recent evidence. Even though information about the specific nature of the visual deficits in amblyopia has greatly expanded, Worth[37] provides a conceptual framework that still guides clinical decisions, for better or worse, and serves as a reference for addressing research questions. (Further discussion of the concepts of arrest and extinction in amblyopia are found in Chapter 6.)

Reduced visual acuity is the best-known clinical feature of amblyopia. There does not appear to be a leveling or dip of acuity at the fovea, as once was believed. In most cases of amblyopia, acuity still peaks at the fovea, as it does in the normal eye, but the resolution capacity of the peak is lower. In contrast, however, the resolution capacity of peripheral retinal regions in an amblyopic eye is approximately the same as in the nonamblyopic eye. The implication is that the foveal receptive field organization in amblyopia is coarser than normal, in part due to lack of development. In other words, amblyopia is fundamentally a defect of central vision.[38]

Reduced visual acuity is not the only visual deficit found in amblyopia (Table 5-9). A large body of research data has accumulated that describes visual characteristics in various types of amblyopia. Cuiffreda et al.[16] wrote an extensive, in-depth analysis of the literature. They regard amblyopia as a developmental anomaly involving primarily those cortical mechanisms involved in form and shape perception. There is insufficient evidence supporting the concept of receptor amblyopia (i.e., a fundamental defect in retinal rods and cones). A defining defect in both strabismic and anisometropic amblyopia is reduced photopic contrast sensitivity for high spatial frequencies (i.e., fine detail), with little or no loss at low spatial frequencies (i.e., coarse forms). This loss of contrast detection for fine detail in central vision increases with the severity of the amblyopia and appears to have a neural basis rather than, for example, an optical or oculomotor basis. In anisometropic amblyopia, this deficit persists throughout the binocular visual field of the amblyopic eye, which is consistent with retinal image defocus. In strabismic amblyopia, however, the deficits in contrast sensitivity are often asymmetrically distributed across the visual field in a way consistent with the pattern of suppression found in strabismics.

According to the review by Cuiffreda et al.,[16] amblyopia is also characterized by marked spatial uncertainty. The amblyopic eye has a relative inability to judge position, width, and orientation of detailed forms. In anisometropic amblyopia, the loss in spatial judgment is consistent with the reduced resolution and contrast sensitivity of the amblyopic eye. In contrast, strabismic amblyopes show an extra loss in positional acuity, often accompanied by monocular distortions (i.e., contractions and expansions) of space perception.[39] The reviewers suggested that this intrinsic cortical spatial distortion in strabismic amblyopia may be due either

Table 5-8. Common Causes of Image Degradation Amblyopia

Congenital cataracts
Ptosis
Corneal opacities
Other media opacities
Occlusion (iatrogenic cause)

to loss of neurons or to scrambling of signals secondary to the abnormal binocular interactions found in constant developmental strabismus. One interesting implication of this concept is that there may be a causal relation among ARC, monocular distortions, and EF in strabismic amblyopia.

A survey of anatomic and physiologic studies of the visual pathways of animals and humans with amblyopia indicates markedly disturbed cortical function.[16] In anisometropic amblyopia, the specific cortical dysfunction appears to be related to those neurons subserving contrast sensitivity. In strabismic amblyopia, there is a dramatic loss of cortical connections of the amblyopic eye. The lateral geniculate nucleus often shows shrinkage of cells in layers connecting the amblyopic eye, a defect believed to be secondary to the cortical changes through retrograde degeneration. Electroretinographic studies suggest that retinal abnormalities are not a fundamental characteristic of amblyopic eyes. Amblyopia apparently results from the effects of at least two mechanisms during early visual development: cortical competition for connections from the two eyes and cortical inhibition (suppression) when there is asymmetric binocular input to cells.

Besides the sensory deficits in visual acuity, contrast sensitivity, and spatial temporal processing, an amblyopic eye has several deficiencies in monocular eye movements, some of which are characteristic of the condition. One characteristic feature found in most amblyopic eyes is an unsteady fixation pattern. Normal fixation appears steady only by gross inspection. With magnification, normal fixation is seen actually to be composed of micro-drifts from perfect fixation, corrective micro-saccades, and physiologic tremor. The abnormal component of microscopic eye movements in an amblyopic eye appears to be the microdrifts having an increased amplitude and velocity.[40] Schor and Flom[41] proposed that there is an increased "dead zone" for corrective saccades in amblyopia: Because there is reduced detection

of a fixation error, the amblyopic eye drifts from foveal fixation farther and faster (due to increasing velocity with distance) than does a normal eye. Therefore, one component to reduced visual acuity in amblyopia might be the reduced and variable resolution of nonfoveal retinal points.

EF is considered to be an extrafoveal time-averaged position of fixation. Rarely does one find a perfectly steady EF pattern in strabismic amblyopia when fixation is attempted with the amblyopic eye. In most cases of strabismic amblyopia, unsteady EF is the usual observation. It is also seen, unexpectedly, in some patients having solely anisometropic amblyopia. In cases of EF, patients believe they are looking directly at the target although they are, in fact, fixating with an extrafoveal point or area: The principal visual direction of the amblyopic eye (also called the *straight-ahead direction*) has shifted away from the fovea. The monocular spatial distortions found in strabismic amblyopic eyes and described by Bedell and Flom[42] may be the pathophysiologic basis for an EF pattern. These monocular spatial distortions occur only when both amblyopia and strabismus are present; they have not been found in amblyopes without strabismus or in strabismics without amblyopia.[43, 44]

Saccadic and pursuit eye movements of an amblyopic eye are usually defective, as one might suppose. In amblyopic eyes, three abnormalities of the saccadic system have been reported: (1) increased latency, (2) reduced peak velocity, and (3) dysmetria (inaccuracy). The increased latency (slower reaction time) often exceeds 100% and is considered by Ciuffreda et al.[16] to reflect a slowing in the sensory pathways that process visual information subsequently used by the oculomotor system in generating saccadic eye movements. Large horizontal and vertical saccades of an amblyopic eye are usually hypometric (undershoots), multiple, and variable. Also, in deep amblyopia, 20% of such eyes make saccades that are unequal in size; the amblyopic eye follows the dominant eye but not to the same degree. These nonconjugancies (lack of exact comitance) often are larger in one direction than in its opposite.[45] Pursuit eye movements of an amblyopic eye often break down into a series of saccades, suggesting reduced and variable gain in the neurologic control process. Consistent with these anomalies, the optokinetic nystagmus (OKN) responses of an amblyopic eye often appear defec-

Table 5-9. Visual Deficiencies Associated with Amblyopia

Sensory testing
Decreased visual acuity
Decreased contrast sensitivity for fine detail
Spatial uncertainty
Monocular spatial distortion
Increased perception and reaction times
Suppression
Reduced stereopsis

Motor testing
Unsteady fixation: increased drift amplitude
Eccentric fixation
Defective saccades: increased latency, reduced peak velocity, inaccuracy
Defective pursuits: jerkiness
Reduced and asymmetric optokinetic nystagmus responses
Subtle afferent and efferent pupillary defects
Defective accommodation: increased latency, inaccurate dynamic responses, inconsistent responses, poor sustaining ability
Deficient accommodative convergence with the amblyopic eye fixating
Deficient or absent disparity vergence

tive, because they are composed of both saccadic and pursuit components. An asymmetry in the OKN responses may be seen in strabismic amblyopia. For example, temporalward stimulation of the amblyopic eye may show a reduced response as compared with nasalward stimulation.

The triad responses of accommodation, pupillary constriction, and accommodative convergence are also affected in amblyopia. Both static and dynamic accommodation demonstrates response abnormalities. One would expect, therefore, that accommodative vergence responses with a fixating amblyopic eye would be correspondingly reduced, and some research evidence supports this prediction.[46] With regard to dynamic accommodation, response abnormalities include increased latency, reduced gain, increased response variability, and poor sustaining ability.[16] The site of the accommodative dysfunction seems to be in the sensory rather than the motor controller. Besides the sensory deficit, accommodation responsiveness is reduced further by such factors as abnormal fixational eye movements, defective contrast sensitivity, and EF. The deficient accommodative responses found in amblyopia can usually be improved significantly with vision therapy.

There are often subtle afferent pupillary defects in many amblyopic eyes; response latencies may be increased and amplitude decreased.[16] Clinical testing with a penlight can, in many cases, indicate an afferent defect, as seen with the swinging flashlight test. There is evidence that these defects normalize with successful amblyopia therapy.[47, 48]

Fusional or disparity vergence often is found to be deficient or absent in cases of amblyopia.[46, 49, 50] The deficient disparity vergence responses appear to be related to the depth and extent of suppression associated with amblyopia and strabismus. Strabismic individuals having defective disparity vergence frequently substitute accommodative vergence to shift their eyes to a new target position.

CASE HISTORY

An in-depth case history should be obtained from every amblyopic patient. Diagnostic conclusions often depend on this evidence. Questioning should relate to strabismic history, refractive history, and social history.

The time of onset of amblyopia often coincides with that of strabismus; therefore, it is vitally important to know the age of onset of the strabismus. It generally follows that the earlier the onset and the later the therapeutic intervention, the deeper the amblyopia and the more difficult it is to treat successfully. Also, eccentric fixation is less likely to develop if the onset is after the child's third birthday.

The mode of onset of strabismus can influence the prognosis. A constant strabismus from the onset is more likely than intermittent strabismus to produce deeper amblyopia. The depth of amblyopia probably is related to both the duration and intensity of suppression, which would be greater in a constant deviation at all distances. Another important question regarding mode of onset is concerned with eye laterality: That is, was the strabismus unilateral or alternating at onset? As a rule, if the child alternates, the likelihood of amblyopia diminishes. Even in some esotropic cases that appear to be unilateral at onset, a child may use a form of alternation. Some esotropic infants and children learn to cross-fixate without any alternation in the primary position of gaze. For example, a left eye with constant unilateral esotropia may be used to view objects in the right field of gaze such that each eye would get adequate visual stimulation monocularly, and the development of amblyopia would be prevented.

Information about previous treatment should be thoroughly and carefully sought. If occlusion was prescribed, the clinician should try to establish whether the patient adhered faithfully to the wearing schedule. Frequently, careful questioning reveals that patching was done only as a token gesture. If extraocular muscle surgery was performed, complete information about the strabismic deviation before and after the operation should be obtained, if possible. The duration of amblyopia can be assumed to be about the same as the length of time the patient has had a constant unilateral strabismus. It is unlikely that amblyopia developed during the period when the strabismus was either intermittent or alternating.

In determining the prognosis for successful treatment of amblyopia, the two most important factors from the case history are

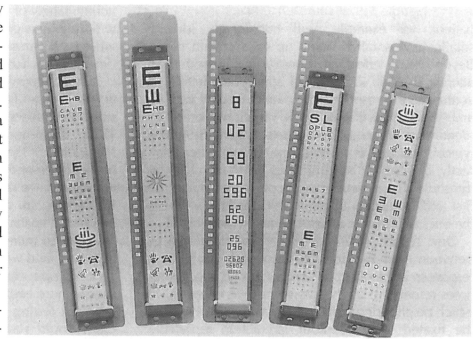

Figure 5-16. Example of Snellen chart designs in which there is neither an adequate number of larger letters as compared with smaller letters nor control for interletter spacing.

the best estimate of the time of onset and the time at which appropriate treatment for amblyopia began. The later the onset of amblyopia, the less profound is the loss of acuity during the critical period of acuity development. The earlier the appropriate treatment begins after the onset of amblyopia, the better and faster is the outcome. The importance of early detection and treatment of amblyopia cannot be overemphasized. We recommend that all children have a complete eye examination within the first year of life to check for the host of visual conditions that can affect visual development.

VISUAL ACUITY TESTING

Departure from customary visual acuity measuring is often required when an amblyopic eye is being tested. This is because of the wide variation of responses when an ordinary chart of Snellen optotype is employed.

Snellen Charts

Snellen tests have remained essentially the same since Herman Snellen devised the first chart in 1862 (see examples in Figure 5-16). A Snellen chart is usually adequate for testing the acuity of nonamblyopic eyes, but it is not designed for reliable interpretation of visual acuity in amblyopia.

A standard clinical criterion for assessing the acuity threshold is that at least 50% of the letters in a particular line on a Snellen chart must be

identified correctly. There is usually no problem in determining this level in a nonamblyopic eye. A myopic patient, for example, will consistently identify smaller and smaller letters up to a certain point. Beyond that, letters are consistently missed if an attempt is made to guess the appropriate letters. In contrast to this response, the patient reading with an amblyopic eye will show wide variation in correctly identifying different-sized letters (Figure 5-17). The typical response is to read one or two letters correctly in each of several lines with no clear-cut threshold. The patient often properly recognizes the first and last letters of any particular line, whereas the ones in between are not correctly recognized.

One reason often given for such differences between amblyopic and nonamblyopic test responses is the effect of contour interaction, sometimes referred to as the *crowding phenomenon*, in which neighboring contours impair the resolution of the fixated letter. Contour interaction reportedly affects amblyopic eyes more than normal eyes.

Using Landolt Cs and movable interacting bars, Flom et al.[51] found that contour interaction started to affect resolution of the gap in the C when the bar spacing equaled the distance of one letter. Maximum effect occurred when the spacings of the bars were 40% of a letter size. Flom et al.,[51] however, challenged the conventional wisdom that

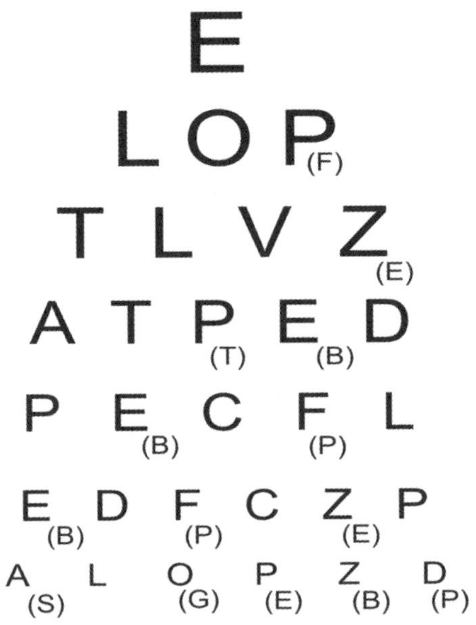

E

L O P (F)

T L V Z (E)

A T P E D (T) (B)

P E C F L (B) (P)

E D F C Z P (B) (P) (E)

A L O P Z D (S) (G) (E) (B) (P)

Figure 5-17. Typical responses during testing of an amblyopic eye. Patient's incorrect calls are shown parenthetically.

DNUP

T E V B C L

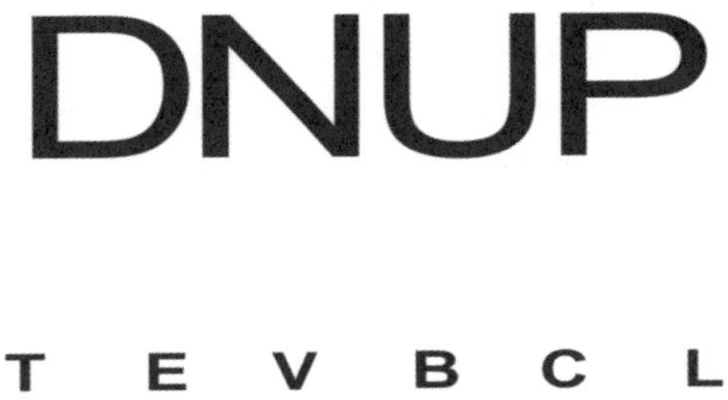

Figure 5-18. Larger Snellen letters having smaller spacing to cause greater crowding effect than the smaller Snellen letters.

amblyopic eyes are more affected by contour interaction. They maintained that the effect is approximately equal at threshold visual acuity levels for both normal and amblyopic eyes.

The letter spacing varies on each line on the Snellen chart and so does the crowding phenomenon. On the 20/20 (6/6) line of a typical Snellen chart slide, the spacing is large, well beyond the distance causing contour interaction. However, the spaces between letters in some Snellen charts are relatively reduced for larger letters in the threshold acuity range of many amblyopes. These patients would show significant contour interaction effect, whereas a person having 20/20 acuity would not. (See Figure 5-18 for clarification.) Standardized acuity charts such as the Bailey-Lovie Chart or The Early Testing in Diabetic Retinopathy Study (ETDRS) logMAR charts and testing protocol addresses many of deficiencies of the Snellen chart. These charts are the generally accepted gold standard of measuring visual acuity in adults and have been recommended for use in clinical research studies.[52] These charts have the same numbers of letters per row, equal spacing of rows on a log scale, equal spacing of letters within the letter rows, and individual rows of letters balanced for letter difficulty. (See Figure 5-19.)

It is commonly observed that amblyopic visual acuity is better for isolated letters or, possibly, for a single line of letters than for full Snellen chart acuity. These differences in acuities were reported by Morad et al.[53] This phenomenon is usually explained on the basis of the impaired "aiming" ability of an amblyopic eye rather than on the basis of contour interaction. In a complex detailed visual field, amblyopic spatial uncertainty and unsteady fixation result in an increased number of fixation errors. A restricted field with fewer letters is less confusing to an amblyopic observer; therefore, each letter can be fixated more easily.

When testing with the Snellen chart, the clinician should suspect amblyopia if (1) letters are missed on several lines using the full chart, (2) letters in the middle of a line are more frequently misread than those at the ends of the line, (3) letters are transposed in position, and (4) isolated letter acuity is better by one or two lines than is single-line or full-chart acuity.

Psychometric Charts

The initial approach to addressing the deficiencies of the Snellen chart was the psychometric chart, also referred to as the *S-chart*, designed by Flom[54] and takes the crowding phenomenon into account as well as the problem of an indefinite acuity threshold in amblyopes. The original S-chart slide series consists of 21 individual 35-mm projected slides. Each slide contains eight Landolt *C*s of a particular size for which the "gap" randomly appears in one of four positions: up, down, left, or right (Figure 5-20). The slides come in graduated sizes from 20/277 to 20/9, descending in 5% visual efficiency increments (20/20 = 100% efficiency; 20/200 = 20%). (See Visual Acuity and Visual Efficiency in Appendix F.) At each of the 21 acuity levels, the interletter spacing is equal to the letter size, and each letter is surrounded by an equal number of contours. Therefore, the contour interaction effects on each slide are constant. At each acuity level, the number of correct responses is recorded on the test form, with eight being the maximum number of correct calls.

The visual acuity threshold for a particular patient is determined by psychometric analysis. After the series is completed, a best-fit sigmoid curve is drawn on a chart (Figure 5-21a) representing the data. (Figure 5-21b illustrates the S-chart visual acuity plot of a normal and an amblyopic eye.) Note that the ordinate of the recording graph represents the acuity threshold and the abscissa, the number of correct responses. The intersection of the sigmoid curve with the abscissa value of 5 determines the visual acuity threshold value. The criterion for acuity is the 50% level of correct responses. Intuitively, four of eight correct responses would represent the 50% level, but this does not take guessing into account. Merely by guessing, the patient has a one in four chance of a correct call for each Landolt C, which is why five of eight represents the adjusted 50% level.

Davidson and Eskridge,[55] to allow ease of use of this test with young children, modified the S-chart test by removing the Landolt Cs but leaving eight Es (Figure 5-22). Less detail is intended to be less confusing. They reduced the interletter spacing to one-half the letter size to increase the effect of contour interaction as compared with the S-chart, which has an interletter spacing equal to the letter size. They reported this test to be reliable in the assessment of visual acuity. It is used in essentially the same way as is the S-chart. A convenient hand-held series of S-charts of this design was devised by Dr. Michael Wesson, University of Alabama, School of Optometry, Birmingham. (This test is available from the Optometric Extension Program Foundation, Inc. See Appendix J for contact information.)

Amblyopia Treatment Study (ATS) Visual Acuity Protocol

The S-chart and the Wesson S-chart may not be practical for clinical practice and with the advent of computer based visual acuity systems it is easier to develop a modified protocol that can accurately measure acuity in the amblyopic eye. A newer approach, developed by the Amblyopia Treatment Study (ATS) group[56], is a visual acuity testing routine based on the ETDRS protocol that was designed for children ages 3 to 10 years of age. The protocol uses an initial screening followed by a modified staircase procedure which has been shown to be a reliable method for measuring acuity in children. In the screening phase the child views

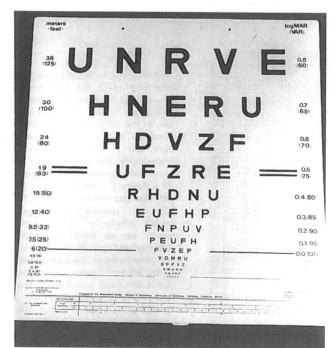

Figure 5-19. Example of Bailey Lovie Chart.

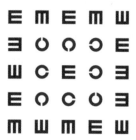

Figure 5-20. Psychometric chart of Flom.

an isolated optotype surrounded by crowding bars at 3 meters and is asked to identify single optotype at each acuity level. The initial acuity value is either 0.7 logmar (20/100) or 1.3 logmar (20/400). Once an error is made the child is asked to identify four optotypes starting at two acuity levels above that found in the initial screening. This phase ends when the child makes two mistakes at a particular acuity level. Next the reinforcement phase begins where the child begins reading a single optotype at 3 logmar values above that found in the initial phase. It is important to remember that the reinforcement phase is not included in the analysis of visual acuity. Following reinforcement, the child reads up to four optotypes starting at the visual acuity level found in phase I. The visual acuity is the level where the child correctly identifies three out of four optotypes.

HOTV and Lea Charts

The two most common and well researched tests of visual acuity in pre-school children are the HOTV

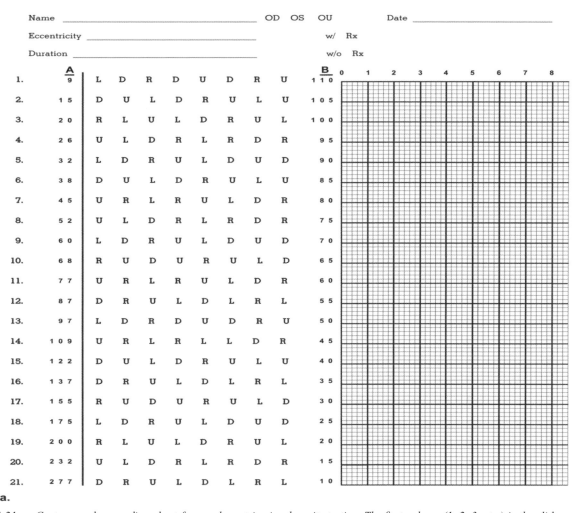

Figure 5-21. a. Custom-made recording chart for psychometric visual acuity testing. The first column (1, 2, 3, etc.) is the slide number. In the second column (A), the numbers (9, 15, 20, etc.) represent 20/9, 20/15, 20/20, and so on, respectively. The next series of columns indicate the correct response (D = down; L = left; R = right; U = up). The last column (B; 110, 105, 100, etc.) represents percentage of visual efficiency.

chart and the Lea symbols (see Figures 5-23 and 5-24). Although, the HOTV letter chart uses letters, children can use a matching procedure to perform the test, since only four letters are presented. The Lea charts use four symbols, square, house, circle, and heart that the child can verbally identify or use a matching procedure. Both charts come in a variety of formats and conform to the standards set forth for accurate acuity measurements. They have equal number of optotypes per row and control for spacing effects. In addition, both tests offer a single optotype presentation mode with surrounding contours bars. Visual acuity threshold is established by finding the threshold distance for a letter of particular size. The practitioner can use a modified ATS protocol if they do not have electronic visual acuity assessment available. For example, the examiner can start testing a child at 3 ft with a 20/100 or higher optotype. The patient is to indicate the correct optotype and the practitioner can have the child identify a single optotype at each level until the child makes mistake. At this point the practitioner would start testing at two lines above the missed optotype and the criterion for determining the threshold distance is at the 75% level (i.e., correct responses to three of four trials).

Amblyopia is suspected if the patient is fully corrected optically and yet shows poorer acuity in one eye than in the other. In a young child, there is often a question whether reduced acuity is due to psychological variables (e.g., inattention, poor cooperation, hysteria). If a child demonstrates relatively poor acuity in one eye, the threshold can be remeasured. If that acuity is reduced significantly both times and an amblyogenic factor is present, it suggests that developmental amblyopia is present and does not have a psychological basis. Contour interaction occurs maximally when threshold letters are used.[51]

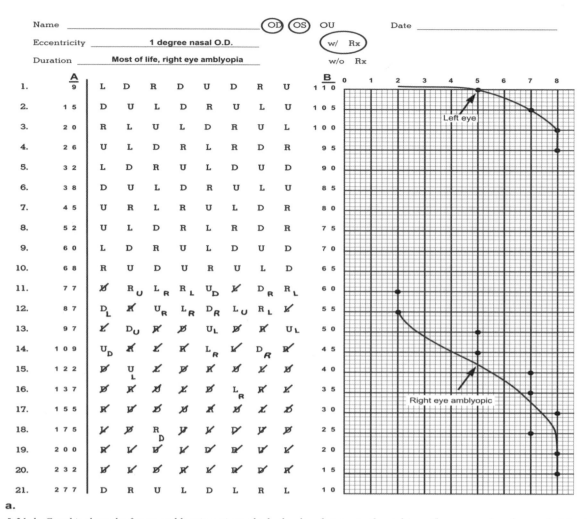

	A									B	0	1	2	3	4	5	6	7	8
1.	9	L	D	R	D	U	D	R	U	1 1 0									
2.	1 5	D	U	L	D	R	U	L	U	1 0 5									
3.	2 0	R	L	U	L	D	R	U	L	1 0 0									
4.	2 6	U	L	D	R	L	R	D	R	9 5									
5.	3 2	L	D	R	U	L	D	U	D	9 0									
6.	3 8	D	U	L	D	R	U	L	U	8 5									
7.	4 5	U	R	L	R	U	L	D	R	8 0									
8.	5 2	U	L	D	R	L	R	D	R	7 5									
9.	6 0	L	D	R	U	L	D	U	D	7 0									
10.	6 8	R	U	D	U	R	U	L	D	6 5									
11.	7 7		R	L	R	U		D	R	6 0									
12.	8 7	D		U	L	D	L	R		5 5									
13.	9 7		D			U			U	5 0									
14.	1 0 9	U				L		D		4 5									
15.	1 2 2		U							4 0									
16.	1 3 7						L			3 5									
17.	1 5 5									3 0									
18.	1 7 5			R						2 5									
19.	2 0 0									2 0									
20.	2 3 2									1 5									
21.	2 7 7	D	R	U	L	D	L	R	L	1 0									

a.

Figure 5-21. b. Graphical results for an amblyopic patient who had reduced vision in the right eye (lower curve) and normal vision in the left eye (upper curve). Large charts are used initially to ensure that two consecutive trials are all correct (i.e., eight of eight calls). Target size is reduced in 5% visual efficiency steps until two or fewer correct calls are made for two consecutive charts. The best-fit curve is drawn for the plotted data. Visual acuity is determined by the place at which the curve crosses the line representing five of eight correct calls. In this example, the left eye has 20/9 acuity (visual efficiency of 110%), and the right eye has acuity between 20/109 and 20/122, with visual efficiency of 42%.

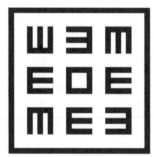

Figure 5-22. Psychometric acuity test design of Davidson and Eskridge of the commercially available Wesson charts.

Infant Visual Acuity Assessment

Amblyopia screening in infants relies primarily on objective methods to identify the specific amblyogenic cause (i.e., usually constant strabismus or anisometropia). However, an informal inferential assessment of visual acuity can also be used for amblyopia screening for infants and children younger than 2 years, in whom visual acuity charts and card sets are inappropriate. The examiner simply observes the infant's behavior when one of the infant's eyes is covered or patched as compared with the behavior when the other eye is occluded. For example, if a child consistently objects to having one eye occluded as opposed to the other, unilateral visual impairment is suspected. If the child's reaching behavior is less accurate with one eye patched as compared with the other, impairment is again suggested.

Some clinicians have advocated fixation preference testing as a qualitative measure of monocular visual function in preverbal children.[57] In this method the clinician compares the fixation of one eye relative to the other and whether the child has a strong preference for fixating with one eye. For strabismic patient's, the practitioner first looks to see if the child spontaneously alternates

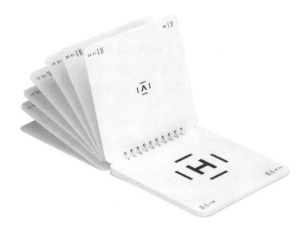

Figure 5-23. HOTV chart. (Courtesy of Good-lite Co.)

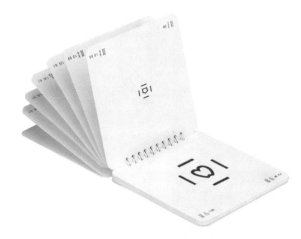

Figure 5-24. Lea Symbols. (Courtesy of Good-lite Co.)

fixation between the two eyes and if alternation is equal. In this case then the acuities are assumed to be approximately equal between the two eyes. If the child prefers one eye for fixating, then the habitually fixating eye is covered and fixation is forced to the other eye, then the cover is removed and the practitioner measures the length of time until fixation shifts back to the habitually fixating eye. (See Table 5-10.) In cases of suspected small angles of strabismus or in suspected anisometropic amblyopia without strabismus a 10Δ or 12Δ base down lens is placed before 1 eye to induce vertical diplopia. This has been called the "induced tropia test". If the child spontaneously alternates between the two targets the prism is placed over the other eye to insure that the response is repeatable. In cases where fixation does not shift between eyes, the practitioner can force fixation with brief occlusion. The prism can again be placed over the other eye to confirm the result. The grade of the occlusion can be derived from Table 5-10.

Recently, the ability of fixation preference testing to identify amblyopia was assessed in a large sample of strabismic and anisometropic amblyopic children ages 30 to 72 months.[57] The results showed that the sensitivity of fixation preference testing among anisometropia amblyopes was 20% and the specificity was 94%. For strabismic children the sensitivity was 69% and the specificity was 79%. The authors concluded that the ability of fixation preference testing to correctly identify amblyopia in preschool children was poor. Thus, relying on fixation preference testing alone in making clinician decisions is problematic and the

clinician should look at both amblyogenic factors along with measures that infer acuity to identify the presence or absence of amblyopia.

Preferential looking methods for visual acuity threshold determination offer a means by which to study or test *behavioral* visual acuity development of the infant. For these techniques, the examiner exposes two targets, side by side, to an infant. One target is a spatial frequency grating of a particular acuity level and the other is a blank gray field that has the same average luminance as the grating. Infants from the time of birth prefer to look at a pattern rather than at a blank field, if they can resolve the pattern. On repeated presentation of the targets, in random left-right order, the examiner watches the patient's eyes and judges whether the infant sees the grating. This is done by observing which target the infant views more frequently. An 80% correct 'looking" criterion often is used to indicate whether the infant does indeed resolve a particular spatial frequency grating. Usually, only monocular testing is undertaken using this technique, which usually works well with infants younger than 1 year, because they innately prefer to look at detail. Older children, however, need more interesting targets or operant conditioning rewards to make reliable responses. The Teller Preferential Looking Cards II—a hand-held series of cards designed for clinical use or other similar tests— are available (Figure 5-25).

OKN has been used to establish visual acuity thresholds in infants, but its validity is questionable. However, directional asymmetries to OKN stimulation have been reported in patients having

Table 5-10.

Grade	Examiner Observations
A	1. Spontaneous alternation between the right and left eyes 2. Switching the prism to the fellow eye causes FP to reverse.

B "Holds Well"	Fixation held with nonpreferred eye under any of the following circumstances before refixation to preferred eye:
	    for > 3 seconds
	    during a smooth pursuit
	    through a blink

C "Holds Momentarily"	Fixation held with nonpreferred eye for 1 to < 3 seconds
D "Does not hold"	Refixation with preferred eye occurs immediately (<1 sec) when the occluder is removed from the preferred eye.

A or B would be considered without strong fixation preference and C or D would be considered strong fixation preference.

Source: Cotter SA, et al Fixation Preference and visual acuity testing in a population-based cohort of preschool children with amblyopia risk factors. Ophthalmology 2009:116;145-53.

infantile strabismus or amblyopia. If visual development proceeds normally, each eye monocularly shows equal amplitude responses to nasalward and temporalward OKN drum rotation by approximately 6 months of age. If the infant develops amblyopia or strabismus, responses are typically less vigorous (i.e., lower amplitude and frequency) when the striped stimuli are moving in a temporal direction as compared with a nasal direction. Schor and Levi[58] investigated this phenomenon and suggested that the asymmetric OKN was due to incomplete development of binocular vision, which may explain why some patients show OKN asymmetry of the nonamblyopic as well as the amblyopic eye. However, there does not seem to be a direct relation between the degree of OKN asymmetry and the depth of the amblyopia, although deeply amblyopic eyes tend to exhibit increased asymmetry.[16]

This observation of OKN asymmetry can be used clinically to screen for amblyopia or strabismus in infants and young children. One eye is occluded while the other is tested using a striped drum rotating at a slow frequency of 8-10 revolutions per minute. The examiner evaluates the responses to nasalward and temporalward stimulation, respectively, while comparing responses of the right eye with the left eye. Although there are pediatric OKN drums with colored pictures, we have found the standard striped drum to be more effective in assessing OKN asymmetries (Figure 5-26).

Visually Evoked Potentials

In infants in whom amblyopia is indicated by these direct observations or by preferential looking methods or other clinical assessments, it may be valuable to access acuity further by visually evoked potential (VEP) methods.

The early works by White and Eason[59] on evoked cortical potentials in the occipital lobe have led to great interest in evaluating vision by electroencephalographic means. By analyzing VEPs displayed graphically as a plot of amplitude against time, visual acuity can be determined. The visually evoked potential is known also as the *visually evoked response* and the *visually evoked cortical potential.*

One of the most important uses of the VEP is determining whether a patient has an organic lesion resulting in decreased visual acuity. Harding[60] believed that organic causes can be ruled in or out by use of formless flash stimuli. A transient VEP, which is a stroboscopically presented stimulus, will elicit a graphical representation of the electrical activity of the visual cortex. This pattern is evaluated in terms of (1) amplitude, (2) latency of occurrence of the major positive peak response, and (3) general waveform morphology. A computerized recording showing a reduced amplitude indicates a lesion somewhere in the visual pathways. Amplitude reduction may indicate optic atrophy (Figure 5-27). Latency differences between eyes in a given patient may indicate optic nerve demyelination, as is found in multiple sclerosis (Figure 5-28).

Another type of VEP is that of pattern stimuli of black and white checks that exchange places at a rapid rate: The black checks become white and vice versa, as in Sherman's procedure.[61] The sustained response with this type of VEP allows assessment of visual acuity and aids in the diagnosis and prognosis of amblyopia. The VEP recording of each eye can be compared for differences in visual acuity to help establish the diagnosis of amblyopia in the absence of an organic lesion, particularly in those patients who do not respond reliably to

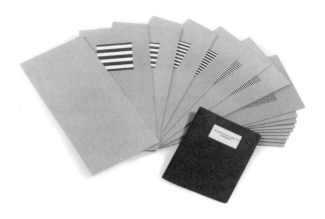

Figure 5-25. Teller Acuity Cards II. (Courtesy of Stereo Optical.)

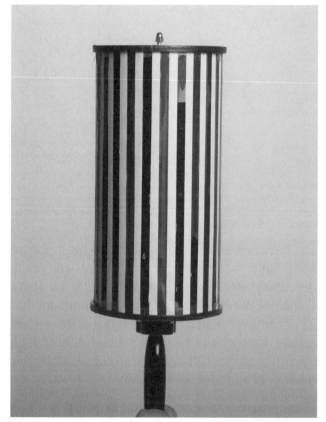

Figure 5-26. Optokinetic nystagmus (OKN) drum used to detect amblyopia.

optotype acuity tests. Figure 5-29 illustrates how visual acuity is estimated by looking at the peak VEP amplitude for different spatial frequency checkerboard patterns. It is a common clinical observation that VEP acuity is often superior to that found using optotype in cases of amblyopia. We consider this observation to be a favorable prognostic sign. This suggests that there is sensory potential for the improvement of visual acuity, often to the level indicated by the VEP. Besides the sensory reduction of acuity, amblyopes often have a motor disorder (e.g., EF). The VEP reveals

the visual acuity independent of the aiming error in the amblyopic eye.

In a recent study, Ridder and Rouse[62] used a sweep VEP to predict the outcome of treatment in 17 patients with amblyopia. The sweep VEP is easier to administer than the pattern VEP and would also help to determine if there is an organic cause to the reduced visual acuity. The subjects viewed a series of spatial frequencies (2 to 24 cpd) that were counterphased at 7.5 Hz with 80% contrast. The correlation between the pre-treatment VEP and the post treatment Snellen acuity was 0.73. The authors concluded that the pre VEP acuity level was a good predictor of post treatment visual acuity level. Thus, the sweep VEP can be useful when the patient or parent want an idea of the potential of improved vision with treatment.

Interferometry

The interferometer is a useful instrument for evaluating the visual acuity of an amblyopic patient. (See Figure 5-30) It uses the principle of interference fringes, as with a laser, to produce a spatial frequency line grating that is projected onto the patient's retina. A dial is turned on the instrument to change the spatial frequency of the grating over a large range, each setting corresponding to Snellen visual acuity. The advantage of using a coherent light source is that the projected image is not affected by minor opacities of the media or by refractive errors. The acuity determination is quick and is obtained by asking the patient to identify the orientation of the grating (vertical, horizontal, or diagonal) at the various acuity settings. The acuity determination is independent of eccentric or unsteady fixation, similar to the VEP. Therefore, in cases of amblyopia, the acuity estimate can be useful in making a diagnosis and, possibly, in estimating the prognosis for success of therapy.

Selenow et al.[63] compared pretherapy interferometry visual acuity with pre- and post-therapy optotype measures of visual acuity in a group of 37 patients with amblyopia. They found that, in most cases, the pretherapy interferometry acuity and the post-training Snellen acuity were in close agreement. Ninety-percent were within two acuity lines of each other and, in 75%, they were within one line. If further investigations support these impressive results, interferometry may prove to be an important prognostic tool in the assessment

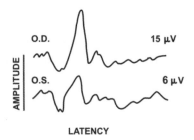

Figure 5-27. Transient visually evoked potentials graph showing normal latency for each eye and normal amplitude for the right eye (oculus dexter [O.D.]) but reduced amplitude for the left eye (oculus sinister [O.S.]), as in optic atrophy.

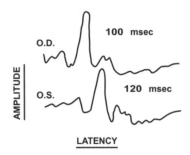

Figure 5-28. Transient visually evoked potentials graph showing normal amplitude for each eye and normal latency for the right eye (oculus dexter [O.D.]) but increased latency for the left eye (oculus sinister [O.S.])., a difference indicative of optic nerve demyelination, as in multiple sclerosis.

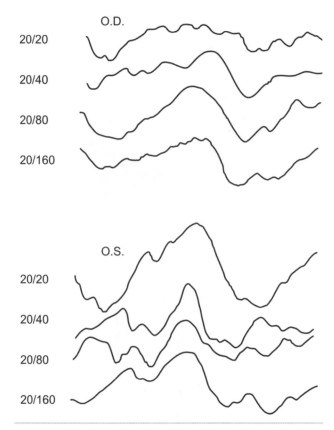

Figure 5-29. Sustained visually evoked potentials graph for visual acuity assessment. Responses indicate visual acuity of 20/80 for the right eye (oculus dexter [O.D.]) and 20/20 for the left eye (oculus sinister [O.S.]), judging from amplitude comparisons.

of amplyopia. Interferometers typically use four-choice targets (Figure 5-31).

FIXATION EVALUATION

Fixation is normal when the center of the fovea is used for fixation and when fixation is steady. If any other area of the retina is used (eccentric fixation), or if there is significant unsteadiness, fixation is considered to be abnormal. *Eccentric fixation*, then, is considered to be an abnormality of monocular fixation in which the time-averaged position of the fovea is off the fixation target. *Unsteadiness* refers to the presence of nystagmus like oscillations (usually irregular flicks and drifts) of the affected eye. These oscillations are often noticeable on careful direct observation but are more easily observed during visuoscopy. An eye with 20/20 (6/6) or better visual acuity necessarily has central fixation that is relatively steady, whereas an eye with poor visual acuity may have eccentric or unsteady fixation.

Ciuffreda et al.[16] considered EF to be caused, in many cases, by a shift in sensory spatial direction away from the fovea and probably was related to the impaired directional sense found in the central retina of amblyopic eyes. Bedell and Flom[42] found monocular spatial distortion, spatial uncertainty,

and direction error to be associated with strabismic amblyopia. Monocular spatial distortion can be described as a monocular asymmetry in spatial values between nasal and temporal retinal loci. This sensory spatial asymmetry and uncertainty results in a motor fixation pattern in which the time-averaged position of the fovea is off the fixation target and appears unsteady.

Description of Eccentric Fixation

The fixation pattern of an amblyopic eye is described with reference to the eccentricity, direction, and degree of steadiness. The classification provided in Table 5-11 can be used to describe centricity in which the fixation point is based on the time-averaged position of an eye.

A description of EF includes reference to the direction and distance from the fovea to the eccentric point (or time-averaged position) located on the retina. The direction of EF is referred to one of eight quadrants: nasal, temporal, superior, inferior, superonasal, inferonasal, superotemporal, and inferotemporal. We have found that nasal EF is generally the rule in strabismic amblyopia, particu-

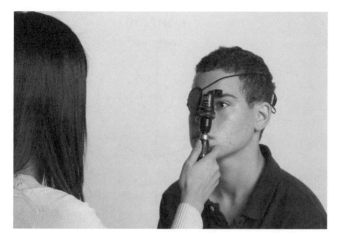

Figure 5-30. SITE IRAS Interferometer.

Table 5-11. Classification of Centricity of Fixation

Central fixation	Foveal
Eccentric fixation (EF)	Parafoveal (between fovea and 2 degrees EF)
	Macular (2-5 degrees EF)
	Peripheral (beyond 5 degrees EF)

larly esotropia, and often has a vertical component, although it is smaller than the horizontal component. Temporal EF is the exception in strabismic amblyopia, even in exotropia.

Unsteadiness of fixation can be associated with central or eccentric fixation. It is clinically relevant to describe the amplitude of unsteadiness if it exists. The degree of unsteadiness is indicated as a plus-or-minus amplitude from the fixation locus (time-averaged position): for example, 3 degrees nasal, unsteady (±1 degree) EF. A more common clinical way of recording this would be unsteady, nasal, 3-degree EF ±1 degree. Note that many clinicians record EF magnitude and amplitude of unsteadiness in prism diopters rather than in degrees.

Visuoscopy

Visuoscopy (formerly known as *visuscopy*) for evaluating fixation is accomplished by using an ophthalmoscope with a graduated reticule in place. The doctor observes a projected image of the reticule on the patient's fundus while the patient is asked to look directly at the center of the projected pattern and to hold fixation as steadily as possible. (Figure 5-32 illustrates commonly used reticules.) The separations in reticules are generally of a magnitude representing 1Δ. This can be verified by projecting the target onto a wall at a distance of 1 m, at which each separation (e.g., circle) would be 1 cm apart. Because fixation must be tested under monocular conditions, one eye of the patient must be occluded during testing. A practical way of accomplishing this is by asking the patient to cover the nontested eye with a hand or an occluder. For very small pupils, dilation (with mydriatic drops) is often necessary to locate the fovea and make visuoscopic observations. A dilated fundus examination should be performed initially in any case of suspected amblyopia, to rule out organic lesions; this is a convenient time during which to perform visuoscopy.

During visuoscopy, four clinical observations are routinely made:

1. Do the fovea and macular areas look normal? The clinician must carefully inspect the fovea and macula for lesions and developmental anomalies. Is there a well-defined foveal light reflex? Are there multiple reflexes? If either area appears abnormal in any way, then a 60- or 90-D lens examination on a slit lamp is recommended to rule out or identify an organic lesion.

2. Is there central or eccentric fixation? If EF is present, what is the direction and magnitude?

3. Is there steady or unsteady fixation? If unsteady fixation is present, what are the amplitude and type of oscillations?

4. Is there faulty localization associated with EF?

Figure 5-33 depicts examples of the visuoscopic patterns of fixation in different cases of EF and their associated clinical description. These examples for the right eye depict nasal and inferior EF, with the fovea (represented by the starlike spot) being temporal to the fixated center of the visuoscopic reticule.

Haidinger Brush Testing

The *Haidinger brush* is a retinal entoptic phenomenon that can be used clinically to indicate whether the fovea is functionally intact and to determine the position and steadiness of the fovea as the patient attempts to fixate a target. The phenomenon is more

Figure 5-31. Typical orientations of grating targets in laser and nonlaser interferometers.

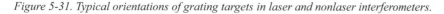

a.

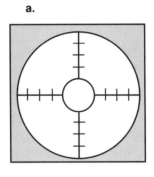

b.

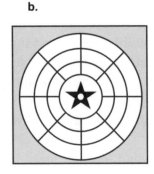

c.

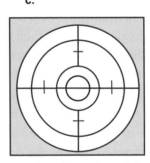

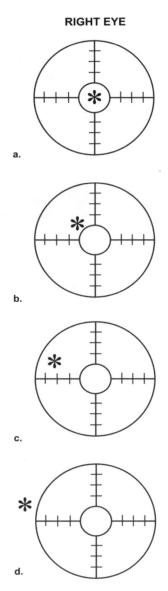

Figure 5-32. Examples of reticules of direct ophthalmoscopes for visuoscopy. a. Welch-Allyn. b. Heine. c. Keeler. These direct ophthalmoscopes are available from local suppliers of ophthalmic instruments.

Figure 5-33. Visuoscopic patterns of fixation in an example of right eye being tested, a. Central fixation, b. Parafoveal eccentric fixation, c. Eccentric fixation within the macular area. d. Peripheral. The direction of eccentric fixation in these examples is nasal and inferior (i.e., projected grid is down and nasal to the fovea [asterisk]).

correctly called *Haidinger's brushes* (plural), but clinicians refer to the entoptic image as a brush. Several instruments are available for producing a Haidinger brush, but the most practical, we believe, is the Bernell Macular Integrity Tester-Trainer (MITT or MITT-2) (Figure 5-34). This instrument has a motor-driven, rotating, polarized filter behind a transparent slide imprinted with fixation targets. Perception of the Haidinger brush requires the patient to look at the rotating polarized filter through a deep cobalt-blue filter in front of the eye being tested. This is a monocular technique; the nontested eye is occluded. The patient should see a brush-like propeller that appears to radiate from, and to rotate about, the point of foveal fixation.

The entoptic image of the fovea is believed to be caused by double refraction by the radially oriented fibers of Henle around the fovea.[64] Because these radial fibers converge on the fovea, the center of the perceived pattern represents the center of the fovea.

In cases of amblyopia, the perception of the Haidinger brush sometimes is difficult to elicit. Evocation of perception of the entoptic phenomenon in the amblyopic eye represents a good prognostic sign. The fovea then is considered to be functionally intact and, practically speaking, a foveal tag is available for training for proper foveal fixation reflexes. Lack of perception of the Haid-

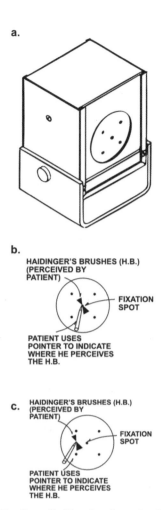

a.

b.

HAIDINGER'S BRUSHES (H.B.)
(PERCEIVED BY
PATIENT)

FIXATION
SPOT

PATIENT USES
POINTER TO INDICATE
WHERE HE PERCEIVES
THE H.B.

c.

HAIDINGER'S BRUSHES (H.B.)
(PERCEIVED BY
PATIENT)

FIXATION
SPOT

PATIENT USES
POINTER TO INDICATE
WHERE HE PERCEIVES
THE H.B.

Figure 5-34. The Bernell Macular Integrity Tester-Trainer, a. Drawing of the instrument; clear slide with fixation spots placed before the illuminated circular window, b. Example of central fixation, in which case the patient sees the Haidinger brush and the fixation spot as superimposed, c. Example of eccentric fixation, whereby the Haidinger brush and the fixation spot are not superimposed. This response would indicate nasal eccentric fixation of the right eye. If this response were found when testing the left eye, temporal eccentric fixation would be indicated.

inger brush does not necessarily mean the macula is dysfunctional or diseased. Some individuals with normal retinas have difficulty seeing this entoptic image. An amblyope may have a particular problem seeing the brush if there is EF, because it does not appear where the patient is fixating. The straight-ahead direction is usually associated with the eccentric point, not the fovea. The brush will appear, when it is perceived, off to one side of the fixation target on the MITT.

When an amblyopic patient is experiencing difficulty in observing the brush, several techniques may help to elicit its perception: First, the appearance of the Haidinger brush can be demonstrated using the patient's non amblyopic eye, for which the entoptic image should be relatively easy to appreciate. Second, the background room illumi-

nation can be lowered to increase the contrast of the MITT screen, and double (two) cobalt-blue filters can be used over the amblyopic eye, occluding the non amblyopic eye, to intensify the perception of Haidinger's brush. A third technique involves placing a high-plus trial-case lens (e.g., +10 D) in front of the cobalt filter, which will blur out all extraneous contours and shadows but leave the entoptic image unaffected. Finally, to confirm that the perceived image is indeed the Haidinger brush, a piece of cellophane or plastic wrap can be inserted before the amblyopic eye to determine whether the direction of brush rotation is reversed. The cellophane acts as a quarter-wave plate and should reverse the perceived direction of rotation of the entoptic image.

Besides establishing macular integrity, the Haidinger brush can be used to evaluate the fixation pattern of an amblyopic eye. Most characteristics of the fixation pattern that are observed by visuoscopy can also be assessed using the brush if the patient is a reliable observer. The patient is instructed to fixate a suprathreshold target on the MITT at exactly a 40-cm distance from the instrument. After the correct perception of the entoptic image is established, the following assessment of fixation can be made: Is there central or eccentric fixation? If there is EF, what is the direction and magnitude? (Note: At a 40-cm fixation distance, 4-mm lateral displacement on the screen represents 1Δ.) Is there steady or unsteady fixation? If there is unsteady fixation, what are the amplitude and type of oscillations? Is the fovea included within the range of unsteadiness? Is there faulty localization associated with EF or is the patient eccentrically viewing?

Visuoscopy, of course, has a major advantage over the MITT as an assessment technique because it is objective; however, the MITT can be immediately employed in the remediation of faulty fixation associated with amblyopia. Both instruments, the visuoscope and the MITT, are important and useful in the management of EF.

Refraction Procedures

Subjective refractive techniques are usually unreliable when testing an amblyopic eye, due to the abnormal fixation pattern and the deficient spatial resolution. Consequently, cycloplegic retinoscopy is often necessary for determining the refractive error. We generally use one drop of 1 % cyclopentolate preceded by a drop of 0.5% proparacaine. In most patients, the cycloplegic effect is sufficiently strong to reveal the full amount of hyperopia, if it exists. We prefer not to rely completely on a phoropter in cases of amblyopia (or strabismus). It is easier to monitor the fixation by directly viewing the patient. The refractive error is determined with trial-case lenses or a lens bar. To ensure accuracy, care must be taken that the retinoscopic beam on the amblyopic eye is directly on axis. The correct visual axis can be estimated with a penlight by moving to a lateral position at which angle kappa of the amblyopic eye equals that of the normal eye. In cases of amblyopia associated with esotropia, on-axis retinoscopy is easily accomplished by scoping the amblyopic eye from the opposite side (e.g., in a case of a right esotropic amblyopic eye, scoping from the patient's left side). In cases of anisometropic or strabismic amblyopia, correction of the full refractive error usually is prescribed even when a patch is to be worn. Undercorrecting hyperopia can be a mistake, because the accommodative responses of an amblyopic eye are usually deficient.

EYE DISEASE EVALUATION

Before the diagnosis of amblyopia is made, the clinician must investigate the possibility that ocular pathology may be the direct cause of the reduction in visual acuity. It is prudent to be suspicious of eye disease or pathology affecting the visual pathways in all cases of unexplained reduction of visual acuity, even in cases associated with anisometropia and strabismus; it is possible for organic eye disease to coexist with amblyopia. The following procedures provide the basis for making a clinical distinction between a pathologic loss of acuity and nonorganic amblyopia.

Ophthalmoscopy

A dilated fundus examination may be necessary for careful inspection of the macular and foveal regions of the amblyopic eye. However, detection of subtle retinal lesions can be difficult. Besides using direct and indirect ophthalmoscopy to examine an amblyopic eye, we recommend a careful slit-lamp inspection of the macula and fovea using high magnification (e.g., a 60D or 90 D lens).

Visual Fields

Automated visual field testing is usually unsuccessful or unreliable due to the poor fixation responses of an amblyopic eye. Ordinary tangent screen field testing has some advantages over the automated techniques. Unsteady fixation of the amblyopic eye can be reduced if no central fixation target is used. As an alternative, four strips of masking tape or paper can be applied to the tangent screen at the 3-, 6-, 9-, and 12-o'clock positions approximately 10 degrees away from the center of the screen; this pattern indicates a virtual fixation point. The patient holds the amblyopic eye steady on the virtual point at which the four lines would theoretically intersect; then the field testing of the blind spot, periphery, and central areas proceeds in the usual manner. Testing with a 1-mm or 2-mm white target at 1 m is generally sufficient to determine whether a scotoma exists. During this procedure, the patient should wear spectacles, contact lenses, or trial-case lenses to correct fully any significant refractive error. The visual field of the amblyopic eye is compared with that of the normal eye.

Amsler grid testing for central field defects is also recommended. As in tangent screen testing, the visual fields of the two eyes are compared for consistency. For testing an amblyopic eye, we recommend that a +2.50-D nearpoint add (a trial-case lens) be used along with any needed spectacle correction, because monocular accommodation of an amblyopic eye is usually deficient. Even if there is significant unsteady EF, the fovea will usually fall somewhere on the grid pattern and a central visual field defect, if it exists, may be noticed by the patient.

Schapero[22] proposed that detection of a central absolute scotoma (no light perception within the scotomatous area) indicates an organic lesion or amblyopia with an organic component and that the prognosis for attaining better acuity is limited by the potential acuity of the retinal area surrounding the absolute scotoma. In contrast, Irvine[65] reported that a relative central scotoma (depressed sensitivity) is an indication of a functional reduction of acuity that is potentially recoverable; this more optimistic view is based on his findings that some nonorganic cases of deep amblyopia apparently exhibited an absolute central scotoma.

Neutral-Density Filters

Ammann[66] proposed that differential diagnosis of organic (pathologic acuity loss) and developmental amblyopia is possible by comparing the visual acuity measured under normal versus reduced illumination. There is an expected decrease of visual acuity when target illumination is reduced for both the normal and the amblyopic eye. Visual acuity normally decreases under mesopic and scotopic conditions. However, if the cause of acuity loss is pathologic (e.g., macular degeneration, optic atrophy, central pathway lesion), the decrease in visual acuity with decreased illumination is sudden and dramatic.

Caloroso and Flom[67] demonstrated that at essentially all luminance levels, visual acuity in the functional amblyopic eye was less than that of the normal eye. At the lowest levels of luminance, however, it was approximately equal. In contradistinction to functional amblyopia, von Noorden and Burian[68] convincingly showed that in cases of macular organic lesions, visual acuity dropped precipitously as illumination decreased, thus confirming Ammann's observations.

Neutral-density filter testing can be used clinically when a patient presents with unexplained monocular reduced acuity and a differential diagnosis is needed. Either a 2.0- or 3.0-log unit neutral-density filter, such as a Kodak Wratten Filter 96, should be used. We recommend measuring the visual acuity of each eye under normal photopic room-lighting conditions by means of visual acuity chart that conforms with psychometric principles of measuring acuity (see earlier section). If a Snellen chart must be used, the acuity thresholds should be converted to the Snell-Sterling visual efficiency scale (e.g., 20/20 - 100%; 20/50 = 76%). The patient's eyes then are partially dark-adapted (for approximately 5 minutes) to a mesopic level. The appropriate neutral-density filter is placed over the projector's objective lens, and the poorer eye is occluded while the visual acuity of the better eye is quickly re-measured. Switching the occluder, the clinician then determines the acuity threshold of the poorer eye. Under mesopic conditions, the visual acuity of the better eye may have decreased from 20/20 to 20/40, approximately a 15% reduction in Snell-Sterling visual efficiency, for example. An organic lesion would be suspected if the visual acuity of the poorer eye decreases from 20/50, for example, to 20/200, nearly a 55% decrease in visual efficiency. The rate of decrease is much faster in cases of macular pathway lesions as compared with functional amblyopia. If the poorer eye, however, showed only a 20% or lesser decrease in visual efficiency with the neutral-density filter, functional amblyopia would be indicated. (See Appendix F for conversion scales.)

Tests of Retinal Function

Two other tests may be helpful in making the distinction between a pathologic reduction of acuity and functional amblyopia. These are monocular color vision and electroretinography. Several diseases of the retina and optic nerve result in subtle monocular color vision defects. Retinal disease tends to produce subtle blue-yellow defects, whereas acquired optic atrophy often results in subtle red-green defects. Monocular color vision can be tested in most children of at least 10 years of age using the Farnsworth panel D-15 test. However, a good blue-yellow differential diagnostic test for younger children may not be available. Using the Farnsworth test, the color vision responses of each eye are inspected for differences that ordinarily are not found. If a defect is found with this test, it represents a strong defect. The desaturated panel D-15 may be necessary to pick up the initial signs of color vision defects attributable to eye disease.

Another test of retinal function that may help in the differential diagnosis is the electroretinogram (ERG). Although the research literature is very mixed. Consistent differences may not be apparent in the ERG responses between normal and amblyopic eyes.[69] If abnormal ERG responses or significant differences between the eyes are found, the condition is unlikely to be functional amblyopia. For example, the *pattern ERG* is abnormal in cases of Stargardt's macular dystrophy (a juvenile rod-cone dystrophy), which may be confused with amblyopia during its early stages. The ERG procedure usually requires referral to a visual functions testing clinic at a medical or optometric center, as most primary care doctors do not have the relatively expensive instruments used for this evaluation. The expense of this test often is justified if there is a reasonable suspicion of retinal disease, because patching of the sound eye can be a very frustrating procedure for a patient, even when the chance of functional improvement is good. Useless patching is to be avoided, within reason

SCREENING FOR AMBLYOPIA

Amblyopia is one of the leading causes of vision loss and monocular blindness and, because it develops in the early years, it affects an individual for life. The earlier amblyopia is identified, the more successfully it is managed. One epidemiologic study found a 1% prevalence of amblyopia in 8-year-old children who had been screened in infancy but a 2.5% prevalence in those children not previously screened.[70] The challenge is to find screening methods that are valid in early childhood, and are time- and cost-effective, and easy to implement.

One of the simplest procedures to apply in infants is for the clinician to watch for avoidance behavior when each eye is occluded in turn. Consistent avoidance when covering one eye is highly suggestive of unilateral vision impairment. If there is strabismus and a child can hold fixation with either eye or can freely alternate fixation, then the patient usually does not have amblyopia; in contrast, those who hold fixation with only a preferred eye tend to be amblyopic. This method should be part of every pediatric health examination.[71]

A more reliable procedure is for a vision specialist to check for the presence of a strabismus using the Hirschberg test or the cover test, followed by objective measuring of the refractive error by retinoscopy. This short screening procedure is effective but expensive, because a doctor's time and skills are involved.

Recently, the Vision in Preschoolers research group conducted a large scale multi-center study evaluating the effectiveness of common screening methods for identifying several visual anomalies in children including amblyopia.[72] In the first phase the instruments were used by highly trained professionals and compared to comprehensive vision examinations performed by optometrists or ophthalmologists. The four best tests were, non-cycloplegic retinoscopy, Retinomax II autorefractor, Suresight vision screener, and Lea symbols for visual acuity. These four tests were 90% accurate to detecting the most severe visual conditions including amblyogenic factors of strabismus and high uncorrected refractive errors. In the second phase nurses and lay screeners administered the following tests; Lea symbols, stereo smile test II, the Retinomax II autorefractor, and the Sure sight vision screener. With these four tests nurses and lay screeners were able to indentify 80% of the most severe vision problems. One conclusion of the study was that the Retinomax II autorefractor and Suresight vision screener were superior to the photorefraction techniques. In addition, nurses and lay screeners would benefit from adding autorefraction to a visual acuity screening for preschool children. Thus, implementing high quality screening practices that combine auto-refractors with visual acuity can identify the majority of amblyogenic conditions.

ANOMALOUS CORRESPONDENCE

Anomalous correspondence is a sensory defense mechanism against diplopia that preserves rudimentary binocular vision in response to a strabismus of early onset. It is defined as the binocular condition in which the two foveas and other homologous retinal loci do not correspond to each other in regard to directional values: The primary visual direction in the deviating eye has shifted to a nonfoveal location to be in accord with that of the fixating eye. This shift of directional value allows at least some sensory integration of the two eyes, so that the strabismic individual is not "monocular." Although the correspondence actually takes place in the cortex of the occipital lobe, clinicians refer to *retinal* correspondence because the retinas are the reference locations for angular measurements. Consequently, the term *anomalous retinal correspondence* is used throughout this book, as is the traditionally recognized abbreviation, *ARC*, although some prefer the designation AC.

Classification

ARC is an anti-diplopic sensory adaptation that is prevalent in developmental strabismus. Its presence indicates a significant difference between the horizontal *objective angle of deviation (H)* and the *subjective angle of directionalization (S)*. The difference between these two angles is the *angle of anomaly (A)*. Some measurement error must be allowed; otherwise, a false-positive diagnosis may result (i.e., a diagnosis of ARC when actually there is normal retinal correspondence [NRC]). In small-angle strabismus, allowance of a 1-2Δ error may be necessary and up to 5Δ should be allowed for large angles of strabismus when comparing

H and *S*. The larger the strabismus, therefore, the more allowance is made for measurement error. In theory, angles *H* and *S* should be exactly the same in NRC (angle *A* being zero in magnitude). Clinical measurements, however, are not always precise, which necessitates the allowance for measurement error. This is particularly so when the patient is an uncooperative child or a poor observer.

An example of NRC is illustrated in Figure 5-35. Angles *H* and *S* are the same in this case of esotropia with NRC:

$$H = 25\Delta \text{ (eso)}, S = 25\Delta \text{ (eso)}$$
$$A = 25\Delta - 25\Delta$$
$$A = 0\Delta$$

In free-space natural viewing, diplopia is likely to occur when there is a strabismus of recent onset and NRC. Point zero, the target point, is stimulated peripherally and produces homonymous diplopia, unless there is strong peripheral suppression. Suppression is likely to take place at the fovea of the deviating eye to prevent overlapping of the two different foveal images (i.e., confusion). ARC would be the more parsimonious anti-diplopic adaptation, as there is the added advantage of preserving rudimentary peripheral binocularity and, possibly, gross stereopsis in small angles of strabismus. However, ARC can probably develop only in response to strabismus during early childhood when there is cortical plasticity with respect to binocular visual direction.

Three angles are involved in ARC. The following relation between these angles applies: $H = A + S$ or, solving for *A*, $A = H - S$. Angle *A* is the angle subtended at the center of rotation of the eye by the fovea (*f*) and the anomalous associated point (*a*) (Figure 5-36). The fovea of the fixating eye corresponds with point a in the deviating eye when there is ARC. Point *a* is strictly functional; there is no retinal landmark as there is for point *f*.

The type of ARC occurring most frequently in natural seeing conditions is harmonious ARC (HARC). An example of this is illustrated in Figure 5-37, in which *S* equals 0^Δ and *A* has the same magnitude as *H*. Such strabismic patients often give orthophoric responses during routine phorometry. This is because point *a* is in the same location as point zero. The fovea of the fixating left eye in this example corresponds to point *a* of the right eye, which happens to be coincident with

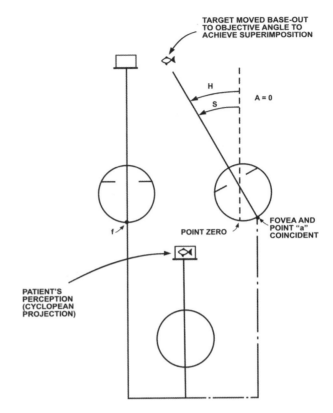

Figure 5-35. Normal retinal correspondence.

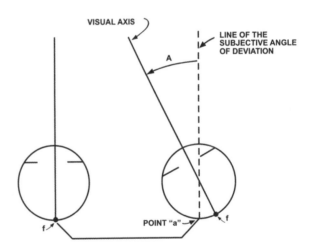

Figure 5-36. The angle of anomaly (A), in which the fovea (f) of the left eye corresponds to point a of the right eye. Angle A is subtended at the center of rotation of the eye by the visual axis and the line of the subjective angle of deviation.

point zero, the target point. Clinicians, therefore, should be on guard if phorometry indicates $S = 0$ (or a value close to zero) when a strabismic deviation is present. HARC is suspected in such cases. An example of HARC is as follows (see Figure 5-37):

$$H = 25\Delta, S = 0\Delta$$
$$A = 25\Delta - 0\Delta$$
$$A = 25\Delta$$

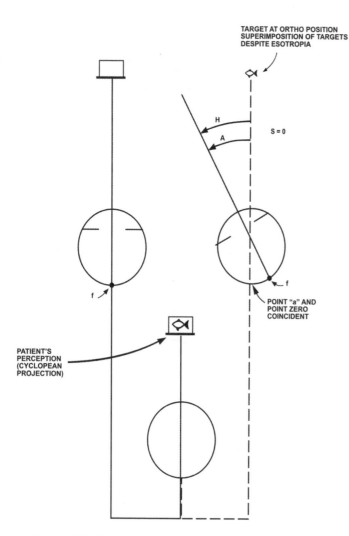

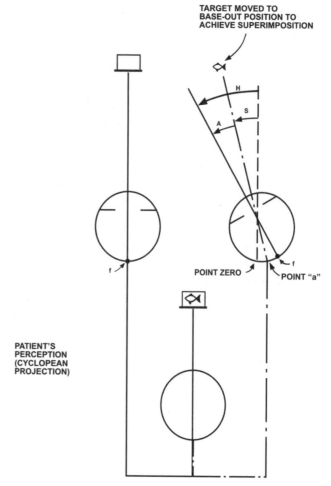

Figure 5-38. *Typical unharmonious anomalous retinal correspondence, (f = fovea.)*

Figure 5-37. *Harmonious anomalous retinal correspondence. (f = fovea.)*

Not all cases of ARC are harmonious. Assume that a patient has an esotropia of the right eye of 25Δ and that *S* equals 12Δ (as measured by subjective tests such as the dissociated red lens test). The fact that *H* and *S* are different suggests ARC. Figure 5-38 illustrates this example by depicting points *f*, *a*, and *zero* (also called *point 0* in the deviating eye). This example represents a case of *unharmonious ARC* (UNHARC), in which *H* is larger than *S*, and point a lies between point *f* and point zero. In the example of UNHARC provided in Figure 5-38, the following values apply:

H= 25Δ, S = 12Δ
A= 25Δ - 12Δ
A= 13Δ

Some relatively rare types of ARC that occur secondary to changes in the angle of deviation (*H*) can result in some unusual measurements of the subjective angle (*S*). An example of paradoxical ARC type one is illustrated in Figure 5-39. In such

a case, the patient has a subjective angle under binocular viewing conditions, as if there were exotropia, even when *H* indicates esotropia. This condition often occurs when the original angle of esotropia was greater before extraocular muscle surgery than afterward. In this example, the deviation was reduced by surgery, but not sufficiently to make the visual axes parallel. Assume that before surgery there had been HARC, so that point *a* was originally at point zero. The outward rotational movement of the deviating eye with surgery caused point *a* to be moved from the ortho demand point to another point farther in the nasal retina. Stimulation of the postsurgical point zero, which is temporal in respect to point *a*, causes *S* to be in the exo direction. For example:

H= 25 (eso), S = -28Δ (exo)
A= 25Δ - (-28Δ)
A= 53Δ

Paradoxical type two ARC often occurs after a surgical overcorrection of exotropia. For example, a patient with an exotropic right eye and HARC

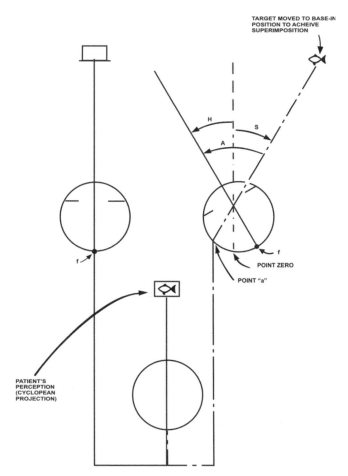

Figure 5-39. Paradoxical type one unharmonious anomalous retinal correspondence. (f=fovea.)

preoperatively may have an esotropic right eye postoperatively (Figure 5-40). Point *a* would be moved from point zero to a location temporalward in relation to point zero. Stimulation of point zero would then cause the patient's angle *S* to be more eso in direction than it was preoperatively. (*S* is more eso in magnitude than is *H*.) For example:

$$H = 17\Delta \text{ (eso)}, \quad S = 30\Delta \text{ (eso)}$$
$$A = 17\Delta - 30\Delta$$
$$A = -13\Delta$$

Causes other than extraocular muscle surgery may alter the magnitude of *H* to result in UNHARC or a paradoxical type of ARC. Plus lenses, for example, may reduce an eso deviation, and minus lenses may reduce an exo deviation. Prisms may optically affect these angular relationships as well as the possibility that vision training techniques will produce changes. There appears to be wide variation in the way that patients in whom HARC is the initial adaptation to their strabismus sensorially readapt to a new angle of deviation postoperatively

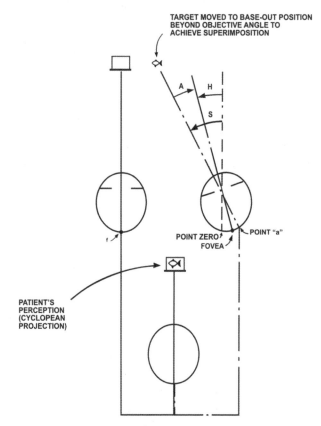

Figure 5-40. Paradoxical type two unharmonious anomalous retinal correspondence, (f = fovea.)

or after optical and training manipulations of the angle *H*. In some cases, HARC and its consequent advantages to fusion re-establish themselves; at other times, paradoxical ARC results, along with the undesirable, but fortunately rare, consequence of intractable diplopia.

In summary, then, the conceptual basis for the classification of NRC and ARC is the location of the anomalous associated point (a) in the deviating eye (Figure 5-41). If point *a* of the deviating eye is anywhere other than at the fovea, then there is ARC. If point *a* is at the target point (zero), there is HARC; if between the fovea and the point zero, there is UNHARC; if nasal to point zero, paradoxical ARC type one; and if temporal to the fovea, then paradoxical ARC type two. See Table 5-12 to review the relations among angles *H*, *S*, and *A* that serve to classify types of correspondence.

Characteristics

Horopter in Anomalous Retinal Correspondence

Flom[73] demonstrated that the identical visual direction horopter in strabismic patients having ARC has an irregular shape that may help to explain

Table 5-12. Classification of Normal and Anomalous Correspondence by Mathematic Formulas

NRC	$H = S; A = 0$
ARC	$H \neq S$
HARC	$H = A; S = 0$
UNHARC	$H > S; H > A$
PARC I	$A > H; S$ opposite direction to H $(S < 0)$
PARC II	$S > H; A$ opposite direction to H $(A < 0)$

A= angle of anomaly; ARC = anomalous retinal correspondence H=objective angle of deviation; HARC = harmonious ARC, NRC = normal retinal correspondence; PARC I (II) = paradoxical ARC type one (two); S = subjective angle of directionalization; UNHARC = unharmonious ARC

many of the characteristics of the condition. The peripheral horopter in ARC cases was similar in shape and location to that in nonstrabismic patients with NRC and, in that sense, these patients can be said to have peripheral fusion (Figure 5-42). The nonstrabismic's horopter goes through the point of fixation. When an intermittent esotrope with NRC lapses into a strabismic deviation, the horopter shifts from the plane of the target to a point where the visual axes cross (the centration point). Images then in the plane of the target, including the target, appear to be diplopic if there is no suppression (see Figure 5-42b). However, if there is esotropia with ARC, the horopter beyond the area between the visual axes remains in the plane of the target of regard, and the world appears fused even though there may be some central suppression (see Figure 5-42c). This is a very convenient adaptation for the strabismic individual, because diplopia is eliminated. Peripheral stereopsis may be present if angle *H* is small (see Figure 5-42d) and fusional vergence eye movements can still occur.

Another remarkable feature of the ARC horopter is its abrupt and radical change in direction within the space subtended between the visual axes (see Figure 5-42c). Flom[73] referred to this area as the "notch" in the horopter. One might ask how the patient processes binocular information within the visual axes when the horopter is so extremely skewed. One possible notion is that this area between the axes is not binocular at all under normal viewing conditions. A skew in the identical visual direction horopter in nonstrabismic subjects usually means there is aniseikonia, and the greater the skew, the greater is the aniseikonia. The radical skew of the central portion of the ARC horopter might mean that aniseikonia is too extreme to

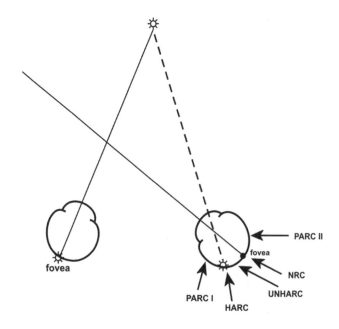

Figure 5-41. Anomalous retinal correspondence (ARC) classification based on the location of point a, indicated by arrows pointing to the retinal site on the right eye. (HARC = harmonious ARC; NRC = normal retinal correspondence; PARC I, PARC II = paradoxical ARC type I, type II [respectively]; UNHARC =unharmonious ARC)

allow binocular disparities to be processed. In this case, the patient may be said to have no central fusion, and the visual information within the axes is processed monocularly. Furthermore, there is usually suppression in the notch area subtended by the angle between the fovea and the target point of the deviating eye.

This interpretation may help to explain the observation by strabismic ARC patients of the Swann *split-field effect*. Red-green glasses are worn by a nonstrabismic subject, and he or she views a detailed target against a white background (Figure 5-43). The usual report in nonstrabismic patients is color fusion (a murky brown) and color rivalry (a percept of alternating, moving red and green areas). However, many ARC esotropic patients report a different percept under similar conditions. Peripherally, there appears to be the melding or rivalry of colors as reported by patients having normal binocular vision, but centrally, ARC patients often describe a split bipartite field in which half is purely red and half purely green. If the red filter happens to be on the right eye and the green on the left, the patient reports seeing the red hemifield to the right and the green to the left. Sometimes a patient will report a seam running down the middle of the split field (Figure 5-44). These central areas

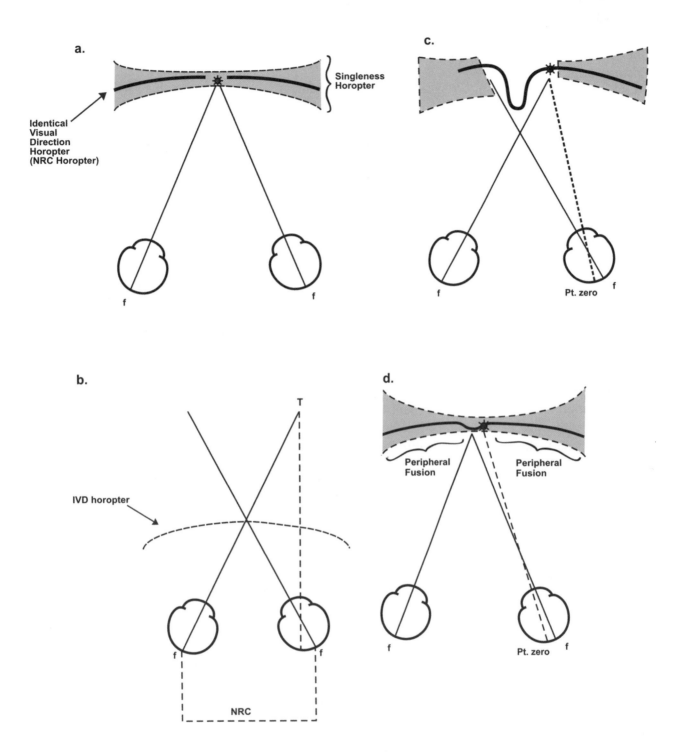

Figure 5-42. Identical visual direction (IVD) horopter, a. Bifixating person, in whom the horopter passes through the centration point and the location of the target, b. Esotropic person with normal retinal correspondence (NRC), in whom the identical visual direction horopter passes through the centration point but not through the location of the target, c. Esotropic person with harmonious anomalous retinal correspondence, in whom the central notch approaches the centration point but the peripheral portion of the horopter passes through the location of the target, d. Same as c, but the magnitude of the esotropia is small, allowing for an almost normal binocular field of fusion. Note that the dashed line is shown crossing anteriorly to the eye: The visual axis and this line should be crossing the center of rotation of the eye but, because of the very small angle of the strabismus, the angles are shown in this manner only for the purpose of illustration, (f = fovea.)

of pure colors represent monocular processing of visual information by each eye within the region between the visual axes under these conditions. Patients with ARC often are described as having peripheral fusion, the implication being that there is no central fusion. The Swann split-field effect is an important example that supports this interpretation of the status of binocularity in strabismic patients having ARC.

ARC appears to be more prevalent in patients having small and moderate angles of constant strabismus (e.g., 30A or less) as compared with those who have larger angles.[74, 75] Some patients with small deviations, usually less than 10Δ, show considerable sensory fusion capability. It is not unusual to find 200 seconds of stereopsis testing with the Titmus animals stereograms but poorer stereoacuity, if any, with the Wirt circles and hardly any with random dot stereograms. Also, fusional vergence ranges may be fairly normal, particularly if prism demands are introduced at a slower rate than in routine vergence testing.[74, 75] Presumably, peripherally sized targets allow for possible motor fusion. In cases of small-angle esotropia with ARC, there is a small notch in the horopter so that the overall shape, location, and thickness of the singleness horopter appears nearly normal (see Figure 5-42d). These clinical observations are consistent with the theoretical concept of peripheral fusion and central suppression as a general mechanism in ARC, whereby the size of the angle of deviation determines, in part, the binocular capabilities of the strabismic patient.

Horror Fusionis

Hofstetter et al.[5] define *horror fusionis* as "the inability to obtain binocular fusion or superimposition of haploscopically presented targets, or the condition or phenomenon itself, occurring frequently as a characteristic in strabismus, in which case the targets approaching superimposition may seem to slide or jump past each other without apparent fusion or suppression." In the past, horror fusionis has been associated with "macular evasion,"[76] patients needing psychotherapy,[77] intractable diplopia,[78] and aniseikonia.[79] Not much has been published on this condition, and the mechanism has been uncertain.

We believe this condition is almost always associated with ARC. An inspection of the horopter in ARC gives a clue to the nature of this binocular anomaly. Aniseikonia, indeed, appears to be a factor. The fovea of the fixating eye seems to be associated with many points in the strabismic eye and vice versa. For example, as shown in Figure 5-42c, it is as though the fovea of the left eye is associated with a series of points between points zero (same location as point a in HARC) and *f* of the right eye, creating an intolerable magnification effect. Flom[73] explained horror fusionis in subjects

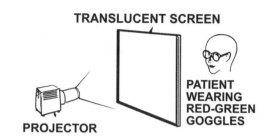

Figure 5-43. Stimulus apparatus for color fusion.

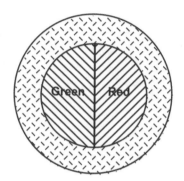

Figure 5-44. Split-field perception.

with esotropia and ARC on the basis of nonuniform, relative distributions of corresponding retinal points (irregularly shaped horopter). He explained the horror fusionis movement of the images when superimposition is attempted, as in the Synoptophore: A sudden movement occurs when the target of the deviating eye is moved across a limb of the notch of the horopter; it is not due to any eye movements. Flom[73] explained, "This jumping phenomenon is commonly observed by strabismics with ARC when viewing constantly illuminated first-degree targets, one of which is moved toward the other to obtain superimposition."

Etiology of Anomalous Retinal Correspondence

The neurophysiologic basis for ARC is unknown, but most authorities assume that the visual cortex mediates binocular visual direction. The binocular striate neurons seem capable of comparing the images from the two eyes, detecting disparities between them, and linking corresponding retinal points.[80] The traditional view is that normal correspondence is innate.[81] ARC is an acquired sensory adaptation to strabismus during early development, when the cortex is still malleable and capable of establishing a new coupling of noncorresponding cortical elements. Visually mature individuals, older than 6 years or so, who acquire a strabismus later in life are almost always incapable of developing ARC. According to Burian,[82] "ARC is acquired by usage ... the acquisition of an anomalous correspondence represents an adaptation of the sensory apparatus of the eyes to the abnormal position of the eyes." The earlier the onset of the strabismus and the longer an individual "practices" ARC (a learned response), the deeper the ARC adaptation is established. This view has come to be known as the *adaptation theory of ARC*. This theory would predict that ARC would tend to be found in early-onset, constant, comitant strabismus and less often in late-onset, intermittent, or noncomitant strabismus. Substantial clinical evidence confirms this prediction.

Morgan[83] proposed that ARC is a motor phenomenon (rather than merely a sensory adaptation) and stated, "Thus anomalous correspondence might depend not on a sensory adaptation to a squint but rather on whether the basic underlying innervational pattern to the extraocular muscles was one which registered itself in consciousness as altering egocentric direction, or whether the pattern was one which was 'nonregistered' in consciousness as altering egocentric direction." A nonregistered innervation would imply NRC, whereas a registered pattern would imply ARC. This notion is called the *motor theory of ARC*. It implies that at the time of strabismus onset, the moment the eye turns, an abnormal neural circuit allows the change in vergence eye position to be "registered" in the perceptual mechanism subserving visual direction. Kerr[84] suggested that the fundamental error in the neural circuitry is a disorder in the disparity detection mechanism, either on the convergent side, yielding esotropia with ARC, or on the divergent side, resulting in exotropia with ARC.

Ordinarily, version eye movements are "registered" and vergences are not, but an abnormal reflex, possibly genetically determined, links vergence to the perceptual apparatus. ARC localization is, therefore, immediate and complete, all or none. This view dispenses with the concepts of depth, learning, and adaptation and suggests that ARC is a neural reflex possibly mediated by the neurology responsible for the well-documented phenomenon of ARC *covariation*. Hallden[85] demonstrated that strabismic patients with ARC have some daily variation in their angle of deviation (H) and that the angle of anomaly increases and decreases in

tandem with it. Co-varying ARC also has been reported in some patients with A and V patterns in which the strabismic angle changes in up- and down-gaze.[86] Correspondence can also be demonstrated to change synchronously with fusional vergence eye position in many cases of strabismus. It is not unusual to find an intermittent exotrope who shows NRC and excellent stereopsis when fusing and ARC when strabismic. As the deviation becomes manifest, angle A increases simultaneously with angle H. Therefore, the subjective angle stays the same (zero) during the motor movement. Far from being a rigid, hard-wired adaptation, ARC is found to vary considerably with changes in vergence eye position.

These two theories of ARC etiology lead to different ideas about its remediation. The adaptation theory suggests that early intervention is critical. NRC must be relearned by realigning the eyes by early surgical and optical means or by stimulating bifoveal localization using vision training techniques, often applied in an amblyoscope. The motor theory, however, suggests that it is necessary to train realignment of the eyes using fusional vergence, thus stimulating covariation. If the eyes can be straightened by fusional vergence, then covariation will change the correspondence from anomalous to normal; NRC will persist as long as the eyes remain straight. This approach is easier to apply to exotropes than to esotropes, because patients can be fairly easily trained in fusional convergence.

Many investigators and clinicians tend to advocate either one etiology or the other. We believe there is reasonable and substantial evidence to support each theory. It may well be that there are two or more etiologies for ARC, and a complete description of the condition will require appreciating at least both developmental sensory and reflex motor aspects. The clinical challenge may be to determine which mechanism is primarily responsible for ARC in a particular patient. Vision therapy related to the cause or causes can then be more appropriately prescribed for efficacious treatment.

Depth of Anomalous Retinal Correspondence
Those who espouse the adaptation theory of ARC believe it is clinically useful to evaluate the depth of the condition. Testing the depth of ARC is analogous to testing the intensity of suppression; if testing conditions are very unnatural, suppression

is not likely to be found. Burian[82] promoted the concept that ARC is an acquired sensory adaptation to a motor deviation and that this adaptation may be either deep or shallow. This may explain the more frequent clinical finding of ARC on Bagolini striated lens testing than on other less natural clinical tests, such as afterimages (AIs). The principle is that the more natural the testing environment, the more likely it is that ARC will be found. Conversely, the more unnatural the environment, the more likely it is that NRC will be found.

Flom and Kerr,[87] espousing the motor theory, rejected the concept of depth of ARC. They contended that disagreement among various tests can be attributed to measurement error, unsteady fixation, or changes in the relative position of the eyes from one test to another. In their study, they employed several different tests, including (1) the Maddox rod cover test, (2) the major amblyoscope, (3) the Hallden test using red-green filters and an AI to measure H, A, and S, and (4) the Hering-Bielschowsky AI test. These testing methods, however, were unnatural in many respects. The Bagolini striated lens test (a relatively natural test) was not included in their study. In contrast, Bagolini and Tittarelli[88] found HARC in 83% of their strabismic patients using the striated lenses but in only 13% using the amblyoscope. von Noorden[69] reported similar results, concluding that ARC has a depth characteristic.

We believe it is prudent to perform several tests for ARC as part of a strabismus examination. If the clinical findings support a depth effect, then this information should be used in determining the diagnosis and prognosis. Prognosis for elimination of ARC and ultimate cure of strabismus is generally more favorable for those patients who demonstrate an ARC response on only one test rather than on all tests. Further research, however, is needed to resolve the issue of depth of ARC.

Prevalence of Anomalous Retinal Correspondence

Statistics on the prevalence of ARC vary, often due to the unanswered questions about which type of ARC was being considered, what testing was done, and who did the testing. In a study of 295 strabismics, ARC was reported in 45% of the cases; of the esotropes, 53% were found to have ARC, as compared with only 16% of the exotropes.[89] These results were based solely on major amblyoscope findings. Possibly, the rates would have been lower if more unnatural tests, such as AIs, had been used and higher with use of more natural tests. Similarly, Hugonnier et al.[90] reported that in 98 cases of strabismus, the Bagolini striated lens test revealed 84 cases of ARC, the Synoptophore yielded 64 cases, and use of AI's identified only 35 cases. In general, ARC is more prevalent in infantile than in late-onset strabismus, in the presence of constant angles versus intermittent and small angles versus large, and in esotropia versus exotropia. ARC due to vertical deviations is possible but, in our clinical experience, rare.

TESTING

Correspondence can be assessed indirectly by comparing the measured angles H and S. The angle of anomaly (A) is simply calculated by subtracting the subjective angle (S) from the objective angle (H). It is often convenient clinically to use the alternate cover test results at farpoint for angle H and the dissociated red lens test results at farpoint for angle S. The angle of anomaly, A, can also be measured directly without reliance on calculation from H and S. Entoptic phenomena, such as the Haidinger brush and Maxwell's spot, may be used, but instruments for these tests are not commonly found in a primary care practice. The most frequently used direct measure of A is done with AIs. Next in frequency is visuoscopy, performed with the patient under biocular viewing conditions (discussed later in the section Bifoveal Test of Cüppers). Most other clinical tests for ARC determine A indirectly by calculating the difference between H and S.

Dissociated Red Lens Test

The dissociated red lens test was recommended by Flom[91] for assessing correspondence as part of the minimal strabismus examination for primary eye care practitioners. This test determines the subjective angle (S) for distant viewing and is compared to the objective angle (H), which is measured by cover test at the same distance and under similar lighting conditions. A red filter and a 10Δ base-down loose prism are held before the dominant eye in a normally illuminated room. The fixation target is a bright "muscle" light (e.g., penlight). Most strabismic patients, even with considerable suppression, will then perceive vertically displaced diplopic images of the light, red on top and white on the bottom. The horizontal angle S is measured using sufficient horizontal prism placed before the non dominant eye until the two images appear to the patient as vertically aligned. The method of limits (bracketing) should always be used to increase measurement accuracy. In the presence of strabismus, if angle S is found to be zero or close to zero, HARC is indicated. If angle S is significantly different from zero but is less than angle H, UNHARC is suggested. If, however, angles H and S are essentially the same (within the limits of measurement error), then NRC is present.

Afterimages

The Hering-Bielschowsky test is the most frequently used AI method of ARC testing and directly measures angle A, the angle of anomaly. An ordinary electronic flash attachment to a camera can be modified to serve as an AI generator (Figure 5-45a). The face of the flash is masked with opaque tape to produce a long narrow slit. A small piece of tape also is placed across the middle of the slit to serve as a fixation target. The unit is held at a distance of approximately 40 cm (16 in.) from the patient when the flash is triggered. A 100-watt light bulb can also be modified if a sustained stimulus is desired (Figure 5-45b). The patient should fixate the masked light bulb for 30 seconds to produce a vivid, sustained AI for each eye. The procedure is as follows:

1. The non dominant eye is occluded while the patient fixates a central mask on a horizontal line strobe flasher or a masked light bulb. The exact center should be opaque to produce a small gap in the AI for purposes of identifying the position of the fovea.

2. After the horizontal AI is applied, occlusion is switched to the dominant eye, and an AI is applied in the same manner to the non-dominant eye, except that now it is oriented *vertically*.

3. The eye is uncovered and the patient is instructed to fixate with the dominant eye a small, discrete target on a blank (e.g., gray) wall so that the gap in the horizontal AI is centered on the target. A recommended testing distance is 1 m to facilitate measurement of angle A.

4. Alternately lowering and raising the room illumination (approximately every 3 seconds) helps the patient to perceive and sustain both the horizontal and vertical afterimages.

5. The negative AI is more reliable in routine testing than is the positive AI. The negative AI is seen in a lighted room, whereas the positive AI is seen in a darkened room. The patient is asked to pay attention to the negative AI as the room illumination is increased.

6. The patient is asked to describe the location of the vertical AI in relation to the gap in the horizontal AI. If the vertical AI is perceived as crossing the horizontal AI any place other than at the exact center of the target, the examiner measures the perceived displacement with a centimeter ruler and converts the measurement to prism diopters.

Interpretation of results is made by measuring the displacement of the vertical AI from the central gap of the horizontal AI. If the patient reports seeing a perfect cross, there is presumption of NRC, as this represents an angle A of zero (Figure 5-46). Whether the eyes are straight (ortho posture) is irrelevant if a perfect cross is perceived and reported: Each fovea was stimulated; if there is normal correspondence between the two foveas, a cross will be perceived regardless of the direction in which each eye is positioned.

An example of a non cross perception is shown in Figure 5-47. The right eye is esotropic with ARC. Point a is the representational point that corresponds to the fovea of the left eye. Cyclopean projection shows the vertical AI being visualized to the left, as point a has the directional value of zero, and the fovea projects as a temporal retinal point.

The Hering-Bielschowsky AI test is not valid unless the effect of a coexisting EF is taken into account. Figure 5-48 illustrates this point by adding to the case presented in the previous examples the condition of nasal EF of the right eye. A perfect cross is perceived if the angle of EF (E) and A are the same in direction and magnitude. Points a and e are in the same location on the retina. In such a case, the patient has point e stimulated with the vertical AI during monocular fixation with the right eye. Because this is the same point on the retina that corresponds to the fovea of the left eye, the patient will project the vertical AI in the same direction as the gap in the horizontal line. This is an exceptional case and not the rule: E and A usually are not of the same magnitude, although they most often are in the same direction (e.g., points a and e at

a.
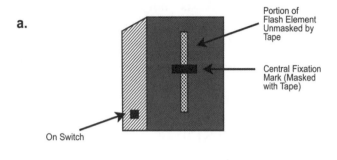

Portion of Flash Element Unmasked by Tape

Central Fixation Mark (Masked with Tape)

On Switch

b.
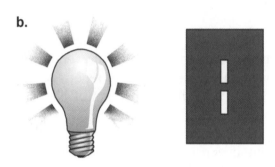

Figure 5-45. Afterimage generators, a. Camera flash attachment, b. Homemade device using light bulb and a mask.

different locations on the nasal retina). Therefore, unless they are in the identical location, a noncross will be perceived.

In an evaluation of correspondence when EF is present, the first step is to measure E using a graduated reticule in an ophthalmoscope. Angle A may then be determined by measuring the separation between the vertical AI and the center of the gap of the horizontal AI and adding to this the magnitude of E. Assume, for example, an E of 5Δ is found (Figure 5-49). If the patient looks at the AI's at 1 m, each centimeter of displacement represents 1Δ. The patient then reports seeing the vertical AI off to the left by 10Δ. This is the measured A but not the true A. The magnitude of E(5Δ in this example) must be added to this measured A to arrive at the true angle of anomaly. It is easily seen that the angle between the fovea and point a is equal to 15Δ (not the 10Δ as measured).

It is not always necessary to use an AI for each eye as in the Hering-Bielschowsky test. The Brock-Givner AI transfer test is another means of measuring A (Figure 5-50). For this test, only one AI is applied to the fovea of the dominant eye, which then is occluded. The projection of the AI

is transferred intracortically to point a of the strabismic eye. Assume, for example, that a strabismic left eye is occluded and the dominant right eye is stimulated with the vertical AI. The occluder is switched to the right eye, and the left eye fixates a black spot on a gray wall at 1 m. The displacement of the fixated spot from the AI represents the angular magnitude of A. It is only when there is no EF (E = 0) that the displacement between the fixated spot and the perceived AI represents true A. Angle E must be added to the measured A to calculate true A. Thus, true A = measured A + the magnitude of EF (At = Am + E).

Conveniently, A and E measurements can be combined into one procedure by using a Haidinger brush (HB) and an AI (Figure 5-50). The separation between the AI and HB represents A. In this example, there is no EF. If there were EF, the HB would be displaced from the fixated black dot, the magnitude representing that of E. In summary, E is measured by the displacement between the dot and the HB, whereas A is measured by the distance between the AI and the HB.

Bifoveal Test of Cüppers

Most tests for ARC have one or more shortcomings, the most common being the contamination of EF. The bifoveal test of Cüppers can eliminate this possibly invalidating factor. It is particularly useful in assessing correspondence in cases of strabismic amblyopia. Testing is done by performing visuoscopy under *binocular* seeing conditions for the measurement of the angle of anomaly (A). This should not be confused with the procedure for measurement of the angle of EF (LE) under *monocular* seeing conditions.

The bifoveal procedure is illustrated in Figure 5-51. Suppose the patient has an esotropia of the right eye. An angled mirror (or a large base-out prism of approximately 40Δ) is placed before the patient's dominant left eye to fixate a penlight off to the side from a distance of 2-3 m (see Figure 5-51a). This is necessary so the patient can maintain seeing under binocular conditions without one eye being occluded by the examiner's head during visuoscopy. The next step is for the examiner to look into the patient's right (amblyopic) eye and observe the image of the star that is projected on the patient's retina. If mydriatics are not used for pupil dilation, a darkened room is recommended.

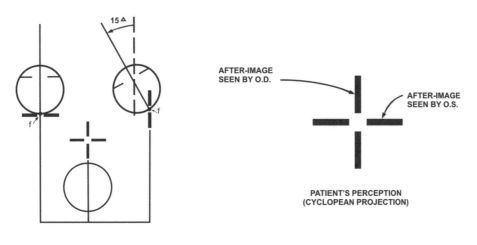

another. If, however, the foveas do not correspond (ARC), as in Figure 5-51c, the patient will report that the star and penlight appear separated in space, even though both foveas are being stimulated. In this case, the examiner should move the star nasalward to find point a so that the penlight and the star are superimposed (see Figure 5-51d). This is necessary because point a corresponds to the fovea of the left eye. The distance from point a to the center of the fovea (f) represents the magnitude of *A*. This distance can be measured by using projected concentric circles of a reticule. If a direct ophthalmoscope without a reticule is used, retinal landmarks, such as the optic disk (or optic disc), can be observed to estimate the magnitude of *A*. Knowing that the center of the disk is normally 15.5 degrees from the center of the fovea helps in estimating the distance from the star to the fovea. Likewise, if the width

Figure 5-46. Hering-Bielschowsky afterimage test in case of esotropia with normal retinal correspondence, (f = fovea; O.D. = oculus dexter; O.S. = oculus sinister.)

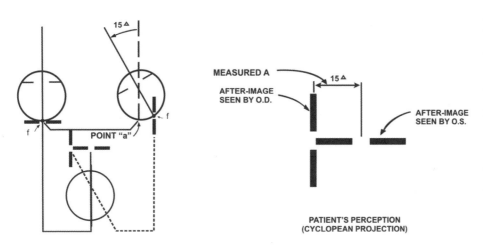

Figure 5-47. Example of harmonious anomalous retinal correspondence, (f = fovea; O.D. = oculus; O.S. = oculus sinister.)

At the same time, the patient is asked to look into the instrument for the star on the grid of the ophthalmoscope (visuoscope). The patient should be aware of both the penlight and the star, unless suppression is very deep and extensive. If so, a red filter can be used to produce a red light stimulus to the left eye. This almost always breaks through any existing suppression.

The examiner's next step is to project the star directly onto the fovea and to ask the patient to report the direction in which the targets are seen. If there is NRC, the patient should report that the penlight and the star are superimposed (see Figure 5-51b), because both foveas correspond to one

of the disk is 5.5 degrees, the first margin of the disk would be 12.75 degrees (23Δ) and the outer margin 18.25 degrees (33Δ) from the center of the fovea (Figure 5-52).

The bifoveal visuoscope test, therefore, takes much of the guesswork out of measuring *A* as compared with other, more subjective methods of testing. In addition to this advantage, the presence of EF does not need to be taken into account (assuming the dominant eye is centrally fixating, which is almost always the case). This is because testing is done under binocular conditions, thereby vitiating any effect of EF that would otherwise come into play if testing were performed under monocular conditions. The disadvantage of the bifoveal visuoscopic test is that a high level of patient cooperation must be maintained; otherwise, either testing is impossible or results are unreliable. Testing is sometimes not feasible in young children.

Major Amblyoscope

The major amblyoscope can be used to detect and calculate angle *A*. The Synoptophore (see Figure 5-12) has a long history in the field of strabismus diagnosis and therapy and is still in use today. Each tube of the Synoptophore has a mirror placed at 45 degrees and a +7-D eyepiece lens. Test targets are placed at optical infinity. (Sketches showing the direction of movement of the carriage arm to create horizontal prismatic demands are presented in Figure 5-13.)

The procedure for measuring the objective angle of deviation (called the alternate exclusion method) using this instrument is as follows:

1. The main power switch is turned on, and the patient is instructed to look into the instrument. The chin and forehead rests and the interpupillary distance setting are adjusted properly for the patient. The illumination for each tube also is adjusted by setting the rheostat to approximately 8.

2. First-degree targets that are central in size are used (see Figure 5-14). For example, the X target may be placed in one tube and the square target in the other. The patient is instructed always to look at the center of each target.

3. Each tube light is alternately doused (occluded) by means of the two small button switches near

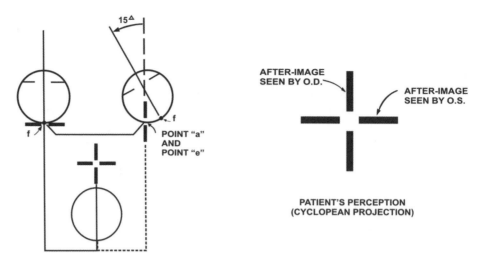

Figure 5-48. Example of esotropia with anomalous retinal correspondence and eccentric fixation. In this particular case, the angle of eccentric fixation is the same as the angle of anomaly, (f = fovea; O.D. = oculus dexter; O.S. = oculus sinister.)

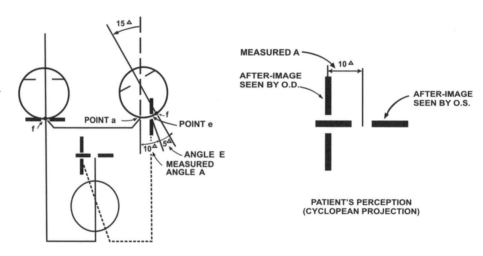

Figure 5-49. Esotropia with harmonious anomalous retinal correspondence and nasal eccentric fixation, in which the angle of eccentric fixation and the angle of anomaly are unequal. Angles A and E must be summed to determine the true angle of anomaly, (f = fovea; O.D. = oculus dexter; O.S. = oculus sinister.)

the front of the control panel. The alternate dousing of each target makes this an alternate cover test in an instrument rather than in true space.

4. The examiner neutralizes the lateral movement of the eyes by adjusting the position of the tube of the patient's nondominant eye. Meanwhile, the tube for the dominant eye is maintained on zero (primary position of gaze). When the conjugate movement is neutralized using a bracketing technique, the objective angle (*H*) is determined. The magnitude is read directly from the prism diopter scale. The direction of

the deviation (eso or exo) is noted by observing the final positions of the tubes, as illustrated in Figure 5-13.

Hirschberg testing can also be performed with a Synoptophore by observing the positions of the corneal reflections of the light from the two tubes. This method is particularly appropriate for determining angle *H* when amblyopia is present in one eye and monocular fixation is inaccurate. For this procedure, the instrument's lights should be turned up to the maximum intensity and the room lights dimmed. The patient must be properly positioned so that the examiner has a good view of the patient's eyes to judge the positions of the corneal light reflexes. The accuracy of the procedure is limited to approximately 5Δ. A recommended procedure follows:

1. Only one target, placed before the dominant eye, is used, and the patient's fixation is directed to the center of that target (e.g., the fish target). The tube must be maintained in the primary position (zero on the scale).

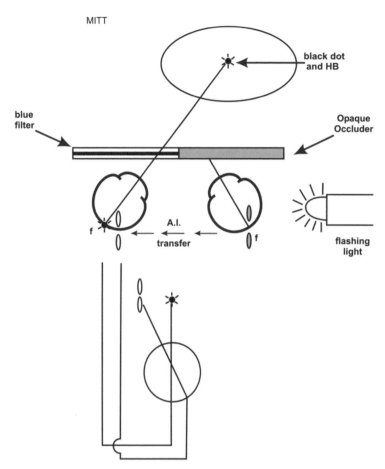

Figure 5-50. Brock-Givner AI Transfer Test. Combination of the Haidinger brush (HB) superimposed on the black dot (seen by left eye) and a vertical afterimage (A.I.; also seen by left eye but transferred from the right eye). Flashing light near right eye enhances the transferred afterimage seen by the left eye. (MITT = Bernell Macular Integrity Tester-Trainer.)

2. Angle kappa (*K*) of the fixating eye is estimated. The tube of the nondominant eye is adjusted so that the corneal reflection is in the same relative position in each eye. (The position of the reflex should look like angle *K*.) The examiner should sight from behind the tube to ensure the greatest accuracy.

3. The method of limits (bracketing technique) is used to determine the symmetric position of the corneal reflections. Then the magnitude of the objective angle (*H*) is read directly from the prism diopter scale of the nondominant eye.

The procedure for finding the horizontal subjective angle (*S*) with the Synoptophore is as follows:

1. After the instrument has been adjusted properly for the patient, the examiner should insert two first-degree targets, one before each of the patient's eyes, of sufficient size to avoid or minimize suppression (e.g., the fish and tank

targets). Because this is a binocular test, neither eye is occluded.

2. The patient is instructed to maintain fixation constantly on the center of the dominant eye's target (e.g., fish), which is set to the zero position on the scale.

3. The patient (or the examiner, if necessary) adjusts the position of the nondominant eye's tube (e.g., with the tank) until the two targets appear superimposed (i.e., the fish inside the tank). If suppression occurs, the illumination can be increased for the suppressing eye or dimmed for the dominant eye.

4. The magnitude of the angle *S* is read directly from the scale, and the measurement is taken several times, approaching angle *S* from both sides (bracketing technique) to increase accuracy.

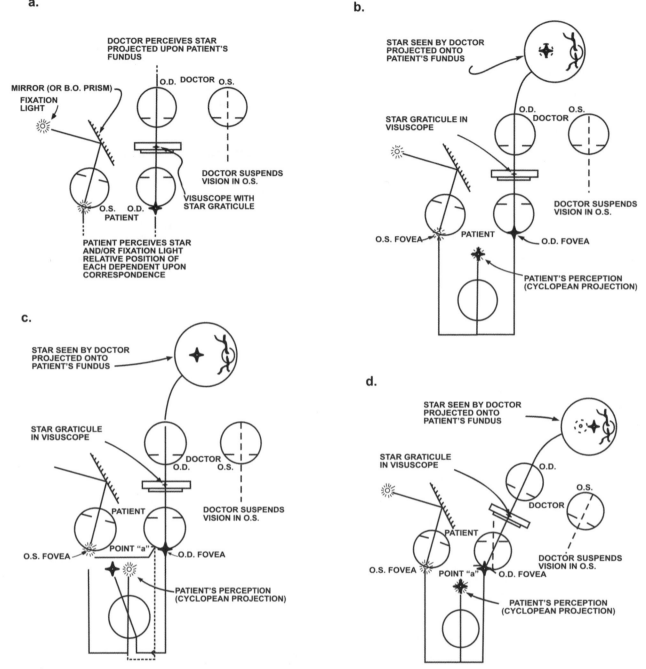

a.

DOCTOR PERCEIVES STAR PROJECTED UPON PATIENT'S FUNDUS

O.D. DOCTOR O.S.

MIRROR (OR B.O. PRISM)

FIXATION LIGHT

DOCTOR SUSPENDS VISION IN O.S.

VISUSCOPE WITH STAR GRATICULE

O.S. O.D. PATIENT

PATIENT PERCEIVES STAR AND/OR FIXATION LIGHT RELATIVE POSITION OF EACH DEPENDENT UPON CORRESPONDENCE

b.

STAR SEEN BY DOCTOR PROJECTED ONTO PATIENT'S FUNDUS

O.D. DOCTOR O.S.

STAR GRATICULE IN VISUSCOPE

DOCTOR SUSPENDS VISION IN O.S.

O.S. FOVEA PATIENT O.D. FOVEA

PATIENT'S PERCEPTION (CYCLOPEAN PROJECTION)

c.

STAR SEEN BY DOCTOR PROJECTED ONTO PATIENT'S FUNDUS

STAR GRATICULE IN VISUSCOPE

DOCTOR O.D. O.S.

DOCTOR SUSPENDS VISION IN O.S.

PATIENT

O.S. FOVEA POINT "a" O.D. FOVEA

PATIENT'S PERCEPTION (CYCLOPEAN PROJECTION)

d.

STAR SEEN BY DOCTOR PROJECTED ONTO PATIENT'S FUNDUS

STAR GRATICULE IN VISUSCOPE

O.D.

O.S.

DOCTOR

PATIENT

DOCTOR SUSPENDS VISION IN O.S.

O.S. FOVEA POINT "a" O.D. FOVEA

PATIENT'S PERCEPTION (CYCLOPEAN PROJECTION)

Figure 5-51. The bifoveal test of Cüppers, a. Doctor's right eye views the patient's right eye by means of visuoscopy. The star is seen by the doctor and the patient. An angled mirror (or a large base-out [B.O.] prism) before the patient's left eye avoids obstruction to seeing by the left eye. b. Example of normal correspondence, c. Example of anomalous correspondence, d. Star must be projected onto point a in order for a patient with anomalous retinal correspondence to achieve superimposition of the pen light and the star. (O.D. = oculus dexter; O.S. = oculus sinister.)

Determining the subjective angle sometimes is difficult, due either to deep suppression or to horror fusionis. Vertical dissociation can sometimes overcome these obstacles, allowing the measurement of angle S. Using the vertical adjustment, the Synoptophore target to the nondominant eye is elevated 10Δ or more above the other target. The nondominant eye's target is then moved horizontally until the one appears exactly above the other. This value represents the subjective angle. Another procedure that is effective is using a large first-degree target before the nondominant eye while the patient is fixating a small target with the other eye (e.g., the X and the sentry box) (see Figure 5-14).

After angles H and S are measured on the Synoptophore, it is a simple matter to calculate angle A ($A = H - S$). Measurement accuracy must be taken into account when determining the presence of ARC.

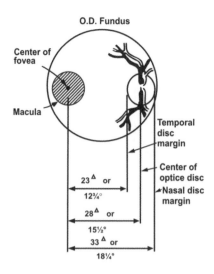

O.D. Fundus

Center of fovea

Macula

Temporal disc margin

Center of optice disc

Nasal disc margin

23△ or

12¾°

28△ or

15½°

33△ or

18¼°

Figure 5-52. Useful dimensions of the fundus for estimating the magnitude of the angle of anomaly when using the bifoveal test. (O.D. = oculus dexter.)

Allowance of 1-2△ error may be necessary for small angles, and up to 5△ should be allowed for large angles of strabismus in comparing *H* and *S*.

Another quick check for ARC on the Synoptophore is the unilateral douse target test. This is done after angle *S* has been measured and the targets appear to be superimposed. The examiner simply shuts off (douses) the illumination to the target of the dominant eye and watches for movement of the nondominant eye. If the nondominant eye makes a horizontal movement to fixate the center of the target, ARC is presumed to be present, and there is a difference between angles *S* and *H*. This test, in effect, is a unilateral cover test. The size of the movement represents the magnitude of angle *A*.

For example, suppose a patient has a 15△ right esotropia (angle *H*; i.e., 15△ base-out by alternate exclusion as measured on the Synoptophore). The fish and the tank, however, appear to be superimposed at 9△ base-out (angle *S*), which represents a significant difference from the measured objective angle. ARC is, therefore, suspected. On the douse target test, when the left eye is doused, the examiner observes an outward movement of the right eye of approximately 6△ to pick up fixation on the target. This is a positive douse target test, confirming the presence of ARC. (As discussed previously, however, any EF must be taken into account.)

Bagolini Striated Lenses

The Bagolini striated lens test is a quick, simple, and informative clinical test for ARC in strabismic patients. Striations in Bagolini lenses are so fine that the patient is unaware of them, therefore making the test a fairly natural one for the subjective angle (*S*). The striations cause a streak of light to be visible when the fixation target is a bright spot of light, similar to the effect of a Maddox rod (Figure 5-53). Various perceptions during this test are illustrated in Figure 5-54. Bagolini lenses do not disrupt binocularity or significantly reduce visual acuity or contrast sensitivity.[92] A patient bifoveally fixating a penlight will see the penlight at the intersection of the streaks, as in Figure 5-54c. If the patient has a manifest strabismic deviation whereby bifoveal fixation is not taking place, diplopic images of the light occur, unless suppression is too intense and extensive. Often, however, only a portion of one line will be missing, as in Figures 5-54d and 5-54e. An esotropic patient is normally expected to have homonymous diplopia and will report seeing the lights above the intersection of the streaks (see Figure 5-54f). In contrast, an exotropic patient with heteronymous diplopia would be expected to report seeing the lights below the intersection (see Figure 5-54g).

The preceding examples presume NRC. However, if an esotrope has ARC of the harmonious type, the patient is expected to report seeing one light centered in the intersection of the streaks (see Figure 5-54c), as would a patient who is nonstrabismic and bifixating. The reason for the strabismic's apparently normal response is that angle *S* is zero in HARC. The clinician will not be misled if the manifest deviation is observed while listening to the patient's report of seeing the light centered at the intersection of the two streaks. This is obviously a case of ARC, because *S* is zero and *H* is of a conspicuous magnitude. If, however, the strabismus is small and difficult to detect by direct observation, the unilateral cover test is necessary. (This is analogous to the douse target test using the major amblyoscope.) The clinician watches for any movement of the uncovered nondominant eye when the dominant eye is occluded. A significant movement means that *H* is greater than zero, which confirms the presence of ARC.

von Noorden and Maumenee[93] suggested that the Bagolini test is not useful in diagnosing cases of UNHARC in which *S* is a magnitude other than zero. We believe, however, that the following procedure is useful in UNHARC cases. The

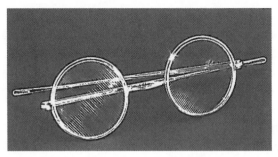

Figure 5-53. Bagolini striated lenses with visible streaks, causing an effect analogous to Maddox rods. (Photo courtesy of Bernell Corporation.)

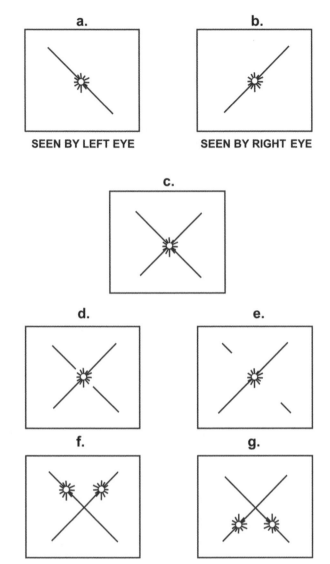

Figure 5-54. Patient's view when looking through Bagolini striated lenses and fixating a penlight. a. Orientation of streak seen by left eye. b. Orientation of streak seen by right eye. c. Perception when the patient is bifoveally fixating, indicating fusion. This same perception indicates harmonious anomalous retinal correspondence if there is a manifest deviation. d. Central suppression of the left eye. e. Peripheral suppression of the left eye. f. Esotropia with normal retinal correspondence is indicated, although this finding may also mean that there is a manifest subjective eso deviation in a case of unharmonious anomalous retinal correspondence. g. An exotropia with normal retinal correspondence is indicated, although this type of response could occur also in an exotropia with unharmonious correspondence.

examiner begins by finding out from the patient where the streaks intersect. If they cross below the lights, as in an eso deviation, base-out prism is increasingly introduced until the patient reports that the light is centered at the intersection of the streaks. At this time, the unilateral cover test is conducted to determine whether there is any movement of the uncovered eye. The patient has UNHARC if there is any significant movement. In this case, S is equal to the base-out prism power necessary for attainment of the centered pattern. (When the patient is strabismic and S is not zero, the ARC is unharmonious.) The estimated magnitude of A is represented by the magnitude of the movement of the uncovered eye on the unilateral cover test during this procedure. This test should be done quickly to avoid possible contamination of prism adaptation.

The great majority of strabismic patients with ARC show HARC on the Bagolini test. HARC is an ideal antidiplopic adaptation for a strabismic individual in natural seeing conditions at school, work, or play; some peripheral binocularity, with its many benefits, often is preserved. The Bagolini test is relatively natural; clinicians find the highest prevalence of ARC using this test as compared with other, less natural clinical methods.

Color Fusion

Color fusion is also known as luster. The most efficacious way to evaluate whether color fusion is present is by having the patient wear colored filters (usually red on the right eye and green on the left eye) while viewing a brightly illuminated, translucent, gray screen containing no contours. Normally, the patient reports a mixture of the red and green, perceived as a muddy yellow or brown, with some color rivalry taking place. Testing at the centration point helps to elicit this response in many esotropic patients. The centration point addi-

tion lens (add) in diopters (D_{cpa}) is calculated by dividing the farpoint horizontal objective angle (H_f) at farpoint (6 m) by the interpupillary distance in centimeters (IPD_{cm}).

$$D_{cpa} = H_f / IPD_{cm}$$

For example, a 24Δ constant right esotropic patient having a 6-cm interpupillary distance would require at least a +4.00-D add to bring targets into focus at the position in space where the eyes cross. Wearing this high-plus add in a trial frame and moving to distance of 25 cm from the screen, this esotropic patient has the optimum conditions to demonstrate true color fusion. (High base-in prisms may help to achieve perception of color fusion in an exotropic patient.) Color fusion is determined by alternately occluding each eye to demonstrate what a monocular response looks like (i.e., purely red or purely green). Under binocular conditions, the patient then is asked if his or her percept looks different as compared with monocular viewing. Color fusion is indicated if the patient reports a yellowish or brownish blending of colors.

A split field is not true color fusion but is indicative of ARC (see Figure 5-44). This is the Swann split-field effect described previously. We have found that patients who give an evenly split response often have HARC, whereas a field not split evenly down the middle suggests UNHARC. Although color fusion testing is not completely reliable, it does seem to have some diagnostic and prognostic value. For example, a patient who shows a Swann split-field effect without contours in the visual field has a poorer prognosis for successful treatment of ARC than does a patient reporting color fusion over the entire field.

REFERENCES

1. Revell MJ. Strabismus: A History of Orthoptic Techniques. London: Barrie and Jenkins, 1971.
2. Hofstetter H, Griffin J, Berman M, Everson R. Dictionary of Visual Science and Related Clinical Terms, 5th ed. Boston: Butterworth-Heinemann, 2000:79.
3. Leske D, Holmes J. Maximum angle of horizontal strabismus consistent with true stereopsis. J AAPOS 2004;8:28-34.
4. Fawcett S, Birch E. Interobserver test-retest reliability of the Randot Preschool Stereoacuity test. J AAPOS 2000;4:354-8.
5. Hofstetter H, Griffin J, Berman M, Everson R. Dictionary of Visual Science and Related Clinical Terms, 5th ed. Boston: Butterworth-Heinemann, 2000:488.
6. von Noorden G. Binocular Vision and Ocular Motility: Theory and Management of Strabismus, 4th ed. St. Louis: Mosby, 1990.
7. Smith E, Levi D, Manny R, et al. The relationship between binocular rivalry and strabismic suppression. Invest Ophthalmol Vis Sci. 1985;26:80-7.
8. Norcia A, Harrad R, Brown R. Changes in cortical activity during suppression in stereoblindness. Neuroreport 2000;11:1007-12.
9. Braddick O. Binocularity in infancy. Eye 1996;10:182-8.
10. Kumagami T, Zhang B, Smith E, Chino Y. Effect of onset age of strabismus on the binocular responses of neurons in the monkey visual cortex. Invest Ophthalmol Vis Sci. 2000;41:948-54.
11. Oguz V. The effects of experimentally induced anisometropia on stereopsis. J Pediatr Ophthalmol Strabismus 2000;37:214-8.
12. Yildirim C, Altinsoy H. Distance alternate-letter suppression test of objective assessment of sensorial status in intermittent exotropia. Eur J Ophthalmol. 2000;10:4-10.
13. Jampolsky A. Characteristics of suppression in strabismus. Arch Ophthalmol. 1955;54:683-96.
14. Pratt-Johnson J, MacDonald A. Binocular visual field in strabismus. Can J Ophthalmol. 1976;11:37-41.
15. Pott J, Oosterveen D, van Hof-van Duin J. Screening for suppression in young children; the polaroid suppression test. J Pediatr Ophthalmol Strabismus 1998;35:216-22.
16. Ciuffreda K, Levi D, Selenow A. Amblyopia: Basic and Clinical Aspects. Boston: Butterworth-Heinemann, 1991:13-17,24,26,43-136.
17. Ciuffreda K, Levi D, Selenow A. Amblyopia: Basic and Clinical Aspects. Stoneham, MA.: Butterworth-Heinemann, 1991:29-37.
18. Schalij-Delfos N, de Graaf M, Treffers W, al e. Long term follow up of premature infants: detection of strabismus, amblyopia, and refractive errors. Br J Ophthalmol. 2000;84:963-7.
19. von Noorden G, Frank J. Relationship between amblyopia and the angle of strabismus. Am Orthopt J. 1976;26:31-3.
20. Helveston E. The incidence of amblyopia ex anopsia in young adult males in Minnesota in 1962-63. Am J Ophthalmol. 1965;60:75-7.
21. Glover L, Brewer W. An ophthalmologic review of more than twenty thousand men at the Altoona Induction Center. Am J Ophthalmol. 1944;27:346-8.
22. Schapero M. Amblyopia. Philadelphia: Chilton, 1971.
23. Flynn J, Cassady J. Current trends in amblyopia therapy. Ophthalmology 1978;85:428-50.
24. Smith E, Hung L, Harwerth R. The degree of image degradation and the depth of amblyopia. Invest Ophthalmol Vis Sci.;41:3774-81.
25. Weakley D. The association between nonstrabismus anisometropia, amblyopia, and subnormal binocularity. Ophthalmology 2001;108:163-71.
26. Tanlamai T, Goss D. Prevalence of monocular amblyopia among anisometropes. Am J Optom Physiol Opt. 1979;56:704-15.
27. Kivlin J, Flynn J. Therapy of anisometropic amblyopia. J Pediatr Ophthalmol. 1981;18:47-56.
28. Ingram R, Walker G, Wilson J, al e. A first attempt to prevent amblyopia and squint by spectacle correction of abnormal refractions from age 1 year. Br J Ophthalmol. 1985;69:851-3.
29. Tomac S, Birdal E. Effects of anisometropia on binocularity. J Pediatr Ophthalmol Strabismus 2001;38:27-33.
30. Agatston H. Ocular malingering. Arch Ophthalmol. 1944;31:223-31.
31. Pratt-Johnson J, Wee H, Ellis S. Suppression associated with esotropia. Can J Ophthalmol. 1967;2:284-91.
32. Fern KD. Visual acuity outcome in isometropic hyperopia. Optom Vis Sci. 1989;66(10):649-58.
33. Pediatric Eye Disease Investigator Group. Treatment of bilateral refractive amblyopia in children three to less than 10 years of age. Am J Ophthalm 2007;144(4):487-96.
34. Brent H, Lewis T, Maurer D. Effect of binocular deprivation from cataracts on development of Snellen acuity. Invest Ophthalmol Vis Sci. 1986;27(suppl):51.
35. Norcia A, Tyler G. Spatial frequency sweep VEP: visual acuity during the first year of life. Vision Res. 1985;25:1399-408.
36. Keech R, Kutschke P. Upper age limit for the development of amblyopia. J Pediatr Ophthalmol Strabismus 1995;32:89-93.
37. Worth C. Squint: Its Causes, Pathology and Treatment. Philadelphia: Blakiston, 1903.
38. Levi D, Klein S. Equivalent intrinsic blur in amblyopia. Vision Res. 1990;30:1995-2022.
39. Yu C, Levi D. Naso-temporal asymmetry of spatial interactions in strabismic amblyopia. Optom Vis Sci. 1998;75:424-32.
40. Ciuffreda K, Kenyon R, Stark L. Increased drift in amblyopic eyes. Br J Ophthalmol. 1980;64:7-14.
41. Schor C, Flom M. Eye Position Control and Visual Acuity in Strabismus Amblyopia. In: Lennerstrand G, Bach-y-rita P, eds.

Basic Mechanisms of Ocular Motility and Their Clinical Implications. New York: Pergamon Press, 1975.

42. Bedell H, Flom M. Monocular spatial distortion in strabismic amblyopia. Invest Ophthalmol Vis Sci. 1981;20:263-8.

43. Levi D, Klein S. Difference in discrimination for gratings between strabismic and anisometropic amblyopes. Invest Ophthalmol Vis Sci. 1982;23:398-407.

44. Bedell H, Flom M. Normal and abnormal space perception. Am J Optom Physiol Opt. 1983;60:426-35.

45. Maxwell G, Lemij H, Gollewijn H. Conjugacy of saccades in deep amblyopia. Invest Ophthalmol Vis Sci. 1995;36:2514-22.

46. Kenyon R, Ciuffreda K, Stark L. Dynamic vergence eye movements in strabismus and amblyopia: asymmetric vergence. Br J Ophthalmol. 1981;65:167-76.

47. Greenwald M, Folk E. Afferent pupillary defects in amblyopia. J Pediatr Ophthalmol Strabismus 1983;20:63-7.

48. Kase M, Nagata R, Yoshida A, Hanada I. Pupillary light reflex in amblyopia. Invest Ophthalmol Vis Sci. 1984;25:467-71.

49. Boman D, Kertesz A. Fusional responses of strabismics to foveal and extrafoveal stimulation. Invest Ophthalmol Vis Sci. 1985;26:1731-9.

50. Boonstra F, Koopmans S, Houtman W. Fusional vergence in microstrabismus. Doc Ophthalmol. 1988;70:221-6.

51. Flom M, Heath G, Takahashi E. Contour interaction and visual resolution: contralateral effects. Science 1963;142:979-80.

52. Ferris FI, Bailey I. Standardizing the methodology for measuring of visual acuity for clinical research studies. Guidelines from the Eye Care Technology Forum. Opthalmology 1996;103:181-2.

53. Morad Y, Werker E, Nemet P. Visual acuity tests using chart, line, and single optotype in healthy and amblyopic children. J AAPOS 1999;3:94-7.

54. Flom M. New concepts on visual acuity. Optom Wkly 1966;53:1026-32.

55. Davidson D, Eskridge J. Reliability of visual acuity measures of amblyopic eyes. Am J Optom Physiol Opt. 1977;54:756-66.

56. Birch E, Strauber S, Beck R, Holmes J. Comparision of the Amblyopia Treatment Study HOTV and the Electronic-Early Treatment of Diabetic Retinopathy Study visual acuity protocols in amblyopic children 5 to 11 years. J AAPOS 2009;13(1):75-8.

57. Cotter S, Tarczy-Hornoch K, Song E, Lin J, Borchert M, Azen S, Varma R, Multi-Ethnic Pediatric Eye Disease Study Group. Fixation preference and visual acuity testing in a population-based cohort of preschool children with amblyopia risk factors. Ophthalmol 2009;116(1):145-53.

58. Schor C, Levi D. Disturbances of small-field horizontal and vertical optokinetic nystagmus in amblyopia. Invest Ophthalmol Vis Sci. 1980;19:668-83.

59. White C, Eason R. Evoked cortical potentials in relation to certain aspects of visual perception. Psychol Monogr. 1966;80(24):1-14.

60. Harding G. The visual evoked response. Adv Ophthal. 1974;28:2-28.

61. Sherman J. Visual evoked potential (VEP): basic concepts and clinical applications. J Am Optom Assoc. 1979;50:19-30.

62. Ridder W, Rouse M. Predicting potential acuities in amblyopia: predicting post-therapy in amblyopes. Doc Ophthalmol. 2007;114:135-45.

63. Selenow A, Guiffreda K, Mozlin R, Rumpf D. Prognostic value of laser interferometric visual acuity in amblyopia therapy. Invest Ophthalmol Vis Sci. 1986;27:273-7.

64. Hallden U. An explanation of Haidinger's brushes. Arch Ophthalmol. 1957;57:393-9.

65. Irvine S. Amblyopia exanopsia. Observations on retinal inhibition, scotoma, projection, sight difference, discrimination, and visual acuity. Trans Am Ophthalmol Soc. 1948;46:531.

66. Ammann E. Einige Beobachtunger bei den Funtion sprufungen in der Spechsturde: Zentrales Sehen-sehen der glau-komatosen-schen der Amblyopen. Klin Monatsbl Augenheilkd 1921;66:564-73.

67. Caloroso E, Flom M. Influence of luminance on visual acuity in amblyopia. Am J Optom Physiol Opt. 1969;46:189-95.

68. von Noorden G, Burian H. Visual acuity in normal and amblyopic patients under reduced illumination: II. The visual acuity at various levels of illumination. Arch Ophthalmol. 1959;62:396-9.

69. von Noorden G. Binocular Vision and Ocular Motility: Theory and Management of Strabismus, 4th ed. St. Louis: Mosby, 1990.

70. Eibschitz-Tsimhoni M, Friedman T, Naor J, et al. Early screening for amblyogenic risk factors lowers the prevalence and severity of amblyopia. J AAPOS 2000;4:194-9.

71. Laws D, Noonan C, Ward A, Chandna A. Binocular fixation pattern and visual acuity in children with strabismic amblyopia. J Pediatr Ophthalmol Strabismus 2000;37:24-8.

72. Vision in Preschoolers Study Group. Findings from the Vision in Preschoolers (VIP) Study. Optom Vis Sci 2009;86:619-23.

73. Flom M. Corresponding and disparate retinal points in normal and anomalous correspondence. Am J Optom Physiol Opt. 1980;57:656-65.

74. Flom M. Treatment of Binocular Anomalies in Children. In: Hirsch M, Wick R, eds. Vision of Children. Philadelphia: Chilton, 1963.

75. Burian H. Fusional movements in permanent strabismus. A study of the role of the central and peripheral retinal regions in the act of binocular vision in squint. Arch Ophthalmol. 1941;26:626.

76. Lyle T, Wybar K. Practical Orthoptics in the Treatment of Squint, 5th ed. In. Springfield, III.: Charles CThomas, 1967.

77. Kramer M. Clinical Orthoptics, 2nd ed. St. Louis: Mosby, 1953.

78. Krimsky E. The Management of Binocular Imbalance. Philadelphia: Lea & Febiger, 1948.

79. Bielschowsky A. Congenital and acquired deficiencies of fusion. Am J Ophthalmol. 1935;18:925-37.

80. Nelson J. Binocular Vision: Disparity Detection and Anomalous Correspondence. In: Edwards K, Llewellyn R, eds. Optometry. Newton, Mass.: Butterworth-Heinemann, 1988.

81. Cleary M, Houston C, McFadzean R, Dutton G. Recovery in microtropia: implications for aetiology and neurophysiology. Br J Ophthalmol. 1998;82:225-31.

82. Burian H. Anomalous retinal correspondence, its essence and its significance in prognosis and treatment. Am J Ophthalmol. 1951;34:237-53.

83. Morgan M. Anomalous correspondence interpreted as a motor phenomenon. Am J Optom. 1961;38:131-48.

84. Kerr K. Anomalous correspondence-the cause or consequence of strabismus? Optom Vis Sci. 1998;75:17-22.

85. Hallden U. Fusional phenomena in anomalous correspondence. Acta Ophthalmol Suppl. 1952;37:1-93.

86. Helveston E, von Noorden G, Williams F. Retinal correspondence in the A and V pattern. Am Orthopt J. 1970;20:22.

87. Flom M, Kerr K. Determination of retinal correspondence, multiple-testing results and the depth of anomaly concept. Arch Ophthalmol. 1967;77:200-13.

88. Bagolini B, Tittarelli R. Sensorio-motorial anomalies in strabismus (anomalous movements). Doc Ophthalmol. 1976;41:23.

89. Enos M. Anomalous correspondence. Am J Ophthalmol. 1950;33:1907-13.

90. Hugonnier R, Hugonnier S, Troutman S. Strabismus, Heterophoria, Ocular Motor Paralysis. St. Louis: Mosby, 1969.

91. Flom M. A minimum strabismus examination. J Am Optom Assoc. 1956;27:642-9.

92. Cheng D, Woo G, Irving E, et al. Scattering properties of Bagolini lenses and their effects on spatial vision. Ophthalmic Physiol Opt. 1998;18:438-45.

93. von Noorden G, Maumenee A. Atlas of Strabismus. St. Louis: Mosby, 1967

Chapter 6 / Diagnosis and Prognosis

Establishing a Diagnosis	165	Other Approaches	181
Prognosis	166	Case Examples	181
Functional Cure of Strabismus	167	Poor Prognosis	182
Prognostic Variables of the Deviation	169	Case 1	182
Associated Conditions	170	Case 2	182
Other Factors	172	Case 3	183
Cosmetic Cure of Strabismus	172	Poor to Fair Prognosis	183
Heterophoria	174	Case 4	183
Modes of Treatment	175	Case 5	184
Lenses	175	Fair Prognosis	184
Prisms	175	Case 6	184
Occlusion	175	Fair to Good Prognosis	185
Vision Therapy	175	Case 7	185
Extraocular Muscle Surgery	176	Case 8	185
General Approach	176	Case 9	186
Adjustable Suture Procedure	178	Good Prognosis	186
Surgical Considerations	178	Case 10	186
Pharmacologic Treatment	179	Case 11	187
Botulinum Toxin	180	Case 12	187

A valid prognosis cannot be made unless there is a complete diagnosis. Most of this chapter is devoted to the diagnosis and prognosis of strabismus rather than of heterophoria, because there is a full range of prognosis, from poor to good, in cases of strabismus (Table 6-1). In contrast, the prognostic range in cases of heterophoria is more limited because there are relatively few complications (e.g., anomalous retinal correspondence [ARC], lack of fusional vergence, and deep and extensive suppression) that adversely affect successful treatment. Because the prognosis for achieving a functional cure is generally good, only a brief discussion is given to the prognosis of heterophoria.

Table 6-1. Range of Prognosis in Strabismus and Chance of Functional Cure

Prognosis	Chance of Functional Cure (%)
Poor	0-20
Poor to fair	21-40
Fair	41-60
Fair to good	61-80
Good	81-100

ESTABLISHING A DIAGNOSIS

The first part of a complete diagnosis of strabismus is the test results of each of the nine variables of deviation of the visual axes: comitancy, frequency, direction, magnitude, accommodative-convergence/accommodation (AC/A) ratio, variability, cosmesis, eye laterality, and eye dominance. The next part includes associated conditions: suppression, amblyopia, abnormal fixation, ARC, horror fusionis, and any visual skills inefficiencies.

A case history also helps establish the exact diagnosis and is necessary for a valid prognosis. Furthermore, time of onset, mode of onset, and duration of strabismus, refractive history, treatment given, and developmental history of the patient are all vitally important in determining the prognosis. The doctor must also assess the results of additional evaluative procedures such as prism adaptation, special cover testing, vertical and cyclo deviation testing, prolonged occlusion, and testing for sensory fusion at the centration point.

A good diagnostic statement is not a listing of clinical data but rather a succinct and understandable account that includes the distinguishing features and nature of the condition. The diagnostic statement must be well written in clinical records and reports, not only for conceptual clarity but also for medicolegal purposes. One acid test of a good diagnostic statement is whether it can be communicated completely and concisely. Examples are given in this chapter to illustrate succinct diagnostic clarity.

PROGNOSIS

Prognosis is the prediction for success by a specified means of treatment. As to binocular anomalies, prognosis pertains to the chance for a favorable outcome by the use of lenses, prisms, occlusion, vision therapy, surgery, medication, mental effort, or any combination of these methods of treatment. After all necessary testing has been completed and a thorough diagnosis has been made, the doctor makes a prognosis of the case. From this, appropriate recommendations for the patient can be made. There are two types of prognoses depending on the goal of treatment. The doctor can describe the chances for either a *functional* cure or a *cosmetic* cure.

Functional Cure of Strabismus

The Flom criteria for functional cure of strabismus has been the standard for assessing success by any or all treatments for many years.[1] Flom's criteria made feasible the comparison of results from various studies. Flom,[2] however, later modified the criteria for clinical purposes. In the past, the criteria for functional cure of strabismus, according to Flom,[1] included the presence of clear, comfortable, single, binocular vision at all distances, from the farpoint to a normal nearpoint of convergence. There should be stereopsis, although Flom[1] did not specify the stereoacuity threshold. The patient also should achieve normal ranges of motor fusion. The deviation may be manifest up to 1 % of the time, providing that the patient is aware of diplopia whenever this happens (i.e., patient knows the deviation is not latent but is manifest at that time). This should mean that the strabismus may occur only approximately 5-10 minutes per day and that the patient has clear, single, comfortable binocular vision during the rest of his or her normal waking hours. Corrective lenses and small amounts of prism may be worn, but prismatic power is limited to 5Δ. In a later publication, Flom[2] dropped the requirement for stereopsis, diplopia awareness, normal ranges of motor fusion, and the limit of 5Δ, stating that "a reasonable amount of prism" meets the criteria.

Flom listed another category of cure that he called *almost cured*. The criteria for this classification allow for stereopsis to be lacking and for the deviation to be manifest up to 5% of the time. Fairly large amounts of prism may be used as long as there is comfortable binocular vision. The remaining criteria for functional cure must be met. The third category was called *moderate improvement*. The stipulation here was that there must be improvement in more than one defect. Flom's fourth category of cure was *slight improvement*, which indicated improvement in only one defect (e.g., amblyopia reduced). A final category was that of *no improvement* as a result of therapy.

Flom's current criteria for functional cure are as follows: (1) maintenance of bifoveal fixation in the ordinary situations of life 99% of the time; (2) clear vision that is generally comfortable; (3) bifixation in all fields of gaze and distances as close as a few centimeters from the eyes; and (4) wearing of corrective lenses and a reasonable amount of prism.[2]

We concur with the new cure criteria set forth by Flom,[2] in which his former category of *almost cured* can be incorporated. We also recommend keeping Flom's categories of *moderate improvement* and *slight improvement*.

Although not included within the stated cure criteria, we believe the level of stereopsis is clinically useful in evaluating functional success. Manley[3] indicated that a stereothreshold of 67 seconds of arc (for *contoured* tests) is the differentiating value between monofixation pattern and bifoveal fusion and, for example, that on the Stereo Fly tests "central fusion (bifixation) must be present for circles 7 to 9 to be answered correctly." This compares closely with the findings on the Pola-Mirror test, in which central suppression was found in all patients whose stereoacuity on *contoured* tests was worse than 60 seconds of arc, whereas all those whose stereoacuity was better than 60 seconds passed the Pola-Mirror test.[4] Therefore, we believe the cutoff value of 67 seconds or arc is reasonable and should be included in the criteria. This stereoacuity criterion can be one of the means of determining whether strabismus is completely eliminated (i.e., when there is bifoveal fixation without suppression). A realistic cutoff for *noncontoured* stereoacuity tests would be 100 seconds of arc. Although there are exceptions, the general rule is that stereoacuity is the "barometer" of binocular status.

It should be pointed out that a patient who has made either moderate improvement or slight improvement may not be much better off from a practical standpoint. These labels are sometimes nothing more than academic, as they are useful only in statistical analyses of reported studies. For example, suppose ARC is temporarily eliminated but the patient still has esotropia, suppression, and the like. The important question that should be answered by the doctor is whether the patient is actually any better off as a result of having had an improvement. There are, however, possible psychological benefits for these patients when they feel they have been helped. These results should be evaluated and put in their proper perspective.

However, most reported studies giving rates of cure have not incorporated such complete and definitive criteria as those of Flom.[1,2] Consequently, it is difficult to evaluate their significance. One of the exceptions, however, is the survey by Ludlam.[5] In this study of 149 strabismic patients, the previous criteria of Flom were followed strictly. Treatment did not include surgery or drugs, which kept the study "clean" as compared to most others, in which the effects of surgery cannot be delineated from nonsurgical methods. According to Ludlam,[5] the reported functional cure rate was 33%, and the almost-cured rate was 40%, with the remaining percentage being distributed among the other categories.

Ludlam's study took place at a large teaching clinic setting with many inherent disadvantages for efficient and effective functional vision training (e.g., frequent change of doctors, poor patient control, group therapy). A higher rate of success was reported by Etting,[6] who surveyed a random sampling of 42 cases reported by an optometrist in a private practice. There were 20 exotropes, 6 of whom had constant strabismus, and 22 esotropes, 18 of whom had constant strabismus. Using Flom's criteria, the overall functional cure rate was 64%: 85% for exotropia and 45.4% for esotropia. Seven patients were known to have undergone surgery prior to training, but there was no subsequent surgery for any of the patients in this study.

A well-documented strabismus report in which surgery was the dominant method of therapy is the study by Taylor,[7] who found that in cases of congenital esotropia, there was not one instance of functional improvement when surgery was accomplished after the second birthday. However, he did believe it possible to achieve functional cure in such cases if surgery was performed early (i.e., before 2

years of age), and particularly if diligent (minimum of 5 years) follow-up care were given. There is no hope for functional results unless surgery results in a deviation that is 10Δ or less horizontally and 5Δ or less vertically. In a selected sample of 50 such patients undergoing early surgery, 30 were later found to have stereopsis ranging from 40 to 400 seconds. Of these 30 patients, 4 had stereoacuity of 40 seconds of arc on the Stereo Fly test. Taylor, therefore, advocated early surgery in cases of congenital esotropia, believing that late surgery is hopeless with respect to achieving a functional cure. Early surgery is currently considered to be the most efficacious means of treatment in cases of infantile esotropia, particularly if the condition is congenital. This applies also to infantile constant exotropia, although this condition is less prevalent than infantile constant esotropia.

Cases of acquired strabismus usually are helped by some or all of the other methods of treatments. The use of surgery for achieving functional cure in cases of acquired strabismus should be considered in patients who fail to respond to nonsurgical means of therapy. Table 6-2 classifies these types of strabismus according *to time of onset*. An expected prognosis is listed for each category, but it is in no way meant to apply to all cases within each category. (Further classification of types of strabismus is discussed in Chapter 7.)

Table 6-2. Classification of Strabismus According to Time of Onset and Prognosis for Functional Cure

Type	Prognosis
Infantile (onset at 4-6 mos of age or earlier)	Poor (unless early surgery)
Acquired (onset after 6 mos of age)	
Nonaccommodative	Fair (depending on circumstances and therapy used)
Accommodative	Good (unless strabismus of long duration)

Most cases of comitant, *nonaccommodative*, acquired strabismus are idiopathic (i.e., unknown cause). Although there are genetic trends in many cases, the etiology of this type of strabismus remains uncertain. Some causes are clinically well established. For example, a sensory obstacle to fusion, such as a unilateral cataract or anisometropia, usually results in an esotropia in young children. In contrast, exotropia is likely in older individuals with sensory obstacles to fusion. Psychogenic causes of strabismus can also occur; these cases are almost always esotropia although psychogenic exotropia is possible. For example, an emotionally disturbed child with a large exophoria may learn how to let his or her deviation become manifest, purposefully, for the sake of gaining attention, recognition, or sympathy.

Accommodative strabismus is usually esotropic, often due to uncorrected hyperopia and a high AC/A ratio. However, there can be accommodative exotropia in cases of divergence excess. This is the condition in which the exo deviation at far is much greater than the exo deviation at near, indicating a high AC/A ratio. For example, a patient with uncorrected moderate hyperopia may be orthophoric at near but exotropic at far. This, therefore, can be thought of as an indirect type of accommodative strabismus.

The prognosis in most cases of accommodative strabismus is usually good, provided that effective treatment is administered without delay. Constant strabismus of long duration makes the prognosis considerably worse. If the sensory adaptive anomalies (e.g., suppression, amblyopia, or ARC) become deeply embedded, the prognosis may be only fair or even poor: An example of a deteriorated accommodative esotropia is the patient in whom the onset of strabismus was at age 1 year. Many years of untreated constant esotropia make it almost impossible to effect a functional cure by means of therapy. When optical therapy is applied later in life, a microesotropia may be the best result that can be attained. Bifoveal fixation achieved in such cases of long duration is the exception. In some cases of untreated accommodative esotropia, the magnitude of the esotropia increases over time; extraocular muscle surgery may be recommended for cosmetic improvement.

The reports on prognosis in strabismus by Flom[1, 2] included certain factors that he found to be favorable and others that he found to be unfavorable for functional cure. A modification of this list, including general rules, is provided in Table 6-3. Flom developed a quantitative scheme for determining the prognosis for a given case (Table 6-4). (Note that his term for *strabismus* is *squint* and for *intermittent* it is *occasional*.) In Flom's scheme, the three most important prognostic factors are (1) direction of the deviation (eso or

Table 6-3. General Rules for Prognosis for Functional Cure of Strabismus by Means of Vision Therapy

Favorable factors
Good cooperation
Intermittent strabismus
Exotropia rather than esotropia
Small rather than large angles of deviation
Comitancy rather than noncomitancy
Family history of strabismus
Patient's age between 7 to 11 yrs
Late onset
Early treatment
Strabismus of short duration
Unfavorable factors
Eccentric fixation
Amblyopia in esotropia (but not as bad in exotropia)
Cyclotropia
Anomalous retinal correspondence in esotropia (but not an unfavorable factor in exotropia)
No motor fusion range (unfavorable in esotropia but not unfavorable in exotropia)
Suppression in esotropia (but not as bad in exotropia)
Constant strabismus
Early onset
Delay of treatment
Strabismus of long duration

Source: Modified from MC Flom. The prognosis in strabismus. Am J Optom Arch Am Acad Optom. 1958; 35:509–514; and MC Flom. Issues in the Clinical Management of Binocular Anomalies. In: Principles and Practice of Pediatric Optometry. AA Rosenbloom, MW Morgan, eds. Philadelphia: Lippincott; 1990:242.

exo), (2) constancy of the deviation (intermittent or constant), and (3) correspondence (ARC or normal retinal correspondence [NRC]). We explain Table 6-4 using the following example: In a case of intermittent esotropia with NRC, the basic probability for functional cure is 60%. If there is good second-degree sensory fusion, a family history of strabismus, and no amblyopia, the prognosis would be improved by 10 + 10 + 10 (total of 30%), yielding a prognosis of a 90% chance for achieving a functional cure by any and all means of treatment, which may include surgery. If, in the given case, there is deep suppression, the prognosis would be lowered to 80%. If there are also marked noncomitancy and deep amblyopia, the prognosis would be 60%. The second significant factor is frequency. For example, intermittent esotropia with NRC would have a 60% chance for functional cure, as compared with 30% for constant esotropia with NRC.

Although this scheme has instructional value for students and can serve as a hypothetical guideline for practitioners, we believe it is unwise to depend entirely on statistical models to make a prognosis for a particular patient with strabismus. Instead, the doctor must take into account all the variables,

Table 6-4. Model for Estimating the Probability of Functional Correction of Different Types of Squint and Associated Factors

Esotropia				Eight Basic Squint Types	Exotropia			
Occasional NRC	Occasional ARC	Constant NRC	Constant ARC		Constant ARC	Constant NRC	Occasional ARC	Occasional NRC
0.60	0.50	0.30	0.10	Basic probabilities	0.40	0.50	0.70	0.80
				+ Factors (add 0.1)				
( )	( )	( )	( )	Good second-degree fusion	(--)	(--)	(--)	(--)
( )	( )	( )	( )	Family history of squint	(--)	(--)	(--)	(--)
( )	( )	( )	( )	No amblyopia	( )	( )	( )	( )
(--)	(--)	( )	( )	Deviation <16Δ	(--)	(--)	(--)	(--)
				- Factors (subtract 0.1)				
( )	( )	( )	( )	Marked suppression	(--)	(--)	(--)	(--)
( )	( )	( )	( )	Marked incomitancy	( )	( )	( )	( )
( )	( )	( )	( )	Deep amblyopia	( )	( )	( )	( )
( )	( )	( )	( )	Estimated probability	( )	( )	( )	( )

ARC = anomolous retinal correspondence; NRC = normal retinal correspondence
Source: From Flom MC. Issues in the Clinical Management of Binocular Anomalies. In: Principles and Practice of Pediatric Optometry. Rosenbloom AA, Morgan MW, eds. Philadelphia: Lippincott, 1990, with permission.

associated conditions, and other factors, and then use professional judgment to arrive at the most correct prognosis for the patient. This requires an item analysis of each factor in the prognosis and evaluation of the total combined effect (possible only after extensive clinical experience).

Prognostic Variables of the Deviation

An important prognostic factor is the *direction* of the deviation. Exo deviations are ordinarily easier to treat than are eso deviations. Vertical deviations present more of a challenge, and treating torsional deviations is even more difficult.

In regard to *frequency* of the deviation, there is general agreement that an intermittent strabismus has a more favorable prognosis than a constant strabismus. However, there are differences in favorability from one intermittent case to another. A deviation that is manifest 95% of the time is obviously more difficult to treat than one that is present 5% of the time. The less time the deviation is present, the better is the prognosis.

The factor of *comitancy* must be considered. Comitant strabismus generally is regarded to carry a better prognosis than noncomitant strabismus, but many exceptions may occur. Noncomitancy caused by a recently acquired paresis in which remission is highly likely would not follow the general rule; the outcome in such a case is usually favorable if the patient's condition is managed properly.

Although there is some correlation between the *magnitude* of the deviation and prognosis, the relationship is not always close. It is generally assumed that the larger the angle, the worse is the prognosis. This rule, however, often is refuted in cases of small-angle strabismus. Wybar[8] stated that "microtropia is unlikely to prove responsive to therapeutic measures." Likewise, Parks[9] concluded that the prognosis for bifoveal fixation in the patient with monofixation pattern is poor.

The effect of the *AC/A ratio* must be considered in regard to the particular case in question. Generally speaking, a normal AC/A ratio is more favorable than either a high or low ratio. However, a high ratio can be either a blessing or a curse, depending on the circumstances. It may be the principal cause of esotropia at near or exotropia at far. However, the mechanical advantage of a high AC/A ratio when wearing lenses may greatly reduce deviations (e.g., plus lenses for nearpoint esotropia and minus for farpoint exotropia). It is difficult, therefore, to make prognostic generalizations about the AC/A ratio.

Variability of the deviation may be favorable if the magnitude of the deviation changes from time to time. As regards the sensory aspect, variation in the magnitude may keep suppression and ARC from becoming too deeply embedded, but such an outcome cannot be assumed in many cases. As regards the motor aspect, however, a widely varying magnitude can be a surgeon's nightmare.

Similarly, the factor of *cosmesis* can be a blessing or a curse. If cosmesis is good, this is a blessing for the patient. However, this causes complacency and is often the reason patients do not enthusiastically seek a functional cure, which creates problems for the doctor treating the strabismus.

As to *eye laterality* traditional thinking is that treatment of an alternating strabismus is more difficult than is treatment of a unilateral condition. This conclusion has been prevalent because alternate fixation is common in cases of infantile esotropia. Findings in this group of patients have led to equating alternation with poor prognosis. Most recent studies show that alternation is not a deterrent to a good prognosis and may be slightly favorable when all types of strabismus are considered.[1,2] This may be true in part because individuals with alternating strabismus usually do not become amblyopes.

Eye dominancy is probably not a factor in strabismus prognosis. However, it can be a consideration in the strabismic's perceptual adjustment to everyday seeing and may be related to certain eye-hand or eye-foot coordination tasks.

Associated Conditions

As with diagnostic variables of the deviation, it is difficult to pin down the influence of each of the associated conditions on the overall prognosis.

Peripheral and deep *suppression* may cause the prognosis to be worse than would be the case for central and shallow suppression. Although this is generally true, there are many exceptions. For instance, there could be an esotropia with ARC in which suppression is very shallow. The prognosis may be poor because of the ARC despite the apparent favorable factor of almost negligible suppression. Because there is always interplay among the many factors that affect a prognosis, it is difficult to speak in terms of absolutes for any one factor. Generally speaking, though, suppression alone is not considered highly unfavorable.

The presence of *amblyopia* is a stumbling block to the successful treatment of strabismus. Fortunately, amblyopia can be detected and treated at an early age. Once amblyopia is eliminated, strabismus therapy is facilitated.

A series of studies by the Amblyopia Treatment Study group has provided direct evidence that treatment for amblyopia is beneficial for children 3 to 7 years of age with mild, moderate, or severe amblyopia. One interesting finding is that part-time occlusion or penalization with atropine appears to work as well as full time patching in most cases.[10-12] A more detailed review of the literature will be given in chapter 10. In children older than 7 years of age, studies have shown improvement with treatment but the success rates are significantly less than for younger children. In one study in children ages, 7 to 17 with acuities ranging from 20/40 to 20/400 in the amblyopic eye were treated with either optical correction alone or optical correction plus part-time occlusion with near activities.[13] Using a response to treatment criteria of a 10 letter improvement the study found a 53% response rate in the 7 to 12 year old group with treatment. One interesting finding was that 25% of children in this group improved with just optical correction. In contrast for children ages 13 to 17 only those children who had not been previously treated showed improvements beyond just wearing spectacle correction.

One factor not adequately addressed by the Amblyopia Treatment Studies is the influence of eccentric fixation (EF) on treatment outcome. The presence of EF have led some to disagree with the contention that direct occlusion is always the best method of occlusion therapy. If a patient older than 5 years has eccentric fixation, direct occlusion is thought to cause the abnormal fixation to become even more deeply embedded. If this happens, very specialized pleoptic therapy using afterimages and entopic foveal "tags" may be necessary to treat the abnormal fixation. The contention is that inverse occlusion would have prevented the degree of embeddedness that resulted from direct occlusion. Kavner and Suchoff[14] reported that prognosis is poorer when there is a stable eccentric fixation as opposed to one that is unstable. They recommended inverse occlusion and specialized pleoptic training when dealing with this type of condition.

We believe that direct occlusion is the procedure of choice in amblyopic patients up to 6 years of age. In patients older than 6, direct occlusion should be tried if fixation is central or if unstable eccentric fixation is present. The prognosis may be fair or good depending on the circumstances. However, in patients older than 5 years who have steady eccentric fixation, the prognosis for eliminating the eccentric fixation and amblyopia by means of direct occlusion alone may be poor. Very often when direct occlusion is used in this type of condition, there is an immediate small improvement in visual acuity but no further gain afterward. This may be so because the eccentric fixation becomes very entrenched, making it difficult to reduce it any further. Therefore, the contention is that the prognosis may be somewhat better if indirect occlusion is tried initially.

Chavasse[15] discussed the concepts of amblyopia of arrest and amblyopia of extinction. *Amblyopia of arrest* is a failure in the development of visual acuity due to strabismus, anisometropia, or other conditions (e.g., cataract). In any event, the development of visual acuity is arrested at the time of onset of the causative condition. The prognosis for improving visual acuity in a documented case of amblyopia of arrest is considered to be very poor. This is probably true if the patient is beyond the developmental age (probably 6 years or older). However, if the same type of case is treated at a much earlier age, the prognosis may be better. Amblyopia of arrest, therefore, is not always a deterrent to treatment if the patient is very young; but if treatment is delayed until the child is older, the prognosis becomes worse.

The prognosis for a case of *amblyopia of extinction* is thought to be good regardless of the age at which treatment is begun. However, an older patient may require a more lengthy therapeutic program than a younger patient. Amblyopia of extinction is a condition in which vision has deteriorated because of suppression resulting from either strabismus or anisometropia. The vision that was once lost can usually be recovered through the re-education process of vision therapy.

Chavasse's concepts[15] are not undisputed. Many authorities have refuted them on the basis of findings that amblyopic therapy results do not always correspond to the level of visual acuity that is traditionally expected. Often in cases of relatively early-onset amblyopia, better acuity is achieved than was believed possible, which would appear to contradict the concept of amblyopia of arrest. However, if modern normative visual acuity levels expected for certain ages are properly matched with the time of onset, the concept of amblyopia of arrest is on solid ground. The apparent mismatch arose because of the old assumption that an infant's vision is poorer than it actually is. Chavasse[15]

believed that the acuity level of a 4-month-old child is normally approximately 20/2500, but research has shown this to be untrue: Infants' visual acuity is much better than was expected in the past. This may explain why treatment in cases of early onset is often successful; perhaps the condition being treated is not amblyopia of arrest but rather amblyopia of extinction.

The presence of ARC is a very unfavorable factor in the prognosis of esotropia. Flom[1] reported that whereas ARC is highly unfavorable in cases of constant esotropia, it is of less significance in cases of constant exotropia. The cure rates of Ludlam[16] were reported to be 23% for esotropes with ARC and 86% for esotropes with NRC. Exotropes with ARC had a cure rate of 62%, as opposed to 89% for those with NRC. Etting[6] reported a cure rate of 10% for esotropes with ARC, as opposed to 75% for esotropes with NRC. The cure rate for exotropes with ARC was 50%. It appears that ARC is a serious factor in cases of esotropia but is less influential in exotropia.

Lack of correspondence is considered to be extremely unfavorable. Current therapies offer no hope for a functional cure in the older child or adult who has a complete lack of correspondence. The best recommendation in such cases is either no treatment or an attempt at cosmetic cure.

In cases of horror fusionis the usual recommendation is no treatment because the prognosis is poor. If the ARC can be broken, however, horror fusionis may not be a significantly adverse factor for functional cure, assuming that the horror fusionis was produced by the ARC. (See Chapter 5.)

Accommodative infacility is not an unfavorable factor in strabismus; however, it frequently accompanies amblyopia with eccentric fixation. Accommodative flexibility training (so-called rock) often is used as part of amblyopia therapy, and considerable time may be required before both the fixation and accommodation improve.

There are poor fusional vergences in strabismus. Sensory fusion must be attained so that disparity vergence can be established. When this is accomplished, fusional vergence ranges can often be increased by means of vision training. The prognosis for functional cure of strabismus, therefore, is not necessarily poor because of poor fusional vergences prior to vision therapy.

Other Factors

The time of onset, mode of onset, and duration of strabismus, previous treatment, developmental history, and additional evaluative procedures all play important roles in determining the prognosis in any case of strabismus. The prognosis is better when the onset of amblyopia or strabismus is later rather than earlier. A short duration is better than a long one, as immediate therapy increases the chance for cure. Existing anomalies that were once successfully treated often are easily eliminated by re-education. Furthermore, developmental history that is normal can be considered favorable in many cases.

Testing for sensory fusion at the *centration point* is another important supplemental prognostic procedure. Plus-power lenses may be efficacious for bringing the eyes to the ortho posture. The appropriate amount of plus-lens power and the centration point distance (the point at which the visual axes cross) must be determined. For example, assume a 15Δ esotropia and an interpupillary distance (IPD) of 60 mm. The centration point would be 40 cm from the patient, which is determined by calculating the lens power that will place the eyes in the ortho posture, using the following formula:

Lens power (in diopters) = H/IPD

where H is the horizontal objective angle of deviation expressed in prism diopters and the IPD is expressed in centimeters. From this example, if 15 is divided by 6, the quotient is 2.50 diopters (D). The distance at the centration point is the focal distance of the lenses (100/2.50 = 40 cm). If 2.50-D lenses are worn, the patient is seeing at 40 cm as though at optical infinity. The horizontal deviation should, therefore, become ortho at the 40-cm test distance with the patient wearing the +2.50-D lenses (Figure 6-1). That being so, various sensory fusion tests can be conducted (e.g., Worth four-dot and stereopsis tests).

The centration point calculation is theoretical, in the sense that the visual system does not always work in a predictable mechanical manner. For example, in some cases of esotropia, plus-power lenses seem to have little or no immediate effect, and only on prolonged wearing (e.g., 1 hour) may there be reduction of the deviation toward the centration point. Furthermore, many esotropic patients (particularly those with ARC) revert to their original angle and over-converge for the concentration point.

Cooperation is a vital factor in treatment when vision therapy techniques are used. A patient must be perceptive and of reasonably good intellect to go through this form of therapy. In addition, genuine interest of the patient and, in the case of a child patient, of the parents is extremely helpful. In fact, cooperation and interest may explain the irony of the favorability of a family history of strabismus: Parents may be motivated to do something about their child's condition because of their familiarity with binocular anomalies.

The age of the patient is an important factor, often dictating what form of therapy the patient will receive. Vision therapy can best be done when the child is 6 years of age or older. Some patients as young as 4 years may be cooperative, but rarely will there be sufficient cooperation for complex vision therapy techniques from those younger than 4 years.

Cure of farpoint strabismus is commonly more difficult than cure of strabismus at near. Treatment of convergence excess is typically easier than is treatment of divergence insufficiency. Similarly, convergence insufficiency (nearpoint exo problem) is less difficult to treat than is divergence excess (farpoint exo problem).

Proper refractive care may prevent some binocular anomalies in strabismics. In this regard, a history of good vision care can be considered favorable to the prognosis in many cases.

Cosmetic Cure of Strabismus

A fault of many reports in the literature is that no distinction is made between functional and cosmetic cure. Many ophthalmic surgeons label the patient as *cured* simply because the eyes appear straight. Studies purporting to give cosmetic cure rates are unreliable, because this is a subjective value judgment for which each reporter uses his or her own criteria.

Certain cosmetic factors have a great effect on the appearance of the strabismic individual (e.g., IPD, eyelid shape, epicanthal folds, facial shape, and symmetry). Another important factor is angle kappa (technically, angle lambda). For example, a negative angle kappa may make an individual with orthophoria appear to have esotropia. Similarly, cosmesis may be good in moderately large

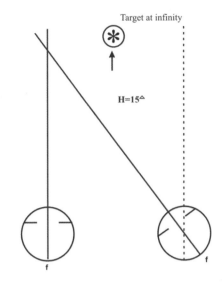

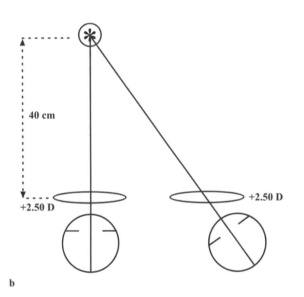

Figure 6-1. Centration point illustration in example of 15Δ esotropia, a. Angle H of 15Δ esotropia of the right eye (esotropia at 6 m, optical infinity), b. Sensory ortho posture at 40 cm with addition of +2.50-D lenses to simulate optical infinity.

angles of strabismus. For instance, a 15Δ esotrope with a positive angle kappa may appear to have no strabismus. Because of the various combinations of cosmetic factors affecting the appearance of the individual, there are no hard and fast rules relating the magnitude of strabismus to cosmesis. In the majority of cases, however, we find that if the strabismic angle is reduced to 10Δ or less, cosmesis usually is good. The esotrope may get by with a larger angle, such as 15Δ or 20Δ, before the deviation is noticeable. This is because most people have a positive angle kappa, which favors the appearance of esotropia. Conversely, an exotropia of the same magnitude will probably be quite noticeable.

Hyper deviations of 5Δ or less are not noticeable. Deviations beyond 10Δ may be unsightly and present a cosmetic problem for patients and parents of young patients. In contrast, cyclodeviations are ordinarily not a cosmetic problem unless they are extremely large. In such cases, usually a vertical and a horizontal deviation are present. These vertical and horizontal deviations, and not the cyclotropia, are usually the cause of the poor cosmesis.

When the goal is only for cosmetic acceptability and not for functional cure, the most frequently used form of therapy is extraocular muscle surgery. Lenses occasionally are used for this purpose, in the form of single-vision lenses for the correction of hyperopia. Plus additions (bifocals) generally serve no purpose in cases in which cosmesis is the sole concern. Minus adds for farpoint exotropia have been used also, although this treatment method is not highly recommended because the cosmetic gain is only transitory. Nothing is achieved in the long run, because the cosmetic problem returns as soon as the individual relaxes accommodation or the overcorrection is removed. Minus lenses do play an important role, however, in certain cases of exotropia in which there is hope for functional cure. Alignment of the visual axes helps to promote sensory fusion.

Inverse prisms have been used for cosmetic improvement, with limited success. The main problem is the thickness and weight factor of glass or plastic prisms. Fresnel prisms eliminate these drawbacks, but they introduce the problem of degraded visual acuity, and the occasional patient reports noticeable lines when looking through the prisms, which becomes a significant problem with powers greater than 15Δ. If, however, all the prism is confined to the deviating eye, the problem of blurred vision is removed. The patient wearing a Fresnel prism may also object to the appearance of the lines to a person looking at him or her. Thus, the use of inverse prism may become impractical because of the objectionable appearance.

In strabismic deviations of moderate magnitude (see criteria listed in Chapter 4) that are just beyond the limit of cosmetic acceptance, a combined method of direct and inverse prism application can be tried. This is illustrated in Figure 6-2 in which the right eye is esotropic (see Figure 6-2a). If a direct prism (base-out) is placed before the left eye, the dextro-

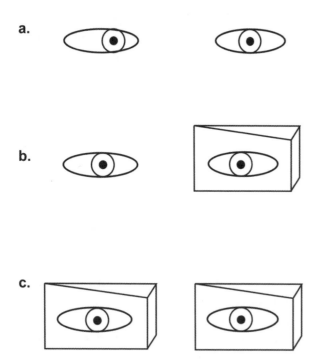

Figure 6-2. The use of prisms to improve cosmesis in an example of esotropia of the right eye. a. Noticeable esotropia of right eye. b. Base-out prism before the left eye causes the left eye to turn in and the right eye out (dextroversion equal to magnitude of prism), c. Yoked prism with base-in before the right eye enhances cosmetic appearance because of the shifting of the palpebral aperture toward the apex of the prism.

version diminishes the esotropic appearance of the right eye (see Figure 6-2b). Inverse prism (base-in) then is placed before the right eye (see Figure 6-2c). Although there probably is no movement of the right eye because of suppression, the optical effect of the prism (image shifted toward the apex) further enhances the salutary cosmetic results. The amount of prism power necessary in this procedure is usually approximately 40% of the magnitude of the strabismus. For example, an esotropic deviation of 20Δ would require 8Δ before each eye (i.e., yoked prisms).

Patients may be taught the tactic of controlling head movements or using specified positions of gaze to minimize a cosmetically noticeable strabismus. This is applicable in cases of comitant as well as noncomitant strabismus. For example, suppose a patient with 20Δ of comitant constant esotropia of the right eye wishes to appear to be orthophoric during a job interview. The effect of "straight eyes" may be accomplished by the individual by making a small dextroversion, such as fixating on the interviewer's left ear, for example, rather than looking directly into the interviewer's face. Such advice can be helpful to patients in their occupational and personal lives.

Heterophoria

The prognosis for improving existing visual efficiency skills in heterophoria is almost always good, provided that there is adequate cooperation and motivation on the part of the patient. If a patient demonstrates outstanding motivation, that patient can be told the prognosis is "excellent." Such superlatives, however, should be used sparingly. Heterophoria therapy is usually effective in abating associated signs and symptoms (Table 6-5). In the sensory realm, stereopsis might be improved by means of vision training, lenses, or prisms. In the motor realm, vision therapy may help to increase fusional vergence ranges, which may be necessary in cases of fixation disparity. Also, the use of prisms is applicable in cases of heterophoria, especially for patients with fixation disparity.

Of the four generally recognized types of vergence—tonic, accommodative, fusional, and proximal—most authorities believe tonic convergence is the least changeable as a result of training. Although there is some dispute over whether the basic deviation can be changed by training, we believe it remains approximately the same in the long run. On immediate testing, however, there may appear to be a post-training difference. However, when there is prolonged occlusion (e.g., several hours), tonic convergence is usually found to be the same as it was before training.

As regards accommodative vergence, Manas,[17] by measuring the AC/A ratio, reported an increase with convergence training. Flom[18] questioned the results of Manas, but in his own study, he found a similar increase. However, after approximately 1 year, Flom found that the AC/A ratio appeared to have decreased and approximated the original values.

Table 6-5. Signs and Symptoms Frequently Occurring in Heterophoria

Blurring of vision at farpoint
Blurring of vision at nearpoint
Frowning or squinting of eyelids
Excessive blinking when reading
Covering or closing one eye during reading
Confusing, omitting, or repeating words when reading
Sustaining nearpoint work with difficulty
Reading at a very slow rate
Losing place when reading a book
Burning, aching, itching, or tearing of eyes, or photophobia

Numerous researchers have reported on the trainability of fusional vergences. Costenbader[19] stated, "In general, the treatment of strabismus includes . . . improving fusion and the fusional vergences." Jones[20] wrote, "In regard to motor fusion, it is the aim of orthoptic treatment . . . to increase them [fusional vergence ranges] sufficiently." Griffin[21] summarized research proving the efficacy of fusional (disparity) vergence training. In general, the prognosis for increasing fusional vergence is good. The fusional vergence that is easiest to treat by training is fusional convergence, followed by fusional divergence. Improving vertical fusional vergence by means of training is the next most difficult. In most cases, torsional fusional vergence is the most difficult to train successfully.

Excessive proximal convergence usually diminishes on familiarity with the testing environment that originally produced the increased vergence. This has occupational importance (e.g., controlling the tendency to overconverge the eyes when using binocular instruments such as a biomicroscope).

For all patients, whether strabismic, heterophoric, or orthophoric, testing for and diagnosing deficiencies of other visual skills (e.g., saccades, pursuits, fixations, accommodation [sufficiency, facility, stamina], and the status of fixation disparity) should be undertaken. The prognosis is generally good for resolving problems in these areas by means of vision therapy.

MODES OF TREATMENTS

Before a prognostic statement for either a functional or cosmetic cure can be considered complete, the doctor must take into account the type of therapy that must be administered to effect the desired results. An overview of approaches to treatments in cases of binocular anomalies is presented in this section. In cases that carry a poor prognosis, the doctor may recommend *no treatment*. This is sometimes the wisest option for certain patients. (See the case examples later in this chapter.)

Lenses

The first consideration in the treatment of any binocular vision condition is full correction of the refractive error, as a defocused or distorted image to either eye (or possibly to both eyes) is an obstacle to fusion. Lens additions (plus and minus) are also used in the treatment of certain types of strabismus and heterophoria. Lens therapy is discussed in Part Two of this book.

Prisms

For more than 100 years, prisms have been used to compensate the angle of strabismus. The primary limitation has been the amount that can be effectively incorporated into spectacle lenses. Prisms often become impractical due to their weight and distortion when more than 10Δ per lens is required. With the advent of Fresnel prisms, the limit has increased to 30Δ per lens which is usually sufficient as most strabismic deviations measure less than 60Δ in magnitude. However, Fresnel prisms appear, at best, to be only a temporary solution because of optical distortion, reduced visual acuity, and loss of contrast. Furthermore, compensating prisms do not help (but hinder) the cosmetic aspect of strabismus, which exacerbates this major concern of most strabismic patients. The use of reverse (inverse) prisms, however, may be attempted to improve the cosmetic appearance in some strabismic cases. When a borderline cosmetic unilateral strabismus is present, small amounts of reverse prism can often mask its appearance. Reverse prisms have also been used to break the adaptations of suppression, ARC, and eccentric fixation in selected cases.

The use of compensating (relieving) prisms in cases of heterophoria has continued to grow in clinical practice, especially in cases of excessive heterophoria. If the angle of deviation does not adapt to the prism power (i.e., phoria increasing in magnitude), asthenopic symptoms usually are resolved or diminished. However, some patients show prism adaptation, which suggests that this is not a viable therapeutic option. (See chapter 3 for discussion of prism in heterophoria.)

Occlusion

Occlusion (i.e., opaque patches or attenuating filters) is used to treat amblyopia (Chapter 10), ARC (Chapter 11), suppression (Chapter 12), and comitant and noncomitant strabismus (Chapters 13-15).

Prognostic considerations regarding occlusion are discussed in the aforementioned chapters.

Vision Therapy

When more than lenses, prisms, and occlusion are necessary to achieve the desired results, vision therapy techniques may be the treatment of choice. Sometimes vision therapy is conducted without other forms of treatment, but other modes of treatment often are included in the vision therapy program. A full discussion of vision therapy approaches and procedures for treating strabismus are presented in the second volume of this book. Vision therapy relative to binocular vision disorders historically has been called *orthoptics*, which etymologically means "straight sight." Orthoptic techniques are usually successful in breaking suppression, building fusional vergence ranges, and improving the reflex aspects of ocular motility. For this reason, orthoptics has the greatest utility in cases of intermittent strabismus, heterophoria, and deficient oculomotor skills.

Many orthoptic techniques (including monocular regimens) are used in the treatment of amblyopia, but *pleoptics* (literally "full sight") is a specific type of training designed exclusively for amblyopia with eccentric fixation. These techniques involve light stimulation techniques to diminish the influence of the eccentric fixation point in the amblyopic eye and enhance foveal fixation. In some cases of severe amblyopia of long duration, both pleoptic and orthoptic techniques, as well as

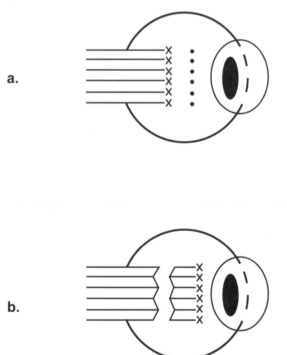

Figure 6-3. Extraocular muscle surgery involving a rectus muscle, a. Recession as a weakening procedure. The insertion of the tendon is removed and reattached posteriorly in the globe, b. Resection as a strengthening procedure. The tendon or muscle is cut and a portion is removed; then it is rejoined.

an aggressive patching (occlusion) program, are required to achieve a successful outcome.

Visual perception training techniques to improve information processing, for certain types of learning disabilities, are not discussed in this text. However, many perceptual training techniques (e.g., figure-ground, visual discrimination, and closure) are used to treat amblyopia.

Extraocular Muscle Surgery

The surgical form of binocular therapy may be necessary in certain cases when the angle of deviation is too large to be consistently and easily overcome by fusional effort or when a significant noncomitant deviation is present. Many different procedures are used by ophthalmologists in extraocular muscle surgery. Some basic principles, however, are accepted by most ophthalmic surgeons. Only those general approaches to correction of deviations of the visual axes are discussed in this book; we do not intend to cover this subject in depth but merely introduce it briefly as one of several alternatives for treating binocular anomalies. Many fine books covering the details of surgical procedures for extraocular muscles and other anomalies affecting ocular motility are available for reference purposes. Particularly good among these are publications by Hugonnier et al.,[22] Hurtt et al.,[23] Mein and Trimble,[24] von Noorden,[25] and Dale.[26] In addition, several case reports are included in the treatment chapters of this book that describe various surgical approaches.

General Approach

The general approach to extraocular muscle surgery is that the action of a particular muscle should be made either weaker or stronger. Examples of weakening procedures include recession, tenotomy, tenectomy, myotomy, and myectomy. When the muscle is *recessed*, the insertion is moved from the original site and transplanted to another location to produce less mechanical advantage (Figure 6-3a). Another weakening procedure is *tenotomy*, either marginal or free (i.e., disinsertion at the scleral attachment). In many varieties of controlled *tenectomies*, the tendon is appropriately cut for weakening the action of an overacting muscle.

Either *myotomy* or *myectomy* is the term used when the muscle, rather than the tendon of the muscle, is altered.

Examples of strengthening procedures include resection, tucking, and advancement. *Resectioning* of a muscle or tendon changes the angle of deviation by shortening it (see Figure 6-3b). The method of *tucking* may involve the tendon or the muscle; it also effectively serves to shorten the muscle. Advancement of the insertion serves to strengthen the action of the muscle by giving it greater mechanical advantage.

The prism adaptation test (PAT) was introduced by Woodward and reported by Jampolsky[27]. Surgeons use this test procedure to estimate the amount of surgery required for alignment. PAT is used to predict success (often when surgery is anticipated) in cases of esotropia. The testing procedure involves the application of base-out prism for the manifest eso deviation. The patient wears prisms for some time, usually an hour, while the clinician measures the angle of deviation at certain intervals, usually every 10 minutes. Jampolsky[27] recommended overcorrecting for the patient's condition by using a prism power that is slightly stronger than the magnitude of the esotropia. For small deviations, an overcorrection of 5Δ is recommended, whereas for larger deviations, a 10Δ overcorrection is suggested. For example, suppose a patient has esotropia of 25Δ. The patient is given 35Δ base-out prisms to wear for 1 hour. Fresnel prisms are more comfortable for the patient than are glass or plastic clip-ons. The immediate measurement on the alternate cover test should show a 10Δ exo movement. In many cases, the exo will decrease in a very short time and, after approximately 10 minutes, the patient will exhibit an eso movement on the cover test. In some cases, the eso deviation becomes larger that the original deviation. Assume that after an hour the alternate cover test shows a 20Δ eso movement of the eyes. The eso deviation is now 35Δ plus 20Δ, or a total of 55Δ. The angle of the deviation has more than doubled in magnitude as a result of the PAT.

Jampolsky[27] believed that this indicated a poor prognosis for cure by surgery and probably by other means as well. If the deviation had remained the same or had increased only slightly, the prognosis would have been considered much better. As a rule, in more than half of the cases of esotropia, after a patient has worn compensating prisms for at least 2 or 3 hours, an increase in the angle of deviation can probably be expected. In a study of 88 patients with esotropia, Aust and Welge-Lussen[28] found that the angle of deviation increased in 71.5% of the patients over a period of 5-9 days. ARC was thought to be more commonly associated with the increase than was NRC.

Alpern and Hofstetter[29] reported a well-documented case of esotropia in which the angle of deviation increased by the same amount as the power of the compensatory prisms. The 14Δ strabismus was constant and unilateral, and the presence of ARC was clearly established. Base-out prisms having a total power of 18Δ were worn for 5 days. The rate of increase of the angle of deviation was rapid within the first 3 hours, with only a slight, gradual increase over the next few days until tapering to the maximum of 32Δ (total increase of angle *H* of 18Δ). After prisms were removed, angle *H* decreased rapidly (within a few hours), but it was approximately 1 week before the strabismus finally was reduced to its original angle of 14Δ.

Postar[30] investigated the use of the PAT for esotropic patients. He concluded that changes in the angle of deviation were related to the status of sensory fusion. The overconvergence reaction to the base-out prisms did not tend to occur when sensory fusion was good, but the tendency was evident when sensory fusion was poor. He advocated improving stereopsis early in the therapy program to keep the deviation from increasing when prisms are applied. He further concluded that the 1-hour testing time was too short and a longer period should be allotted for evaluating the effects of prism adaptation.

In taking a different approach to prism adaptation testing, Carter[31] found that heterophoric individuals with good binocularity and without symptoms showed the same magnitude as the original heterophoria before prisms were worn. Thus, a 5Δ esophore, corrected with 5Δ base-out prisms, still showed 5Δ of esophoria by cover test through the prisms that were worn for approximately 30 minutes. In contrast, individuals who had heterophoria and asthenopia (possibly with fixation disparity) accepted compensatory prisms. Their symptoms were relieved, and there was no prism adaptation effect.

From the preceding reports, we can conclude that prism compensation should be considered in cases of heterophoria with symptoms. In contradistinction, the magnitude of deviation in heterophoric patients without symptoms will likely increase as a result of the wearing of compensatory prisms. In the case of esotropia, the deviation is likely to increase when sensory fusion is poor (e.g., ARC and suppression). If, however, sensory fusion is good, the strabismic deviation is likely to stay the same or increase only slightly. On rare occasions, the basic deviation appears to be reduced in magnitude as a result of wearing prisms.

It is generally agreed that little or no increase (or, as occasionally happens, a decrease) in the angle of strabismus on the PAT is an indication of a good prognosis. However, there is incomplete agreement as to the interpretation of the results of the PAT when the angle increases significantly. The majority opinion holds that the prognosis is unfavorable in these instances, but some authorities believe there may be exceptions to the rule. Some cases result in a functional cure despite dismal expectations that were derived from the PAT. This points out the need for practitioners to be cautious when making a prognosis and not to rely too much on any one test.

Adjustable Suture Procedure

Jampolsky[32] pioneered the adjustable suture technique for extraocular muscle surgery, which allows a surgeon to refine the surgical result within 24 hours after the operation. Many surgeons find that this procedure improves their long-term results. At the very least, the adjustable suture procedure helps to avoid large overcorrections and undercorrections[33]. The severed muscle tendon is not reattached tightly to the sclera at the time of the operation. After the muscle is resected or recessed by the necessary amount, long sutures in the tendon are passed through the superficial sclera and are secured externally with a slipknot. Under a local anesthetic, the final adjustment of alignment can be made on the same day of the operation or the next day while the patient is awake. Most adults and many school-aged children can cooperate adequately with the procedure.[34] Using the cover test to check alignment, the surgeon loosens the slipknot and repositions the muscle insertion as needed. The loose ends of the sutures are pulled to advance the insertion (a strengthening procedure) or are pulled in the opposing direction to achieve more recession (a weakening procedure). There is a linear relationship between the millimeters of adjustment and the change in the strabismic deviation.[35] The adjustment procedure can alter the deviation by up to 23Δ.[36] The dissolvable sutures then are secured in position externally with surgeon's knots and the muscle tendon adheres permanently to the sclera during the healing process.

This procedure can be used with any of the rectus muscles and the superior oblique tendon. Both vertical and horizontal muscles can be put on adjustable sutures when strabismus is present in both directions. Adjustable sutures are particularly appropriate when the outcome is not readily predictable (e.g., cases of previous unsuccessful surgery) or when the patient has fusion potential and precise alignment is critical to a successful outcome, as in cases of thyroid ophthalmopathy. Some strabismus surgeons use adjustable sutures in nearly every case of rectus muscle surgery. Efforts have been made to extend the time between the operation and the postsurgical adjustment using medications,[37] but there is little change in the final outcome by delaying the adjustment until 24 hours as opposed to only a few hours postoperatively.[38] The reoperation rate after conventional surgery is estimated to be 19-35%, as compared with 4-10% using the adjustable suture technique.[39]

Surgical Considerations

Most patients and parents are naturally apprehensive about undergoing strabismus surgery. The doctor must give realistic information regarding the potential complications and what is involved in the procedure. This information usually relieves some anxiety. The patient should be encouraged to ask all possible questions during the preoperative visit. For medicolegal purposes, the surgeon should document in the patient's record the specific complications that were discussed. Not every potential complication need be mentioned, however. According to Helveston,[40] preoperative informed consent requires a discussion of at least three possibilities: diplopia, loss of vision, and need for reoperation.

Depending on the age and sensory status of the patient, diplopia is a common occurrence during the initial postoperative phase of healing. Most patients experience only transient diplopia that disappears within a week or so after the operation. Older patients tend to notice diplopia more often, as one might expect. If the diplopia is debilitating, the patient can wear a patch or be given a Fresnel prism in an attempt to achieve sensory fusion. Many patients will notice diplopia only if they consciously look for it in some extreme field of gaze; this behavior should be discouraged. Diplopia that disrupts the normal course of daily activities is cause for concern.

An extremely rare but serious complication of strabismus surgery is loss of vision. This devastating complication can be caused by perforation of the sclera and retina with a surgical instrument or needle. Loss of vision in this event occurs subsequent to retinal detachment, vitreous hemorrhage, cataract, glaucoma, optic nerve incision or transection, endophthalmitis, or other damage. Some patients have an unusually thin sclera, which makes them vulnerable to this complication and, of course, there is the ever-present possibility of human error.

Patients usually want to know about the need for reoperation. They often ask whether the results will be permanent. In any case, this issue must be discussed prior to surgery. The possibility of additional operations at some future time depends primarily on the type and characteristics of the strabismus and the skill of the surgeon. The surgeon should discuss with the patient his or her success rate in similar cases. For example, in cases of congenital esotropia, Helveston[40] informs his patients that the motor alignment achieved is considered acceptable by doctor and parents 90% of the time. He also tells his patients that between 10% and 20% of children will need one or more additional surgical procedures months to years later for new problems such as secondary exotropia, overacting oblique muscles, an A or V pattern, dissociated vertical deviation, or recurrent esotropia, even when alignment is perfect after surgery.

Some other complications that can occur and that may be discussed with patients are (1) postoperative nausea and vomiting due to anesthesia and, possibly, traction on the extraocular muscles; (2) acute, allergic suture reaction, which can occur in approximately 10% of cases in which organic absorbable suture material is used and for which topical steroids are given for 7-10 days; and (3) ptosis of the upper eyelid (which can occur after excessive recession of the superior rectus muscle) or of the lower eyelid (with large recession of the inferior rectus muscle).

Besides learning about the potential complications of surgery, patients generally want to know about several other practical issues relative to the operation. In most cases, strabismus surgery is a 1-day, "in-and-out" procedure. An overnight stay at the hospital is not usually required, except for general health considerations or when other surgical procedures are being performed. The patient registers with the selected hospital, and standard blood tests are completed. The anesthesiologist usually meets with the patient or parents immediately before the operation to check the patient and to ensure that the preoperative instructions from the hospital have been followed. The strabismus operation itself usually takes only 1 hour, give or take 15 minutes. Some surgeons work with an assistant surgeon in addition to a scrub nurse. During the immediate postsurgical phase, many doctors bandage the operated eye for a short time, usually 1 day, to help to prevent infection and to increase patient comfort due to photophobia. A topical, wide-spectrum antibiotic is usually given for daily instillation for the first week to 10 days. Conjunctival injection usually disappears in a month or two. The frequency of postoperative visits varies widely depending on the case and the surgeon, but a typical schedule might consist of 1-day, 1-week, and 6-week follow-up examinations. After these visits, if no complications develop, the patient is placed on a standard recall schedule or is instructed to return to the referring doctor for comanagement (e.g., vision training) and shared responsibility relative to the strabismus.

Pharmacologic Treatment

Although numerous pharmaceutical agents have been used at one time or another for the treatment of binocular anomalies, those in use today are relatively few. Cycloplegics may be used for purposes of occlusion. Miotics for accommodative esotropia are sometimes used. The two more popular anticholinesterase drugs are diisopropylfluorophosphate (DFP) and echothiophate iodide (Phospholine). These two agents greatly increase accommodation, without a significant increase in accommodative convergence, which results in a lower AC/A ratio.

Abraham[41] pioneered the use of DFP to reduce esotropia. A report by Gellman[42] summarized the effectiveness of DFP by citing case reports in which the nearpoint eso deviation was reduced by use of this drug. However, Phospholine has become the more popular of these two agents, as it apparently causes fewer side effects (e.g., formation of iris cysts) than does DFP. One effect that should always be avoided is the cardiovascular or respiratory failure that may occur when a drug of this type is combined with those used for general anesthesia. Bartlett and Jaanus[43] emphasized that Phospholine and DFP are very stable complexes and produce action of long duration. Manley[3] warned of the danger of giving general anesthesia in surgical cases of esotropia when the patient has previously been taking one of these anticholinesterase drugs. If succinylcholine chloride is used before endotracheal intubation, a drug overeffect will occur if the patient has been taking anticholinesterase drugs, and cessation of respiration may result. A case history should be carefully obtained to determine whether any such drug was used within several months of the scheduled time of extraocular muscle surgery.

The use of drugs in the treatment of binocular anomalies appears to be somewhat limited and may be on the decline. There are times, however, when their use may be advantageous in the treatment of accommodative esotropia. They may be effective when the AC/A ratio is high, in cases of significant hyperopia, and when wearing lenses is not tolerable. Under most of these circumstances, it is feasible to prescribe bifocals but, in the case of infants and some children, drugs may be a means to reduce an eso deviation.

Systemic medications that have generated interest and clinical research lately, such as levodopa, are designed for use in Parkinson's disease and are now being tried in the treatment of adult amblyopia. However, the results to date provide more questions than answers.

Botulinum Toxin

Chemodenervation using botulinum toxin A injection is another nonsurgical approach in strabismus management that is gaining respect and widening applications. Alan Scott et al.[44] developed this procedure as a method for weakening extraocular muscle function as though a surgical weakening procedure had been performed. The toxin prevents release of acetylcholine at the muscle-nerve junction, producing a temporary paralysis of the ipsilat-

eral antagonist. In right esotropia, the right medial rectus muscle usually is injected, and for a few weeks, the patient experiences a right exotropia that gradually resolves over 1-2 months to result in a smaller-angle eso deviation. The therapeutic effect comes more from the stretching and relaxation of muscles as they assume a new position than from any prolonged toxic effects.[45] Botox, Allergan's form of botulinum toxin A (Dysport injection, Porton Laboratory Supplies, Salisbury, England), has now proven its worth over the last few years in selected patients. It has been used with good effects in unilateral fourth and sixth nerve palsies of acute onset.[46, 47] The best results tend to occur for smaller angles of strabismus and shorter time intervals between onset and Botox injection.[48]

Chemodenervation also has a role in cases of surgical overcorrection of strabismus (e.g., when an exotrope has been converted into an esotrope). Rather than risk another operation, Botox injection serves as a conservative option, and the results are encouraging, particularly if there is fusion potential.[49,50]

Botox has been used with some success in nystagmus associated with esotropia, congenital nystagmus, and complex forms of nystagmus. All of these conditions usually require three or four muscle injections or retrobulbar injections (see Chapter 8).[51,52] Better visual acuity is usually the result but lasts for only 3-4 months before further injections are necessary.

Although still controversial, chemodenervation has been used as an alternative to surgery in cases of developmental comitant exotropia and esotropia, even infantile esotropia.[53,54] In patients older than 18 months, in one study, the overall success rate was 58%, which is fairly good for infantile esotropia with abduction nystagmus.[55]

Chemodenervation is not nearly as invasive as is extraocular muscle surgery. It often can be performed without general anesthetic for infants younger than 1 year or patients 6 years of age and older. A local anesthetic is used, of course, as are oral sedatives such as diazepam for the very apprehensive patient. The needle-electrode is connected to an amplifier to ensure proper placement in the muscle body; there is a crackling electromyographic signal when the needle is in position, and then the toxin is slowly injected. Injection is easiest in the lateral and medial recti, but the inferior rectus and inferior oblique muscles also can be readily accessed. The superior rectus and oblique muscles can be injected, but the levator usually is affected by diffusion and produces a full ptosis that can be expected to last for 2 months. Hence, the superior oblique muscle has not proven to be a good site for injection, yielding disappointing results.[45]

Chemodenervation has many advantages over strabismus surgery, not the least of which is convenience for the doctor and patient.[56] The in-office procedure is quick, relatively easy, and less expensive in comparison to surgery. Botox rarely overcorrects the deviation after the adjustment period. There is less chance of infection and serious complications with chemodenervation. Botulinum toxin A has no systemic side effects when used for strabismus.

Nonetheless, the agent has some negative attributes that the patient or parents need to know and accept before proceeding. Diplopia, some spatial disorientation, and a large-angle eye turn can be expected for 1 month or so after successful injection. A patch can be worn if these results are intolerable; children usually adapt quickly and well. Transient partial ptosis and a transient vertical deviation are fairly common side effects of even horizontal recti injection. In many patients, particularly those with large angles of deviation, multiple injections are needed to achieve the desired effect or maintain the result after 4 or 5 years. The doctor should wait for 5 or 6 months for complete stabilization before reinjecting the same muscle. Although rare, there is always the possibility of perforation of the globe; highly myopic eyes are the most vulnerable. Despite these potential drawbacks, in many cases the positive attributes outweigh the negative features of chemodenervation, and so this procedure is gaining in popularity.

Other Approaches

The doctor must serve his or her patients as a counselor regarding visual health and welfare. Sometimes, the best interest of the strabismic patient is served by doing nothing except monitoring the condition for changes over time. For example, if the spectacle lens prescription is current, the deviation is cosmetically and functionally stable, and the patient is satisfied with the status of the strabismus, then the doctor should not recommend treatment but rather should describe to the patient the condition, its prognosis for long-term changes, and any other practical considerations. Sometimes patients cannot follow through on a recommended vision therapy program for several reasons and prefer simply to live with the condition for the time being. The clinician has a duty to explain, in a sensitive manner, any consequences that may result from that decision and how best to manage the situation. It remains imperative for the doctor to make recommendations based on the best interest of the patient rather than to promote a particularly preferred mode of treatment.

The vision specialist must be sensitive to the need for referral when it arises. Many types of strabismus and other binocular vision conditions can be subtle indicators of active ocular or systemic disease. Patients should also be encouraged to seek a second opinion if any questions remain in the mind of the clinician or the patient. Occasionally, vision specialists examine patients in whom the binocular vision condition is of psychogenic origin (e.g., hysterical amblyopia, or esotropia following emotional trauma). The professional services of a psychologist or psychiatrist may be necessary for resolution of the condition.

Hypnosis is an alternative mode of therapy that has some applications within the field of binocular vision therapy. Kohn[57] stated that vision therapy lends itself ideally to hypnosis because it is "focused attention" that helps patients to achieve functional cure. Hypnosis has been used to motivate patients for vision training as well as to increase patient acceptance of occlusion, spectacle lenses, surgery, and many techniques in vision training. Hypnosis may be considered in cases of intractable diplopia.

When one mode of treatment is inadequate, others may be used. It is possible that any combination of the basic methods outlined here may be employed, and some cases require them all. The treatment section of this book (Part Two) contains further discussion of the uses of these treatment modalities and suggests various combinations in case studies.

CASE EXAMPLES

The previous discussions focused on generalities regarding the favorability of various prognostic factors. In this section, we present 12 specific cases that illustrate typical diagnostic groups having a prognosis for functional cure ranging from poor to good. Some clinicians may disagree with our prognostic judgments because of differences in clinical experience. We tend to be slightly conservative, as conventional wisdom dictates. A surprisingly successful cure after therapy is never unappreciated by patients. The same cannot be said when therapeutic results do not match the expectations of patients.

Poor Prognosis

Case 1

The patient is 10 years old with a history of esotropia of the right eye since birth. The strabismus has been constant since then, although the magnitude is lower now than in infancy. No previous treatment has been given. Further history reveals possible traumatic injury during delivery. Developmental history appears to be normal, other than that the child always has difficulty abducting the right eye. The refraction is

OD: plano, 20/400 (6/120)

OS: plano, 20/20 (6/6)

The deviation is a noncomitant, constant, unilateral esotropia of the right eye of 15Δ at far and near, with a normal AC/A ratio (6/1), and good cosmesis. The associated conditions include lack of any fusion; deep amblyopia; nasal, unsteady, parafoveal, eccentric fixation; complete lack of correspondence; poor accommodative facility in the amblyopic eye; no motor fusion; and slightly noticeable facial asymmetries. Muscle testing indicates a complete paresis of the right lateral rectus. Cosmesis is not a concern to the patient or parents.

The basic esotropia of this 10-year-old patient is congenital. The prognosis for a functional cure by any or all means of therapy is poor. Flom's prognosis chart for a functional cure of the strabismus would indicate 0% chance of success (see Table 6-4).

It is also probable that the prognosis is poor for any significant change in the status of the amblyopia, because the deviation has probably been unilateral since birth; therefore, it can be speculated that the reduced visual acuity is due to amblyopia of arrest. The ultimate differential diagnosis would be made by treating the condition to find out whether there is any improvement. If there is enhancement of visual acuity, the amount of improvement represents that portion of visual loss due to amblyopia of extinction. If there is no improvement, the presence of amblyopia of arrest is confirmed, assuming any organic cause of reduced visual acuity has been ruled out. Predictive testing such as interferometry and visually evoked potentials could also be recommended.

No treatment for the strabismus is recommended in this case if the cosmesis is acceptable to the patient. Because the deviation is not large, the appearance of the eyes is fairly good in the primary gaze; however, the esotropia may become noticeable on right gaze because of the right lateral rectus paresis. Cosmesis is acceptable otherwise.

Direct total occlusion should be recommended except when the patient cannot see well enough in school with the amblyopic eye. Occlusion should continue for 1 or 2 months to determine whether there is any improvement. If visual acuity improves in the right eye, pleoptics to treat the eccentric fixation may be advised. If there is no change in visual acuity after that, further vision therapy is not indicated. The patient would then be advised to have a routine follow-up examination in 1 year.

Case 2

The patient is 9 years old with a history of constant esotropia since the age of 1 year. No previous treatment has been given. The patient does not report diplopia. Refraction is

OD: +2.50 -0.50 x 180, 20/40 (6/12)

OS: plano, 20/20 (6/6)

Vision at near was commensurate with that at far.

The deviation is a comitant, constant, alternating, esotropia, with the left eye being preferred. The deviation is 45Δ at far and 35Δ at near, with a low AC/A ratio (2/1). Cosmesis is poor. The associated conditions include deep peripheral suppression; shallow amblyopia with unsteady central fixation; probable harmonious ARC; horror fusionis; and no motor fusion or stereopsis.

This case can be described as divergence insufficiency esotropia because of the larger deviation at far. The prognosis for a functional cure by any or all means of therapy is poor. The Flom prognosis chart would indicate only a 10% chance for success (see Table 6-4). However, the prognosis for a partial cure is poor to fair, meaning that the large manifest deviation could be converted into a smaller deviation by means of surgery. This implies that peripheral fusion might be developed or reeducated, thereby helping the patient to hold the eyes relatively straight. The patient would technically be strabismic but, if motor ranges could be developed, the patient could function with at least some degree of binocularity. This would be a monofixation pattern. With a history of no previous treatment and a duration of 8 years of constant esotropia, there is little hope for anything beyond this expectation.

The shallow amblyopia is probably due to the anisometropia rather than the strabismus, as the deviation is alternating and not unilateral. The prognosis for cosmetic cure by means of extraocular muscle surgery is fair to good. Prism adaptation testing would be useful in this case to predetermine whether the angle of deviation would be stable after the operation. The patient should be advised that several appointments are needed for further evaluation and that vision training will be tried on a short-term basis, approximately 5 weekly visits, to determine whether there is any improvement in visual acuity. Correcting lenses should be worn during this time, along with constant patching of the left eye in an attempt to improve the acuity of the right eye. After lenses and vision training have achieved the maximum results, surgery should be recommended for cosmetic and, it is hoped, functional improvement. A contact lens for the right eye may be considered as an alternative to the spectacles at a later time.

Case 3

The case history reveals that the onset of esotropia for this 7-year-old patient was at approximately 3 months of age. Examination at age 4 years found a refractive error of +0.75-D sphere in each eye. Lenses of this power were prescribed at that time but were worn only a few days before being rejected by the patient. Present refraction is plano and 20/20 in each eye.

The deviation is a comitant, constant, alternating (right-eye-dominant), esotropia of 15Δ at far and 13Δ at near. There is also a large, double-dissociated hyper deviation (dissociated vertical deviation). The AC/A ratio is normal, and cosmesis is good because angle kappa is positive. There is harmonious ARC and shallow central suppression, and the patient has no demonstrable fusion range.

The prognosis for a functional cure by means of any or all methods of vision therapy is poor. The Flom chart, however, would indicate a chance of cure of 20-30% (see Table 6-4). The reason for a poor prognosis in this case of infantile esotropia is that the onset was very early and of long duration. Also, the constant deviation and ARC are negative factors, and the dissociated vertical deviation may be negative as well. If treatment had been attempted soon after the onset of strabismus, there might have been a chance for bifoveal fusion.

Because there is no cosmetic problem, no treatment should be recommended. Furthermore, onset of amblyopia is unlikely to occur, considering the age of the patient and the fact that the strabismus is alternating. The patient should be advised to have a routine follow-up examination in 1 year.

Poor to Fair Prognosis

Case 4

The patient is 10 years old and has a history of exotropia of the right eye that was intermittent, beginning at 7 months through 1 year of age. The strabismus has been constant since then. Direct patching was attempted for a few weeks at age 3, but only token occlusion was accomplished. No other treatment has been given since. Refraction is

OD: -1.00 -1.00 x 180, 20/100 (6/30)

OS: plano, 20/20 (6/6)

Vision at near was commensurate with that at far.

The deviation is a comitant, constant, unilateral exotropia of the right eye of 25Δ at far and 15Δ at near with a high AC/A ratio (10/1). Cosmesis is poor due to the magnitude of the deviation and to a large positive angle kappa (+1.5 mm). The associated conditions include deep peripheral suppression; moderate-to-deep amblyopia; unsteady, temporal, parafoveal eccentric fixation; harmonious ARC; and no evidence of motor fusion (i.e., lack of disparity vergence). No stereopsis response could be elicited.

This patient has divergence excess exotropia. The prognosis for a functional cure of the strabismus by means of therapy is poor to fair. The Flom chart would indicate a 30% chance for success (see Table 6-4). However, the prognosis for achieving a monofixation pattern is fair, and the chance of partially ameliorating the amblyopia is also fair, because of the history of intermittence. Some of the amblyopia may be of extinction rather than arrest. It is unlikely that 20/20 (6/6) vision will be attained, although some improvement can be expected.

Assuming the amblyopia can be effectively reduced, minus-lens overcorrection may be used initially in an attempt to align the visual axes. The high AC/A ratio is useful for accomplishing this. The ARC probably is not as unfavorable as is the deep suppression in this case of exotropia. A surgical overcorrection (resulting in a small eso deviation) may be called for, both for functional outcome as well as for ensuring a good cosmetic result in the event vision training fails to effect a functional improvement or cure. It is hoped that good fusional (disparity) vergences can be developed and that the patient will at least achieve gross stereopsis.

The patient should be advised that approximately 25 office appointments and intensive home training will be recommended. Surgery may also be needed, and the patient would be given postsurgical vision therapy.

If the parents and the patient do not elect vision therapy with the possibility of surgery and are concerned only with cosmesis, an optical approach can be tried. A 10Δ base-in prism can be worn over the dominant left eye. The left eye would then fixate 10Δ to the left, and the strabismic right eye would appear straighter, possibly within the cosmetic limit. If, however, cosmesis remains unacceptable, yoked prisms may be tried. In this case, a 10Δ base-out prism would be worn over the right eye in addition to the 10Δ base-in prism over the left eye.

Case 5

The patient is a 5-year-old strabismic with a history of constant esotropia that began at age 2. No previous examination or treatment has been given. The present refraction is

Dry retinoscopy:

    OD: +2.00 DS, 20/40 (6/12)

    OS: +1.00 DS, 20/20 (6/6)

Wet retinoscopy (1% cyclopentolate):

    OD: +2.50 DS, 20/40 (6/12)

    OS: +1.50 DS, 20/20 (6/6)

The deviation is a comitant, constant, unilateral esotropia of the right eye of 10Δ at far and 20Δ at near with a high AC/A ratio. Cosmesis is good because of a large positive angle kappa (+1.5 mm). The associated conditions include deep suppression; shallow amblyopia; nasal, inferior, unsteady, paramacular, eccentric fixation; and no fusional (disparity) vergence. Correspondence is normal, and there is no evidence of horror fusionis. Neither gross nor fine stereopsis could be elicited.

This patient has convergence excess esotropia. The prognosis for complete functional cure is poor to fair. The Flom chart would indicate a prognosis of 30% for success (see Table 6-4). However, the prognosis for a partial cure, whereby a monofixation pattern is to be achieved, is fair to good. The chief reason that a complete cure (in which there is exact bifoveal fixation) is difficult to achieve in this case is that the duration of constant strabismus is 3 years.

There are many cases in which regaining bifoveal fixation is difficult after the patient has lost it for a relatively long period of time. This is particularly true in very young patients.

In this case, however, the prognosis for cure of amblyopia by means of constant occlusion, pleoptics, and other monocular training activities is good because of the patient's young age and relatively late onset of the amblyogenic strabismus.

The patient should be advised that bifocal spectacles lenses will be necessary and that approximately 25 weekly office training sessions, along with home training, are needed to develop peripheral fusion and good fusional vergence ranges. Because cosmesis is good and functional results can be expected without surgical intervention, there is probably no need for an operation in this case. However, prisms may be required during and after vision training.

Fair Prognosis

Case 6

The patient is 9 years old and has had a slightly noticeable esotropia of intermittent onset of the right eye since the age of 3. The strabismus is occasionally observed by family members when the patient is looking far away. No previous treatment has been given. Refractive history is incomplete, but the patient was taken for an eye examination at age 5. No treatment was given then, and the advice was that the strabismus would "eventually go away" The present refraction is

Dry subjective:

OD: +1.00 DS, 20/30 (6/9)

OS: +1.00 DS, 20/20 (6/6)

Wet subjective (1 % cyclopentolate):

OD: +1.50 DS, 20/30(6/9)

OS: +1.50 DS, 20/20 (6/6)

Vision at near was commensurate with that at far.

The deviation is a comitant, intermittent (constant at far and estimated 75% of the time at near), unilateral esotropia of the right eye of 15Δ at far and 4Δ at near. Cosmesis is good because of a positive angle kappa and a relatively wide IPD of 65 mm. The AC/A ratio is low (2/1). Associated conditions include intermittent, deep, central suppression; shallow amblyopia; small (foveal off-center) nasal eccentric fixation; harmonious ARC (covariation at near); and good second-degree fusion but limited motor range. Some peripheral stereopsis was occasionally elicited at near.

This patient has a divergence insufficiency esotropia. The prognosis for functional cure by means of therapy is fair. The Flom prognosis chart would indicate a 50% chance for functional cure (see Table 6-4). Although there is deep central suppression, the factor of intermittence helps the prognosis immensely. The primary purpose of vision therapy in this case is to improve the presently existing visual skills that are at play at least some of the time at near distances. Binasal occlusion for farpoint seeing may be tried, as well as the possibility of base-out prisms, followed by antisuppression training and the development of adequate fusional divergence. A certain amount of training to improve monocular fixation and accommodative facility would be helpful prior to the binocular therapy regimen.

The prognosis must remain somewhat guarded because of the long duration of strabismus and lack of previous treatment. The patient should be advised of the need for spectacles, occlusion therapy, and approximately 30 weekly office appointments along with intensive home vision training. Surgery should be recommended only if it is absolutely required for functional results.

Fair to Good Prognosis

Case 7

The patient is 6 years old and has had an exotropic deviation of the left eye since the age of 4 years. Since then, the strabismus has been intermittent. No previous treatment has been given. The present refraction is

OD: plano, 20/20 (6/6)

OS: plano, 20/30 (6/9)

Vision at near was commensurate with that at far.

The deviation is a comitant, intermittent, unilateral exotropia of the left eye of 20Δ at far and 5Δ at near, with a high AC/A ratio (12/1) and poor cosmesis. The appearance of the strabismus is very noticeable because of the intermittence and a positive angle kappa (+1.5 mm). The exotropia is estimated to be present 90% of the time at far and 10% of the time at near. Associated conditions include deep peripheral suppression when the deviation is manifest; shallow amblyopia with unsteady central fixation; and covariation between harmonious ARC and NRC. An exo fixation disparity is detected when there is bifixation at the nearpoint with an associated exophoria of 4Δ. Motor fusion (disparity vergence) ranges are very limited, being from 22-18Δ base-in at far and from 8Δ base-in to 1Δ base-out at near.

This case is a classic example of divergence excess exotropia. The prognosis for a functional cure by means of lenses and vision training is fair to good. The Flom prognosis chart would indicate a 70% chance for success (see Table 6-4). The prognosis must be guarded because of the larger deviation at farpoint and the intense and extensive suppression when the deviation is manifest. ARC is not a significantly adverse factor with which to be concerned, because normal correspondence predominates while there is fusion.

Monocular vision therapy should be done in conjunction with binocular sensory and motor fusion training in order to eliminate the amblyopia as quickly as possible. The patient should be advised that spectacles, probably bifocals (see Chapter 14 for explanation), and approximately 25 weekly office visits and diligent home training are recommended.

Case 8

The patient is 8 years old with a history of exotropia since the age of 3 years. The onset was intermittent, and the condition has been so ever since. An examination was performed at age 4 years. No significant refractive error was found, and lenses were not prescribed. There has been no other examination since that time. The present refractive error is

OD: plano, 20/20 (6/6)

OS: plano, 20/20 (6/6)

Vision at near was commensurate with that at far.

The deviation is a comitant, intermittent (25% of the time at far and 95% at near), unilateral exotropia of the right eye of 15Δ at far and 25Δ at near. Cosmesis is fair. The associated conditions include moderately deep peripheral suppression when the deviation is manifest; covariation between harmonious ARC and NRC; a limited motor fusion range; and poor stereopsis.

This patient has convergence insufficiency exotropia. The prognosis for a functional cure by means of vision training is fair to good. The Flom prognosis chart would indicate an 80% chance for success (see Table 6-4). Other supplemental testing, such as the prolonged occlusion test, could help to make the prognosis more decisive. It would also be helpful to know the patient's stereoacuity, if that can be elicited at times when the patient is fusing.

Surgery is probably not called for in this case. All that may be required to cure this patient with convergence insufficiency is vision training that emphasizes antisuppression and fusional convergence training.

The patient should be advised to plan for 25 weekly vision therapy appointments and vigorous home training, with the remote possibility of extraocular muscle surgery.

Case 9

The patient is 35 years old and is reporting intermittent diplopia of sudden onset after trauma to the head in an automobile accident 3 weeks ago. This resulted in a mild paresis of the left superior oblique muscle. The refractive history is unremarkable with the exception of a small myopic refractive error. The present prescription being worn is

OD: -1.00 DS, 20/20 (6/6)

OS: -1.00 DS, 20/20 (6/6)

Vision at near was commensurate with that at far.

The deviation is a noncomitant, intermittent, unilateral hypertropia of the left eye of 6Δ at far

and near. Also, there are deviations of 1 degree excyclodeviation, 4Δ of eso at far, and 7Δ at near. Cosmesis is good in the primary position and on levoversion, but the hyper deviation is quite noticeable on dextroversion. The frequency of the manifest deviation is approximately 50% of the time in the primary position and 100% on dextroversion. There is a vertical fixation disparity, and the associated phoria is a 4Δ left hyperphoria that is measurable only when the patient is fusing.

Additional information (e.g., stereoacuity and motor fusion ranges) would be helpful before the final prognosis is made. Assuming these additional test results are relatively normal, the prognosis for this adult patient is fair to good for a functional cure by any means of therapy. There is a good chance of spontaneous remission of the superior oblique paresis with the passing of time, and so approximately 6 months should be allowed to determine whether the paresis will resolve. The Flom chart is not applicable in this case, but we believe the overall prognosis is fair to good.

Management of the noncomitancy should emphasize the prevention of extraocular muscle contractures (see Chapter 15). The patient should be advised to make follow-up appointments as necessary for evaluation and training involving occlusion, prisms, and fusional vergence improvement. Communication with other specialists, particularly the neurologist, should be maintained. The patient should be advised of the eventual possibility of extraocular muscle surgery, although the necessity for this seems unlikely.

Good Prognosis

Case 10

The patient is 7 years old with a history of esotropia since the age of 4 years. The onset was intermittent, and the condition has remained so. The patient was examined at age 5, at which time a small amount of hyperopia was found in each eye, but no lens prescription was given. Diplopia is noticed occasionally during near-point tasks. Cycloplegic and manifest refraction results are

OD: plano, 20/20 (6/6)

OS: plano, 20/20 (6/6)

Vision at near was commensurate with that at far.

The deviation is a comitant, intermittent (10% of the time at far and 90% at near), unilateral esotropia of the right eye of 6Δ at far and 16Δ at near. Cosmesis is good. There is NRC. Associated conditions include shallow central suppression; eso fixation disparity (associated esophoria of 5Δ at far, but nearpoint findings could not be obtained); and a fair motor fusion range. Stereoacuity with contoured targets was 120 seconds of arc at far and 60 seconds of arc at near when +2.00-D addition lenses were worn.

This patient has an accommodative esotropia of the high AC/A type. The prognosis for a functional cure by means of lenses (bifocals) and vision training is good. According to the Flom chart, the prognosis for functional cure would be 80% (see Table 6-4). This is a classic case of convergence excess being caused by a high AC/A ratio. The far deviation may be partially alleviated by incorporating base-out prism (less than 6Δ) in the patient's spectacles. This together with bifocal additions will partially alleviate the deviation at near.

The prognosis must be slightly guarded because of the possible unacceptability of the spectacles by this 7-year-old child. Otherwise, the prognosis is theoretically good. As in other cases, treatment depends on good patient motivation and cooperation. These factors must always be taken into account.

The patient should be advised to have five weekly office appointments for vision therapy after the bifocal spectacles have been dispensed. The patient will be taught to accept and properly use the spectacles. Some antisuppression training and a great deal of fusional vergence training is required. Fortunately, much of this can be done at home, assuming the patient and parents are motivated and cooperative.

Case 11

The patient is 8 years old and has a history of intermittent exotropia at near that was first noticed at age 6 years. The frequency of the deviation has increased somewhat since that time. No previous treatment has been given. Refraction is

OD: -1.00 DS, 20/20 (6/6)

OS: -0.25 DS, 20/20 (6/6)

Vision at near was commensurate with that at far.

The deviation is a comitant, intermittent (5% of the time at far and 40% at near), unilateral exotropia of the right eye of 8Δ at far and 20Δ at near. The AC/A ratio is very low (1.2/1.0). Cosmesis is good with far fixation but is noticeable at times with near face-to-face viewing. NRC is present. Associated conditions include shallow central suppression when the deviation is manifest; fixation disparity (associated exophoria of 1Δ at far and 5Δ at near); and poor motor fusion ranges. Stereoacuity is approximately 60 seconds arc at far and near during fusion.

The prognosis for a functional cure by means of lenses and vision therapy is good—90% according to the Flom prognosis chart (see Table 6-4). This case of convergence insufficiency exotropia should be aided by the wearing of lenses that correct the myopic anisometropia. Also, fusional vergence ranges can most probably be expanded by means of vision training. The patient should be advised to make ten weekly office appointments and plan on an intense home vision training program.

Case 12

The patient is a 22-year-old college student who is reporting blurring of vision and asthenopia during prolonged reading. The refraction is

OD: plano, 20/20 (6/6)

OS: plano, 20/20 (6/6)

Vision at near was commensurate with that at far.

The deviation is a comitant exophoria of 5Δ at far and 10Δ at near. The AC/A ratio is normal (4/1). Motor fusion ranges are fair (vergences at far of 11Δ base-in to 4Δ base-out and nearpoint vergences of 16Δ base-in to 3Δ base-out). The nearpoint of convergence is 12 cm. Associated conditions include accommodative infacility (able to clear only three cycles of ±1.00-D lenses in 1 minute) and an exo fixation disparity at near (associated exophoria of 2Δ). Noncontoured (random dot) stereoacuity was 20 seconds of arc at near. The only other abnormal clinical findings were low positive and negative relative accommodation.

The prognosis for a functional cure by means of vision therapy is good. Even though this is a case of heterophoria and not strabismus, the patient does not meet the criteria of Flom as being functionally cured because of the blurring of vision and discomfort and the inadequate nearpoint of convergence. (Note that in cases of strabismus in which the patient is cured, the patient then is treated as in heterophoria therapy to effect a cure of any deficient binocular visual skills and, it is hoped, to enhance binocularity for efficient visual skills.)

The patient should be advised to make 10 to 15 weekly office appointments for vision therapy and to plan on home training for approximately 30 minutes per day during this time. Afterward, 5-10 minutes per day of continued home training may be recommended as a home maintenance program, until a progress evaluation is conducted in 4 months.

REFERENCES

1. Flom M. The prognosis in strabismus. Am J Optom Arch Am Acad Optom. 1958;35:509-14.

2. Flom M. Issues in the Clinical Management of Binocular Anomalies. In: Rosenbloom A, Morgan M, eds. Principles and Practice of Pediatric Optometry. Philadelphia: Lippincott, 1990.

3. Manley D. Symposium on Horizontal Ocular Deviations. St. Louis: Mosby, 1971.

4. Griffin J, Lee J. The Polaroid mirror method. Optom Wkly. 1970;61:28-9.

5. Ludlam W. Orthoptic treatment of strabismus. Am J Optom. 1961;38:369-88.

6. Etting G. Visual training for strabismus: success ratio in private practice. Optom Wkly 1973;64:23-6.

7. Taylor D. Congenital Esotropia: Management and Prognosis. In. New York: Intercontinental Medical Book Corp, 1973.

8. Wybar K. The Use of Prisms in Pre-Operative and Post-Operative Treatment. In: Fells P, ed. First Congress of the International Strabismological Association. St. Louis: Mosby, 1971.

9. Parks M. The Monofixation Syndrome. In: Mosby CV, ed. Symptoms on Strabismus, Transaction of the New Orleans Academy of Ophthalmology. St. Louis, 1971.

10. The Pediatric Eye Disease Investigator Group. A randomized trial of patching regimens for treatment of moderate amblyopia in children. Arch Ophthalmol. 2003;121:603-11.

11. The Pediatric Eye Disease Investigator Group. A randomized trial of prescribed patching regimens for treatment of severe amblyopia in children. Ophthalmology 2003;110:2075-87.

12. The Pediatric Eye Disease Investigator Group. A randomized trial of atropine vs patching for treatment of moderate amblyopia. Arch Ophthalmol. 2008;126(8):1039-44.

13. The Pediatric Eye Disease Investigator Group. Randomized trial of treatment of amblyopia in children aged 7 to 17 Years. Arch Ophthalmol. 2005;123:437-47.

14. Kavner R, Suchoff I. Pleoptics Handbook. New York: Optometric Center of New York, 1969.

15. Chavasse F. Worth's Squint, 7th ed. Philadelphia: Blakiston's, 1939.

16. Ludlam W, Kleinman B. The long term range results of orthoptic treatment of strabismus. Am J Optom Arch Am Acad Optom. 1965;42:647-84.

17. Manas L. The effect of vision training upon the ACA ratio. Am J Optom. 1958;35:428-37.

18. Flom M. On the relationship between accommodation and accommodative convergence. Am J Optom. 1960;37:630-1.

19. Costenbader F. Diagnosis and clinical significance of the fusional vergences. Am Orthop J. 1965;15:14-20.

20. Jones B. Orthoptic handling of fusional vergences. Am Orthop J. 1965;15:21-9.

21. Griffin J. Efficacy of vision therapy for nonstrabismic vergence anomalies. Optom Vis Sci. 1987;64:411-4.

22. Hugonnier R, Hugonnier S, Troutman S. Strabismus, Heterophoria, Ocular Motor Paralysis. St. Louis: Mosby, 1969.

23. Hurtt J, Rasicovici A, Windsor C. Comprehensive Review of Orthoptics and Ocular Motility. St. Louis: Mosby, 1972.

24. Mein J, Trimble R. Diagnosis and Management of Ocular Motility Disorders, 2nd ed. Oxford: Blackwell Scientific, 1991.

25. von Noorden G, Campos E. Binocular Vision and Ocular Motility: Theory and Management of Strabismus, 6th ed. In. St. Louis: C.V. Mosby, 2002.

26. Dale R. Fundamentals of Ocular Motility and Strabismus. In. New York: Grune & Stratton, 1982.

27. Jampolsky A. A Simplified Approach to Strabismus Diagnosis. In: Symptoms on Strabismus, Transaction of the New Orleans Academy of Ophthalmology. St. Louis: C.V. Mosby, 1971.

28. Aust W, Welge-Lussen L. Pre-operative and post-operative changes in the angle of squint following long-term, preoperative, prismatic compensation. In: Fells P, ed. First Congress of the International Strabismological Association. St. Louis: Mosby, 1971.

29. Alpern M, Hofstetter H. The effect of prism on esotropia: a case report. Am J Optom. 1948;25:80-91.

30. Postar S. Ophthalmic Prism and Extraocular Muscle Deviations: The Effect of Wearing Compensatory Prisms on the Angle of Deviation in Cases of Esotropia. On file in the M.B. Ketchum Memorial Library. Fullerton, Calif.: Southern California College of Optometry, 1972.

31. Carter D. Effects of prolonged wearing of prism. Am J Optom. 1963;40:265-72.

32. Jampolsky A. Adjustable Strabismus Surgical Procedures. In: Symptoms on Strabismus, Transaction of the New Orleans Academy of Ophthalmology. St. Louis: C.V. Mosby, 1978.

33. Wygnanski-Jaffe T, Wysanbeek Y, Bessler E, Spierer A. Strabismus surgery using the adjustable suture technique. J Pediatr Ophthalmol Strabismus. 1999;36:184-8.

34. Chan T, Rosenbaum A, Hall L. The results of adjustable suture technique in pediatric strabismus surgery. Eye 1999;13:567-70.

35. Bacal D, Hertle R, Maguire M. Correlation of postoperative extraocular muscle suture adjustment with its immediate effect on the strabismic deviation. Binocul Vis Strabismus Q. 1999;14:277-84.

36. Rosenbaum A, Metz H, Carlson M, et al. Adjustable rectus muscle recession surgery: a follow-up study. Arch Ophthalmol. 1977;95:817.

37. Hwang J, Chang B. Combined effect of Interceed and 5-fluorouracil on delayed adjustable strabismus surgery. Br J Ophthalmol. 1999;83:788-91.

38. Spierer A. Adjustment of sutures 8 hours vs 24 hours after strabismus surgery. Am J Ophthalmol. 2000;129:521-4.

39. Siegel L, Lozano M, Santiago A, Rosenbaum A. Adjustable and Non adjustable Recession and Resection Techniques. In: Rosenbaum A, Santiago A, eds. Clinical Strabismus Management. Philadelphia: Saunders, 1999.

40. Helveston E. Surgical Management of Strabismus: An Atlas of Strabismus Surgery 4th ed. St. Louis: Mosby, 1993.

41. Abraham S. The use of miotics in the treatment of convergent strabismus and anisometropia. Am J Ophthalmol. 1949;32:233-40.

42. Gellman M. The use of miotics for the correction of hypermetropia and accommodative esotropia. Am J Optom. 1963;40:93-101.

43. Bartlett J, Jaanus S. Ocular Pharmacology 4th ed. Boston: Butterworth-Heinemann, 2001.

44. Scott A, Rosenbaum A, Collins C. Pharmacological weakening of the extraocular muscles. Invest Ophthalmol Vis Sci. 1973;2:924-9.

45. McNeer K, Magoon E, Scott A. Chemodenervation Therapy: Technique and Indications. In: Rosenbaum A, Santiago A, eds. Clinical Strabismus Management. Philadelphia: Saunders, 1999.

46. Garnham L, Lawson J, O'Neill D, Lee J. Botulinum toxin in fourth nerve palsies. Aust NZ J Ophthalmol 1997;25:31-5.

47. Ohba M, Nakgawa O. Treatment of paralytic esotropia by botulinum type A toxin. Nippon Ganka Gakkai Zasshi. 1999;103:112-8.

48. Quah B, Ling Y, Cheong P, Balakrishnan V. A review of 5 years in the use of botulinum toxin A in the treatment of sixth cranial nerve palsy at the Singapore National Eye Center. Singapore Med J. 1999;40:405-9.

49. Dawson E, Marshman W, Lee J. Role of botulinum toxin A in surgically overcorrected exotropia. J AAPOS 1999;3:269-71.

50. Lawson J, Kousoulides L, Lee J. Long-term results of botulinum toxin in consecutive and secondary exotropia: outcome in patients initially treated with botulinum toxin. J AAPOS 1998;2:195-200.

51. Carruthers J. The treatment of congenital nystagmus with Botox. J Pediatr Ophthalmol Strabismus. 1995;32:306-8.

52. Lennerstrand G, Nordbo O, Tian S, et al. Treatment of strabismus and nystagmus with botulinum toxin type A. An evaluation of effects and complications. Acta Ophthalmol Scand. 1998;76:27-37.

53. Rayner S, Hollick E, Lee J. Botulinum toxin in childhood strabismus. Strabismus 1999;7:103-11.

54. Robert P, Jeaneau-Bellego E, Bertin P, Adenis J. Value of delayed botulinum toxin injection in esotropia in the child as first line treatment. J Fr Ophthalmol. 1998;21:508-14.

55. Ruiz M, Moreno M, Sanchez-Garrido C, Rodriguez J. Botulinum treatment of infantile esotropia with abduction nystagmus. J Pediatr Ophthalmol Strabismus 2000;37:196-205.

56. McNeer K. An investigation of the clinical use of botulinum toxin A as a postoperative adjustment procedure in the therapy of strabismus. J Pediatr Ophthalmol Strabismus. 1990;27:3-9.

57. Kohn H. Clinical hypnosis as an adjunct in vision therapy. Optom Monthly. 1983;74:41.

Chapter 7 / Types of Strabismus

Accommodative Esotropia	190
Refractive Accommodative Esotropia	190
Characteristics	190
Management	191
Optical Treatment	191
Other Approaches	192
Non-Refractive Accommodative Esotropia	192
(High Accommodative-Convergence/	
Accommodation Ratio)	
Characteristics	192
Management	193
Optical Treatment	193
Vision Therapy	193
Miotics	193
Surgery	194
Infantile Esotropia	195
Characteristics	195
Management	197
Optical Treatment	198
Vision Therapy	198
Surgery	198
Primary Comitant Esotropia	199
Characteristics	200
Management	200
Primary Comitant Exotropia	201
Characteristics	201
Management	203
Optical Treatment	203
Occlusion	204
Vision Therapy	204
Surgical	204
A and V Patterns	204
Characteristics	205
Management	205
Microtropia	206
Clinical Characteristics	206
Management	208
Cyclovertical Deviations	209
Comitant Vertical Deviations	209
Dissociated Vertical Deviations	210
Sensory Strabismus	210
Consecutive Strabismus	211

Several types of strabismus occur in young patients during their early formative years. If the deviation is caused primarily by genetic factors or developmental anomalies in oculomotor control, it can be described as a developmental strabismus. This chapter discusses the clinical characteristics and management principles of common developmental deviations that are usually comitant. Paralytic strabismus and oculomotor restrictions, although they often occur during childhood or may be congenital, are discussed in Chapter 8.

Classification of types of strabismus has not been uniform across different clinicians, researchers and textbooks. Recently, the National Eye Institute sponsored a workshop on classification of eye movement abnormalities and strabismus. The purpose of the workshop was to create a uniform classification system that can be used in clinical research.[1] We have attempted to mention the various terms used to describe the different types of strabismus in this chapter.

ACCOMMODATIVE ESOTROPIA

The two general types of accommodative esotropia that often require different optical treatment approaches are refractive (normal accommodative-convergence/accommodation [AC/A] ratio) and nonrefractive (high AC/A ratio). There exists an accommodative component to most eso deviations that occurs during the early developmental years; in that sense, most cases of esotropia can be considered partially accommodative in etiology. In addition, not all cases of accommodative esotropia will be resolved with correction of the hyperopia with or without additional plus lenses for near. In these cases the deviation is considered to be partially accommodative esotropia and may need additional management with prisms, vision therapy, or surgery. Our discussion begins with the characteristics of accommodative esotropia and an overview of management when the mechanism is primarily accommodative, causing excessive accommodative convergence.

Refractive Accommodative Esotropia
Characteristics

Both types of accommodative esotropia usually occur between the ages of 2 and 3 years, concurrently with the development and increased use of accommodation. However, the range of onset is broad, extending from infancy into young adulthood.[2] The strabismus can become manifest with illness, extreme emotion, or eye fatigue. The etiology of refractive accommodative esotropia is better understood than that of all other developmental types of strabismus. Moderate or high

Table 7-1. Characteristics of Accommodative Esotropia

	Refractive Esotropia	High AC/A Esotropia
Mechanism	Uncorrected hyperopia Limited divergence	High AC/A ratio Limited divergence
Onset	Most often at 2-3 yrs old	Most often at 2-3 yrs old
Refractive error (Mean Value)	+4.75 DS	+2.25 DS
Constancy	Usually intermittent	Often constant at near distances
Correspondence	Usually normal retinal correspondence	Usually normal retinal correspondence
Amblyopia	Rare	Rare
AC/A ratio	Normal	High
Prognosis	Good with correction of hyperopia	Fair with plus-addition lenses and vision training

AC/A = accommodative-convergence/accommodation; DS = diopters sphere

uncorrected hyperopia, usually between 2 and 6 diopters (D), forces an individual to accommodate sufficiently to attain clear retinal images. An average hyperopia of +4.75 D was reported for accommodative esotropes.[3] There is usually a normal AC/A ratio, but excessive accommodation, which is required to overcome the hyperopia, evokes excessive convergence. If compensating fusional divergence is insufficient, a latent eso deviation becomes manifest, due to the combination of uncorrected hyperopia and inadequate fusional divergence ranges. The onset of accommodative esotropia is usually gradual and intermittent. Because of its intermittent nature, there is usually normal retinal correspondence (NRC) and seldom any amblyopia. If the manifest deviation becomes constant at an early age, amblyopia, anomalous retinal correspondence (ARC), or a microtropic component can develop. Older children may report intermittent diplopia, blur, and eyestrain, particularly when performing near tasks. In some cases of high uncorrected hyperopia (e.g., more than 6 D), the eyes may remain straight much of the time when the individual is not using accommodation; however, the consequence may be bilateral amblyopia (i.e., isometropic amblyopia) if the retinal images remain blurred most of the time. Characteristics of accommodative esotropia (refractive and high AC/A types) are listed in Table 7-1.

Management
Optical Treatment
With early treatment, the prognosis is good for complete resolution of the strabismus, particularly if normal binocularity existed prior to the onset of the deviation. Usually all that is necessary is a prescription of lenses for the full optical correction of the uncorrected hyperopia (and any significant astigmatic component) as verified by cyclo-

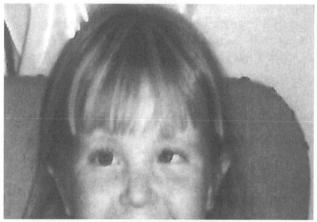

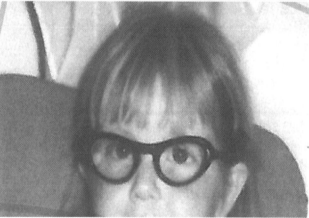

Figure 7-1. Refractive accommodative esotropia without spectacle lens correction (top) and with lenses that fully correct the manifest deviation (bottom).

plegic refraction (Figure 7-1). The goal of optical treatment is not necessarily orthophoria. Some authorities recommend leaving the patient slightly esophoric so that there is a continuing demand for fusional divergence.[4] If the patient's accommodation does not relax fully after the prescription lenses are worn for a few days and if there is significant blurred farpoint vision, the doctor should also recommend accommodative rock training or administer a cycloplegic drug (atropine) if absolutely necessary. The purpose would be to reduce an accommodative spasm. Occasionally, even after these measures have been applied, the patient is unable to relax accommodation sufficiently to achieve the full ametropic correction. If the accommodative spasm persists for weeks, power of the plus lenses must be reduced accordingly.

Soft contact lenses have proven particularly useful and acceptable to patients for alleviation of accommodative esotropia.[5,6] The optical properties of contact lenses may be beneficial as compared with spectacle lenses. Slightly less accommodation is required to focus an image at near using plus contact lenses as compared with plus-lens spectacles, due to the difference in vertex distance. Grisham et al.[6] found that contact lenses were more effective than spectacle lenses in reducing residual angles of eso deviation (either esophoria or esotropia). Wearing of contact lenses also resulted in better fusional control in cases of NRC.

For patients younger than 1 year, retinoscopy should be repeated every 3 months, because refractive changes during infancy are frequent. New lenses are indicated if there is a change of at least 1 D. Follow-up examinations should be performed at least every 6 months in these children from ages 1 to 5 years to ensure that the lens prescription is current and fusional control of the deviation is maintained.

Other Approaches

In cases where spectacle lenses do not resolve the esotropia or when associated sensory anomalies are still present, vision therapy is useful if the child can cooperate. Patients who undergo vision therapy tend to maintain a good result longer than do patients who do not receive vision therapy. If there is NRC, the goals of vision training are to eliminate any amblyopia, break suppression, and build fusional divergence ranges with reflex control. (Refer to Chapter 13 for vision training techniques for eso deviations.) Often a patient who has completed vision therapy can remove the lenses for brief periods, such as for swimming or other sports, and still maintain fusional control of the deviation.

The use of miotics or surgery in cases of refractive accommodative esotropia is strongly discouraged. Miotics are only a temporary solution at best and are associated with many possible undesirable side effects. They should be tried only after complete optical treatment has failed to achieve alignment and fusional control. For example, some children initially refuse to wear the prescribed lenses. Later, however, they may prefer the optical treatment to daily instillation of eye drops.

Surgery may be indicated in cases of partially accommodative esotropia in which there remains a conspicuous residual strabismus after full correction of the refractive error. Surgery for any significant associated hyper deviation or marked A-V pattern may also be necessary and appropriate. In postsurgical cases of refractive esotropia, consecutive exotropia is a common finding and has been reported in as many as 44% of cases.[7] In such cases undercorrection of the hyperopic correction is straightforward and can be an effective management strategy.

Non-Refractive Accommodative Esotropia (High Accommodative-Convergence/Accommodation Ratio)

Characteristics

Accommodative esotropia may occur even when there is little or no hyperopia. This can be due to a high AC/A ratio, in which there is an excessive amount of accommodative convergence with a relatively small amount of accommodation. In this situation, an esotropia may occur at near fixation distances when fusional divergence is insufficient to compensate for the excessive accommodative convergence. This type of accommodative strabismus, called *high AC/A accommodative esotropia*, is known also as *convergence excess esotropia* in the Duane-White classification system. The main distinguishing feature of high AC/A accommodative esotropia is that the magnitude of the deviation at near exceeds that at far distance. This stands in contrast to *refractive accommodative esotropia*, in which the near and far deviations are approximately equal (i.e., a *basic* eso deviation). As in refractive accommodative esotropia, high AC/A accommodative esotropia is usually intermittent with NRC.

High AC/A accommodative esotropia is relatively independent of refractive error. High hyperopia is possible but rare. However, many patients have mild to moderate degrees of hyperopia. In one series of patients with high AC/A accommodative esotropia, the average refractive error was +2.25 D,[2] which is approximately half the average amount of hyperopia found in refractive accommodative esotropia. There is, however, wide variability in

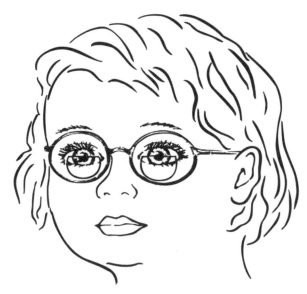

Figure 7-2. Proper segment height for a child with accommodative esotropia with a high accommodative-convergence/accommodation ratio.

refractive error, with some patients presenting with emmetropia and even myopia. In those cases of moderately high hyperopia in combination with a high AC/A, treatment must address both causes of the deviation.

Management
Optical Treatment

Because of the high AC/A ratio in this type of strabismus, it is usually necessary to correct any manifest hyperopia with lenses. Cycloplegic refraction should be performed to reveal any latent hyperopia. In addition, the optimum bifocal lens power should be determined to promote fusion at the patient's nearpoint working distance. This amount is, of course, determined under noncycloplegic testing conditions. Plus-lens additions are used for the patient's preferred working distance to determine empirically which power will best align the eyes. In effect, this technique uses the measured AC/A ratio (i.e., lens gradient method) to determine the optimum bifocal power. When prescribing a bifocal lens for very young children, it is important to fit the bifocal line high, at mid-pupil, if the lens is to be used properly (Figure 7-2). For older children and adults, the segment height can be slightly lower. By age 8 years, the segment line can be at the lower edge of the pupil. By teenage years, the line can be at the lower eyelid margin. For progressive addition lenses, the fitting would be approximately 2 mm higher than a linear segment bifocal lens.

For older children and adults, bifocal contact lenses may be considered as an alternative to bifocal spectacles in the high AC/A type of accommodative esotropia. The added near power is useful in all fields of gaze, unlike spectacle bifocals, and many patients do not report difficulty with the slight decrease in contrast inherent in the bifocal contact lens design.[6] One longitudinal study, however, indicated that more than 40% of optically aligned accommodative esotropes did not remain so over a 7-year period.[8] This finding illustrates the importance of close follow-up examinations and subsequent refractive and vision training management of such patients.

Another consideration that clinicians should keep in mind when a previously corrected accommodative esotropia deteriorates at near is the possibility of a psychological etiology resulting in a spasm of the near reflex triad.[9] Such patients may require palliative therapy, such as a reading add, and professional counseling.

Vision Therapy

After the optimum bifocal correction has been prescribed to promote alignment at far and near, vision therapy may be necessary to build a reserve of fusional vergence function or treat associated sensory anomalies. Vision therapy should be programmed to eliminate amblyopia and suppression and then to develop and improve fusional divergence. Adequate fusional vergences serve to improve control of the deviation at all viewing distances, which is important because the deviation varies in magnitude from far to near. (See Chapter 13 for vision training techniques.) Without adequate vision training, these patients tend to lose control of the deviation at near, and suppression can recur at near fixation distances. The higher the AC/A ratio, the more a patient tends to lose control of the deviation over time.[10] We do not recommend combining miotic therapy with a vision training program. Although some clinicians may disagree, our experience indicates that vision training progress is erratic when miotics are used simultaneously. It is unclear why this is so, but results are better when one or the other therapeutic method is applied alone.

Miotics

If the nearpoint deviation cannot be adequately controlled using bifocals and vision training, miotics may be considered as a treatment option. We believe that topical anticholinesterase drugs have been overused in the treatment of accommodative esotropia. Because they have significant side effects and do not offer a long-term solution, it seems prudent to try to control the near deviation by other means, if possible. Miotics, however, may be effective initially to achieve temporary ocular alignment when other methods have failed. Introduction of more conservative vision therapy methods for long-term management of the deviation can then be made.

Common anticholinesterase eye drops such as diisopropylfluorophosphate (DFP 0.025% ointment) and echothiophate iodide solution (Phospholine Iodine [PI], 0.03%, 0.06%, or 0.125%) produce an accumulation of acetylcholine at the myoneural junction of the ciliary muscle. This acetylcholine buildup results in a decrease in the innervation necessary for effective accommodation and, therefore, in a corresponding decrease of accommodative convergence. Vergence is effectively decoupled from accommodation, so an increasing eso deviation at near does not occur with accommodative effort. An additional factor responsible for the reduction of accommodation and accommodative convergence is the miosis itself. Small pupils increase the depth of focus so that near objects can be seen clearly with much less accommodation than is needed by normal-sized pupils. Of the two commonly used agents, DFP is the most effective miotic and is associated with less systemic absorption. However, PI is readily available in different concentrations and, therefore, has greater versatility in clinical management. DFP often is preferred for preschool children and PI for older children and adults. The miotic agent is given one time daily, often at night, before sleep.

Clinicians must be aware of the complications associated with the use of miotics (anticholinesterase agents), some of which are serious. The most hazardous complication occurs when a patient taking topical miotics is given a depolarizing muscle relaxant, such as succinylcholine, during general anesthesia. This drug combination can result in a prolonged, even fatal, apnea. Consequently, patients taking a topical miotic should carry a card clearly identifying its use, in case of emergency surgery. A patient should discontinue the use of miotics for at least 6 weeks before succinylcholine can be used safely. Another potentially fatal mistake is the oral ingestion of topical miotics. These agents must be kept securely out of the reach of children. Death is caused by a cholinergic crisis resulting from blockage at motor end plates of the heart and lungs.

Although uncommon, serious systemic toxicity resulting from the use of miotics has been reported, manifesting in the gastrointestinal system as nausea, abdominal discomfort, and diarrhea.[11] Manual depression of the lacrimal canaliculi during and after topical administration should prevent, or minimize, these systemic side effects.

The most common ocular side effect is the development of iris cysts at the pupillary margin, which occurs in approximately 50% of children taking PI. The cysts can grow large enough to obscure vision, but these usually are reversible by discontinuing the use of the miotic. The development of such cysts can be minimized by instilling a drop of 2.5% or 10% phenylephrine (Neo-Synephrine) concurrently with the miotic. Iris cysts occur less often as a side effect with the administration of DFP than with PI.

Miotics cause other ocular side effects including ciliary spasm with brow ache, conjunctival injection, and iritis. These are usually transitory, but more serious complications can occur such as angle-closure glaucoma, retinal detachment, and anterior subcapsular cataracts (usually reversible in children). Because of these possible side effects, we recommend the initial use of optical treatment and vision training techniques rather than miotics in most cases of high AC/A accommodative esotropia.

In summarizing his clinical impressions, Raab[12] spoke disparagingly of the results of miotic management of accommodative esotropia. He has found that compliance with miotics has been inadequate in patients in whom compliance with bifocal lenses has faltered. This finding suggests that the real problem is one of parent-child conflict over therapy and that this issue needs to be resolved rather than substituting one therapy for another.

Surgery

An operation may be indicated if the AC/A ratio is extremely high (e.g., $10\Delta/1$ D or higher) or if the deviation at near is not adequately controlled by optical means or vision training. If the deviation

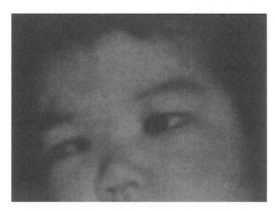

Figure 7-3. Infantile esotropia in a 4-month-old patient.

occurs intermittently and infrequently at near, the operation should be deferred until age 5 or 6 years, at which time the patient is usually able to cooperate with preoperative and postoperative vision training. The conventional surgical procedure is a recession of both medial rectus muscles (e.g., 5 mm, each eye), because this operation reduces the deviation more at near than at far.[13] Semmlow et al[14] reported good long-lasting reductions in the AC/A ratio of 21 patients having this surgical procedure. In cases of very large esotropic angles at near (e.g., more than 45Δ), other surgical procedures may also be required for adequate reduction of the eso deviation. If the patient has fairly good fusional abilities preoperatively, the surgical results are usually good. In some surgical cases, however, the long-term result is a microtropia with only peripheral fusion.[15]

INFANTILE ESOTROPIA

In the past, the term *congenital esotropia* was applied to those cases of primary comitant esotropia (PCE) that developed within the first 6 months of life (Figure 7-3). The term *congenital*, however, literally means "existing from birth" and does not adequately describe most of the esotropia cases occurring at an early age that have many of the same clinical characteristics. Therefore, the term *infantile esotropia* is preferable and connotes a period of onset from birth to 6 months. Nixon et al[16] reported that only a fraction of cases of infantile esotropia are reliably observed to originate at birth. Furthermore, the eyes of a neonate rarely are aligned exactly and consistently during the first week of life; the deviation usually is variable, sometimes aligned and other times convergent or divergent. Normally, alignment and coordinated oculomotor control is not rudimentarily estab-

lished until the age of 3 months.[16, 17] Nevertheless, the specific age of onset in constant esotropia is fundamentally important in establishing the prognosis for treatment when the patient is first examined months or years later. The more time that normal binocular vision has had to develop prior to a constant manifest deviation, the better is the prognosis for cure of the strabismus. Recently, some practitioners have recommended the term infantile esotropia syndrome or essential infantile esotropia to describe a spectrum of eso deviations and associated characteristics that occur during the first 6 months of life. We have chosen to use infantile esotropia to describe esotropia occurring within the first 6 months of life.

The term *infantile esotropia* is somewhat ambiguous in that the etiology of the strabismus, often innervational, seems to be the same as that in primary comitant esotropia. von Noorden[18] suggested that the primary etiology of infantile esotropia is either delayed development of fusional vergence or a primary defect of fusional vergence. However, associated clinical features (e.g., dissociated vertical deviation, inferior oblique overaction, and latent nystagmus) tend to occur in infantile esotropia but not in esotropia of later onset.

Characteristics

Approximately half of all infantile esotropia patients have hyperopic refractive errors of at least +2.00 D.[19] Ingram and Barr,[20] however, reported a study of 1-year-old infants from a general pediatric practice in which only 11% of patients had hyperopia in this range. Although accommodation may be a factor in the etiology of infantile esotropia, most infantile esotropia cases are not exclusively accommodative. The angle of deviation is usually large (30Δ or more), stable, comitant, and approximately the same magnitude at all distances (which indicates a normal AC/A ratio). Characteristics of infantile esotropia are listed in Table 7-2.

Clinicians frequently observe crossed fixation in infantile esotropia. The child uses the right eye for targets in the left visual field and the left eye for objects in the right field. This crossed fixation behavior accounts for an apparent limitation of abduction of each eye that is often observed. Testing ocular rotations adequately in extreme fields of gaze is difficult in infants, particularly if they have developed the habit of crossed fixation.

Table 7-2. Characteristics of Infantile Esotropia

Mechanism	Innervational; familial tendency (genetic)
Onset	Birth-6 mos
Refractive error	In approximately 50%, <2 D of hyperopia
Constancy	Usually constant angle, >30Δ
Comitancy	Usually comitant
Eye laterality	Often either alternating or crossed fixation pattern
Correspondence	Usually anomalous retinal correspondence; in some cases, lack of correspondence
Amblyopia	Approximately 40% of cases
AC/A ratio	Usually normal
Symptoms	Usually cosmetic concerns only
Long-term prognosis	Poor if treated after age 2 yrs; fair if treated before age 2 yrs
Long-term associations	Overacting inferior oblique muscles, dissociated vertical deviation, latent nystagmus
AC/A = accommodative-convergence/accommodation	

Repeat testing and observation may be needed to differentiate a true paresis from an apparent abduction limitation resulting from habitual crossed fixation. Observing abduction during the doll's-head maneuver, left and right, may help one to make the distinction between a lateral rectus paresis and a pseudoparesis. The examiner holds the infant directly in front and makes eye contact while rotating the patient's head to the left and right. For example, the examiner should look for abduction of the patient's right eye as the head is rotated to the patient's left. If the right eye is seen to abduct, pseudoparesis is indicated. The unaffected, or less affected, eye should be patched for a few days to determine whether abduction rapidly develops in the other eye. If it does, then pseudoparesis is confirmed. If, however, paresis is present, there will be little or no abduction.

Amblyopia often is associated with infantile esotropia if the child habitually fixates with only one eye. Two large clinical surveys of children with infantile esotropia found amblyopia in 35% and 41% of the samples, respectively.[19, 21] Established amblyopia in infancy, if not identified and treated early, will most likely become deep and may become unresponsive to subsequent therapy at ages 5-7 years or older.

Vertical deviations often are associated with well-established infantile esotropia, but their etiologies are not well understood. One common condition is overaction of one or both inferior oblique muscles (Figure 7-4). The clinician may observe an increasing hyper deviation of an eye as it moves nasally during versions. The other eye is similar as this inferior oblique overaction is usually bilateral. In one series of 408 infantile esotropes, overaction

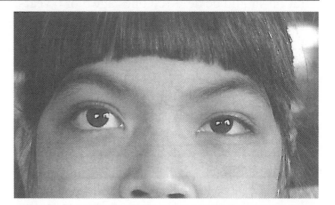

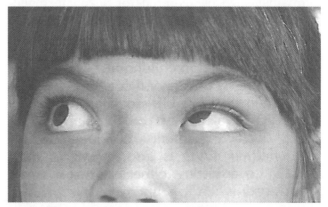

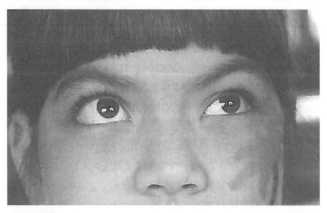

Figure 7-4. Overacting inferior oblique muscle, Top. Primary gaze. Middle. Right gaze with large overaction of the left inferior oblique muscle. Bottom. Left gaze with smaller overaction of the right inferior oblique muscle.

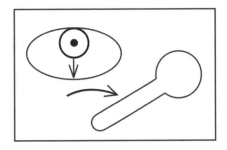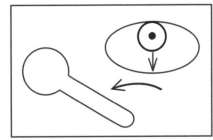

Figure 7-5. Dissociated vertical deviation as seen on the alternate cover test.

of the inferior oblique muscles was found in 68% of the sample.[22] For unknown reasons, the condition usually is not present during the first year of life but appears later in childhood.

Another poorly understood condition associated with infantile esotropia is dissociated vertical deviation (DVD), which must be distinguished from bilateral overacting inferior oblique muscles in young children. DVD is also known as *double hyper*. On cover testing, either eye that is covered drifts upward; when it is uncovered, a downward movement is observed (i.e., either eye is hyper on the cover test) (Figure 7-5). This is the opposite of the usual hyper-hypo relationship seen in most vertical deviations. One eye may show a larger hyper deviation than the other, which suggests the presence of an ordinary hyper deviation component that is obscured by the double hyper.

In contrast to overacting inferior oblique muscles, DVD is usually evident in all fields of gaze. The prevalence of DVD in infantile esotropia is high, ranging from 51% to 90% depending on the patient series.[22, 23] The onset of DVD is usually after age 2 years, and it may occur years after successful surgical management of the esotropia. It is advisable to discuss this possibility with the patient's parents so that, if DVD should occur in the future, it would not be completely unexpected. It is noteworthy that we have seen DVD in orthophoric (or nearly orthophoric) patients who have normal binocularity in all other respects.

Another fairly common feature of infantile esotropia is nystagmus, both latent nystagmus and manifest nystagmus with a latent component. Reported prevalences range from 25% to 52% depending on the particular patient series.[22, 23] Many nystagmus patients with esotropia have an abnormal head posture in an unconscious attempt to dampen the nystagmus. Lang[23] proposed that the reason nystagmus and DVD are associated with infantile esotropia is the presence of a midbrain lesion disrupting both vestibular and oculomotor control centers.

Infantile esotropia is also associated with other abnormal eye movement patterns including nasotemporal asymmetries of optokinetic nystagmus (OKN), and smooth pursuits.[24] The development of ocular motor systems are quite sensitive to the effects of abnormal binocular visual experiences. In normal infants up to 6 months of age, the OKN response favors nasalward over temporal movement but the asymmetry disappears after 6 months. In children and adults with infantile esotropia this response can persist beyond 6 months of age. (See Chapter 5 for discussion.) In a similar vein, infantile esotropes may show nasotemporal asymmetry when making pursuit eye movements favoring nasalward movement during monocular eye movements.

Management

A cardinal principle in the management of infantile esotropia is early intervention. Generally, the longer effective therapy is delayed, the worse is the long-term prognosis (see Chapter 6). The ideal time at which to initiate treatment is at the onset of the condition. Prognosis for a functional cure of very early infantile esotropia approaches zero if treatment is delayed beyond the age of 2 years. Early treatment is not merely important; it is essential. In addition, due to the large angle of deviation surgical intervention is usually required.

Since eye turns can be variable, especially during the first 6 months of life, it is important to identify when the esotropia is stable in infants. The characteristics and stability of the deviation in the first 6 months of life was investigated by the Congenital Esotropia Observational Study (CEOS).[25] In this study, 175 infants between 4 and 20 weeks of age were enrolled and the primary outcome measure was ocular alignment at 28 to 32 weeks of age. The esotropia was classified as resolved if the deviation was less than 8 prism diopters at the outcome visit. The results showed that 27% of patients had spontaneous resolution of the esotropia and this tended to occur in cases where the deviation is less than 40Δ and is intermittent and variable. In contrast, the

CEOS study found that infantile esotropia persists in most infants who have a constant large angle of deviation ($\geq 40\Delta$) with onset after 10 weeks of age and a refractive error ≤ 3.00 D of hyperopia. Thus, frequent examinations of the infant are necessary, because the visual status can change dramatically and rapidly during the first year of life. General principles of clinical management are as follows.

Optical Treatment

Corrective lenses to cover full cycloplegic, retinoscopic findings should be prescribed if there is a significant refractive error. In general if the hyperopia is ≥ 2.50 then correction of the hyperopia should be prescribed. Spectacle lenses are intended to correct any accommodative component of the deviation as well as any significant astigmatism or anisometropia. Prescription for even small amounts of hyperopia may be warranted if the lenses are intended also to provide a platform on which to mount Fresnel prisms. The prism power should be equal to or greater than the amount of the residual deviation. Prism spectacles should be worn at least 3 hours daily in an attempt to provide normal binocular stimulation during the critical developmental period. Retinoscopy should be repeated at least every 3 months during the first 2 years of life, as changes in refractive status can occur frequently and rapidly.

Occlusion Therapy

In cases of suspected or confirmed amblyopia, treatment should begin with monocular occlusion. Even in cases of no amblyopia, part-time patching ensures that amblyopia will not develop. Appropriate patching builds monocular fixation, prevents suppression and the development of ARC, and promotes abduction. Patching should be constant if there is constant esotropia. If the strabismus is intermittent (a rare occurrence in cases of infantile esotropia), patching should be intermittent during those times that the patient is likely to have a manifest deviation (e.g., fatigue in afternoons or evenings). Since acuity measures can be difficult to obtain at this age, unless the clinician has access to preferential looking procedures, the practitioner typically uses alternation of fixation as a guide to monitor amblyopia improvement. The alternation can either be spontaneous or demonstrated by forcing fixation to the amblyopic eye during cover testing. Care must be taken to avoid occlusion amblyopia when patching a patient younger than 5 years. Infants younger than 2 years should receive daily alternate patching even in cases of unilateral amblyopia. (Refer to Chapter 10 for a discussion of occlusion.)

Parents and caregivers should be instructed about active stimulation of fixation and abduction of the child's strabismic eye. To build fixation and eye-hand coordination skills, small toys, candies, and other objects can be offered to the child to touch, while the child's dominant eye is patched. To stimulate abduction, interesting and desired objects can be slowly introduced into the child's restricted field of gaze. However, many vision training techniques for building binocularity are not practical for children younger than 2 years. The goals of vision training, however, are to establish equal and normal visual acuity, free alternation of the eyes (to prevent recurrence of amblyopia), and good ocular motility. The next step is eye alignment to promote development of normal binocular vision.

Surgery

If the residual angle of deviation after full correction of the refractive error is too large to be managed practically with prisms (greater than 20Δ), surgery is necessary before the age of 2 years to ensure a reasonable chance for normal binocular vision. In a now classic study, Taylor[26] demonstrated the advantage of early surgical intervention (see Chapter 6). Subsequent studies have also confirmed this advantage but, even so, the best result that can be expected in many cases appears to be peripheral, but not central, fusion. Often there remains a microtropia (monofixation syndrome), reduced stereopsis, and ARC. Nevertheless, there may be fairly good motor vergence ranges. Normal stereoacuity should not be expected in many cases of infantile esotropia.

A controversial issue is the timing of surgery in infantile esotropia within the first two years of life. It is generally accepted that surgery by 2 years of age results in improved outcomes. However, the earliest age at which surgery should be performed remains controversial. In the past, there appeared to be little advantage for a successful outcome in performing surgery in patients younger than age 1.[27] In addition, the risks of general anesthesia may be enhanced in this very young population. However, there has been a recent trend toward earlier surgical intervention in cases of infantile esotropia. The rationale for very early intervention is to provide ocular alignment during the critical period when stereopsis develops (4 to 6 months of age).[28] In addition, recent advances in pediatric anesthesia and surgical techniques have made it possible to obtain eye alignment in the first few months of life.[24] One primary issue in very early intervention is the stability of the esotropia. The data from the CEOS[25] study described above showed that infants with <+3.00 D refractive error and $\geq 40\Delta$ of esotropia on at least 2 visits at an age > 2.5 months are very unlikely to show resolution of the esotropia via optical intervention. These infants would be candidates for very early surgical intervention. In a recent study Birch and Stager[28] compared very early surgery (surgery by 6 months of age) to early surgery (7 to 12 months of age) in a group of 128 children. The very early surgery group had a higher prevalence of fusion and stereopsis without adverse motor outcome when compared to the early surgery group. Thus, it is very important to determine the refractive status and stability of the esotropia along with treating amblyopia in infantile esotropia in order to determine which cases require surgical intervention. However, the timing of surgery in the first 2 years of life remains somewhat controversial.

Figure 7-3 depicts a case of infantile esotropia that was present at birth; the photograph shows a large constant deviation at age 4 months.[29] At age 13 months, this baby girl underwent bilateral medial rectus and lateral rectus resections. At age 2.5 years, penalization (attenuation) therapy with atropine was given to treat amblyopia of one eye. By age 6, the visual acuity of the amblyopic eye had improved from 20/60 to 20/30, at which time vision training techniques were initiated and continued for 2 years. At age 11, the patient's visual acuities were 20/20 and 20/25, but there was constant 20Δ unilateral exotropia at far and intermittent 20Δ exotropia at near, DVD, covarying retinal correspondence with intermittence of the exotropia, shallow suppression, and no stereopsis. After 1 year of vision training, stereoacuity varied from 50 to 200 seconds of arc on contoured targets, but there was no stereopsis on noncontoured (random dot) testing. The unilateral cover test revealed 2Δ of esotropia, in which the exo deviation was latent most of the time. The angle of anomaly on the Cüppers bifoveal test was approximately 2Δ, which suggested harmonious ARC

centrally, although peripheral sensory and motor fusion seemed normal, which probably kept the exo deviation latent. Best corrected visual acuities were 20/20 and 20/25+. Although not completely cured, this patient with congenital esotropia was able to achieve a satisfactory monofixation pattern with the help of several modes of vision therapy.

The recommended type of operation varies from one authority to another. The most common procedure is recession of both medial rectus muscles.[30] In cases of very large deviations some surgeons will operate on 3 or even 4 horizontal rectus muscles. Cases with associated overaction of the inferior oblique muscle are usually treated by the same surgery with using procedures to weaken the oblique muscle.

Although it is beneficial in establishing some degree of binocularity, early alignment does not guarantee stability over the long term. Amblyopia, secondary overactions of the oblique muscles, and accommodative esotropia can all develop; therefore, vigilant subsequent examinations and management are necessary.[31-34]

Botulinum injection into the medial recti is not recommended in cases of infantile esotropia, for several reasons: Frequent injections are needed under general anesthesia, transient vertical deviations and ptosis are common complications, and research has not demonstrated better results than with conventional surgical techniques.[18]

PRIMARY COMITANT ESOTROPIA

Primary comitant esotropia (PCE) is also known as *acquired nonaccommodative esotropia*. Under the Duane-White classification system, there are three subclasses: basic eso deviation (BE), convergence excess (CE), and divergence insufficiency (DI). This simplified classification is based on the farpoint deviation in relation to the AC/A ratio. (See Chapter 3, as this classification also applies to heterophoria.) The category of convergence excess, or high AC/A esotropia, was discussed earlier in this chapter; hence, only basic esotropia and DI esotropia are discussed here.

PCE occurs in early childhood, as does infantile esotropia. The distinguishing feature of PCE, however, is a later onset of the manifest deviation, after 6 months of age but usually before 6 years. Presumably, a child with PCE has had at least 6 months of normal binocular development, during

Table 7-3. Characteristics of Primary Comitant Esotropia

Mechanism	Innervational; familial tendency (possibly genetic)
Onset	6 mos-6 yrs of age; can be rapid or gradual
Refractive error	Some hyperopia in most; wide variation, approximately 5% myopic
Constancy	Usually constant angle, 20-70Δ; initial stage possibly intermittent
Comitancy	Comitant horizontally; A or V pattern in many cases
Correspondence	Usually anomalous retinal correspondence if early onset and normal retinal correspondence if late onset
Amblyopia	Approximately 30% of cases
AC/A ratio	Usually normal, low in some cases
Symptoms	Usually none
Prognosis	Good if normal retinal correspondence; poor if anomalous retinal correspondence
AC/A = accommodative-convergence/accommodation	

which the neurologic architecture that supports normal binocular vision has matured to a considerable degree. Generally speaking, subsequent associated conditions such as suppression and amblyopia may be absent or only mild in severity. For example, ARC may or may not be present, depending largely on the age of onset of a constant deviation. In contrast, it is almost always present in cases of untreated infantile esotropia.

Characteristics

The most important feature of PCE is patient age at onset. (See Table 7-3 for characteristics of PCE.) The later the onset, the better is the prognosis. Onset is often gradual, and the child may pass through a period of intermittent esotropia before the strabismus becomes constant. The size of the deviation is usually between 20Δ and 70Δ, and the magnitude may slowly increase over time. Refractive error often is independent of the onset of the deviation, because many affected patients have little or no ametropia. However, there can be a partially accommodative component to the strabismus that requires optical compensation.

The cause of PCE is believed to be a developmental innervational anomaly, possibly a multifactorial genetic trait, but the specific pathogenic mechanism is unknown. A small number of PCE cases originate from a supranuclear tumor that may be life-threatening.[35] In most tumor cases, however, the deviation is noncomitant and conspicuous. The clinician must be a very conscientious observer in cases of strabismus that develop early in life, to ensure immediate detection and appropriate referral for imaging studies and neurological evaluation.

Most cases of PCE are basic eso deviations, which means they are characterized by a normal AC/A ratio and approximately equal deviations at far and near. A common exception, however, is DI esotropia, in which the AC/A ratio is low; the near eso deviation is significantly less than that at far. It is important for the clinician to distinguish DI from divergence paralysis, which has serious neurologic implications. Divergence paralysis originating from a midbrain lesion often presents with a greater eso deviation at far than at near, as in DI. However, the deviation is usually noncomitant initially but may gradually evolve toward comitancy over time. This feature can complicate the differential diagnosis between divergence paralysis and DI. Therefore, clinicians should closely monitor all new patients presenting with characteristics of DI. Neurologic examination and neuroimaging can usually be deferred in the initial presentation of low AC/A esotropia that is associated with farpoint diplopia, unless there are other neurologic signs or symptoms.[2, 22]

Management

Prognosis is generally good in cases of PCE if there is early intervention with vision therapy (often including surgery). The later the onset of PCE, the better is the prognosis. Lang[36] reported that an onset of PCE after 1.5 years of age indicates a good prognosis after surgical alignment; many patients can develop good random dot stereopsis. If therapy is delayed, however, patients often develop amblyopia, ARC, suppression, increased magnitude of the esotropia, and other problems that adversely affect the prognosis for later improvement.

The surgical approach in PCE usually relies on recession and resection procedures. Adjustable sutures frequently are used to fine-tune the surgical results on the day of, or after, the operation. Also, botulinum toxin injections into the medial recti to weaken them sometimes are used in older children

Table 7-4. Characteristics of Primary Comitant Exotropia

Mechanism	Innervational; familial tendency; female-male ratio 2 to 1
Onset	Birth-8 yrs; usually gradual
Refractive error	Wide variation, same as general population
Constancy	Approximately 80% intermittent; tendency to become constant over time; angle, 20-70Δ
Comitancy	Comitant horizontally; A or V pattern in many cases
Correspondence	Usually normal retinal correspondence; frequent covariation of anomalous retinal correspondence cases with the intermittent deviation
Amblyopia	Approximately 5% of cases
AC/A ratio	Usually normal or low; high in approximately 10% of cases
Symptoms	Frequent photophobia, squinting (eyelids), or asthenopia
Long-term prognosis	Good if intermittent; poor if constant with anomalous retinal correspondence
AC/A = accommodative-convergence/accommodation	

and adults. (Detailed discussions of vision therapy for eso deviations are provided in Chapter 13.)

The immediate postsurgical goal is to position the eye slightly on the esotropic side of straight alignment, approximately 10Δ eso, because the eyes typically diverge with healing. The best long-term results are found in cases that show ortho alignment or a small eso deviation 1 month postoperatively. The worst stability occurs in patients showing consecutive exotropia at the 1-month checkup.[37]

When treating acquired esotropia, some surgeons will use the prism adaptation test. This test requires that the patient is prescribed the full hyperopic correction, if significant, and then Fresnel prisms that neutralize the eso deviation are worn over the glasses for 1 or 2 weeks. The patient is then re-examined and if the deviation increases with the prisms by more that 8Δ, then the residual deviation is neutralized with an increase in prism power. The process continues until there is an 8Δ or less increase in the deviation. Those exhibiting fusion with the adapted amount of prism are considered responders. In these cases the surgeon then plans the operation for the full prism adapted angle of deviation. In patients who do not have fusion or who build an angle greater than 60Δ without fusion or who develop exotropia with the prisms are classified as non-responders. In these cases the surgeon plans the operation for the original amount of the deviation. A large scale clinical trial using the prism adaptation method showed improved surgical outcomes with a significant reduction in the undercorrection rate when performing surgery for the larger prism adapted angle of deviation in responder patients.[38]

PRIMARY COMITANT EXOTROPIA

Under the Duane-White classification of primary comitant exotropia (PCX), there are three subclasses: basic exo deviation (BX), divergence excess (DE), and convergence insufficiency (CI). This simplified classification is based on the far-point deviation in relation to the AC/A ratio. (See Chapter 3, as these classifications also apply to heterophoria.)

Characteristics

Primary Comitant Exotropia has an etiology similar to that of PCE, an innervational anomaly probably of multifactorial genetic origin. Table 7-4 lists some of the features of PCX. This condition is less prevalent than PCE (approximately 33% as frequent) and reportedly occurs more often in girls than in boys (66% more frequent) for unknown reasons.[39,40]

Unlike esotropes, most exotropes are intermittent (approximately 80%) throughout life. Jampolsky[41] pointed out that the progression of exotropia is usually gradual, starting with an exophoria, then evolving to an intermittent strabismus, with only a small portion of patients becoming constant exotropes. He suggested that suppression is the mechanism of decompensation from exophoria to exotropia.

Infantile presentations of exotropia, before age 6 months, are very rare (1 in 30,000) as compared with infantile esotropia (0.5-1.0%).[42] Nevertheless, these few cases are not usually referred to as infantile exotropia, because of the common intermittent nature of exotropia as compared with constant esotropia. Also, the sequelae of the two conditions differ. In these cases of early-onset constant exotropia there is a high prevalence (67% in one study)[43] of other coexistent ocular and systemic conditions (e.g., ptosis, congenital nystagmus, prematurity, neurologic and genetic diseases).

Exotropia is more likely to manifest at a later age than is true of esotropia. Late-onset intermittent exotropia often is associated with illness, fatigue, and other precipitating factors such as daydreaming, inattentiveness, and photophobic reactions. All these factors can disrupt fusional control of an exo deviation. Clinicians have traditionally associated exotropia with myopia. The implication was that myopia played some part in the etiology of exotropia. However, most studies indicate that the distribution of refractive error in exotropia resembles that in the general nonstrabismic population, and so myopia does not appear to play any special role in the etiology of exotropia.[44,45] Anisometropia, however, can hinder the control of exophoria and can be a precipitating factor.

The intermittent nature of exotropia causes some special problems. Constant strabismus of developmental origin rarely results in subjective reports of asthenopia from patients, but patients with an intermittent deviation, even with deep suppression when strabismic, frequently experience symptoms. Many individuals with intermittent exotropia manifest their deviation mostly at far and maintain fusion (with effort) at near. Besides the common symptoms associated with excessive heterophoria at near (i.e., tired eyes, sleepiness, eyestrain, intermittent blurring of vision, reading difficulties, and headaches), the intermittent exotrope seems unusually predisposed to photophobia. It is common to see an individual with intermittent exotropia close one eye or lapse into the deviation when stimulated by bright light (e.g., as when walking from inside a darkened theater into full sunlight). This "dazzle" effect disrupts fusional control of the latent exo deviation when fusional amplitudes are restricted, whereas patients with adequate fusional amplitudes are not greatly affected in this manner.[46] The reason for this higher sensitivity of intermittent exotropes as compared with other strabismics is unknown.

Intermittent exotropia also presents the examiner with some unique difficulties in establishing the correct diagnosis. The measured angles of deviation at far and near are often not the true angles of deviation. The farpoint deviation often is less when measured in a small, narrow examination room as compared with that measured in the open environment. Burian and Smith[47] reported significantly larger exo deviations in 31 of 105 patients when measured at 30 m (100 ft). For this reason, a questionable exotropic magnitude at far should be remeasured while the patient is outdoors or looks at a distant target through a window.

The measured deviation at near, where the exotropic patient is usually fusing, can also be erroneous. Many exotropes fusing at near present with a smaller measured nearpoint deviation than at far. Frequently, however, patching one eye for approximately 30 minutes results in an increased near deviation that equals the farpoint magnitude.[48]

These patients have simulated (pseudo) divergence excess. Any patient presenting with a larger exo deviation at far than at near should be patched to break down any spasm of fusional convergence, which can mask the true magnitude of the deviation at near. The examiner must take care not to allow any binocular fusion before the nearpoint angle is remeasured. The cover paddle should be placed before the patient's occluded eye as the patch is removed. If the near-point deviation is not influenced by occlusion, the patient can be considered to have true divergence excess and should be treated accordingly. Another test used to identify simulated divergence excess is the gradient AC/A ratio. The angle of deviation at near is remeasured with plus sphere lenses in place (+2.00 D is recommended) to find the gradient AC/A ratio. This gradient ratio then is compared with the calculated AC/A ratio based on the initial cover test findings for far and near. If the calculated AC/A ratio is high and the gradient ratio is relatively low, then the implication is simulated divergence excess. However, if the calculated and gradient AC/A ratios prove to be high, true divergence excess is indicated. For example, if the calculated AC/A is 10/1 and the measured gradient AC/A is 7/1, both are considered to be high and the difference between them is as expected for the two different procedures. Thus, a true divergence excess is indicated. However, if the calculated AC/A ratio is 10/1 and the gradient test measures 4/1, the difference between the two is relatively large, and simulated divergence excess is indicated. Whenever simulated divergence excess is suspected, a prolonged cover test should be performed, as it is the definitive diagnostic procedure for far and near deviation measurements.

Kushner has argued that many cases of divergence excess are the result of "tenacious proximal fusion" (TPF) and that divergence excess with a high AC/A ratio is rare.[49] He states that measuring the AC/A with a +2.00 or +3.00 add at near without first occluding the patient for approximately 1 hour will lead to inaccurate results. The 1 hour of patching allows the TPF response to dissipate and then eliminates this contaminating factor. To support his argument he has published results showing that the gradient AC/A ratio is normal in the majority of divergence excess patients as long as the AC/A testing at near is done following 1 hour of monocular occlusion.

Another important clinical feature of intermittent exotropia is variable diagnostic findings, day to day and hour to hour. The amount of fusional vergence available to compensate for a deviation varies from time to time depending on a given patient's state of fatigue, alertness, and general health. Patients tend to lapse into their exotropic deviation when inattentive, daydreaming, or gazing at the ceiling or sky. The time of day of the visual examination can influence the measured clinical features of the condition. Early in the day, the patient may present with exophoria with excellent stereopsis, whereas in late afternoon, the same patient may have exotropia with deep suppression. Since the deviation tends to occur more frequently at distance viewing than near viewing the use of distance stereotests can aid in determing the patient ability to maintain alignment.

For this reason, it is often advisable to examine patients with intermittent strabismus late in the day, for comparison with results found earlier in the day.

Over time, there is a tendency for intermittent exotropia to worsen; the condition is usually progressive, von Noorden[18] followed up 51 young patients with intermittent exotropia for an average of 3.5 years without treatment; 75% of the cases were found to worsen, often becoming a constant deviation. No change occurred in 9%, and 16% improved without therapy. The practitioner needs to take this into consideration when making recommendations for treatment. When feasible, we recommend early and aggressive treatment, especially with vision training, as soon as the condition is identified.

Management

Prognosis for recovery of binocular function in exotropia is good in patients who experience a long period of intermittence, as compared with a child who has a constant deviation from early childhood. Amblyopia is relatively rare in PCX unless there is significant anisometropia. Likewise, ARC is usually not a serious clinical problem, because the angle of anomaly can covary with the magnitude and intermittence of the exo deviation. (See the discussion of covariation of correspondence in Chapter 5.)

Optical Treatment

Any significant refractive error should be corrected. Unequal visual inputs can have an adverse impact on intermittent exotropes and any significant astigmatism or anisometropia should be corrected. One optical approach to treating exotropia is either undercorrection of hyperopia or an over-minus correction in cases of myopia or ametropia can promote alignment in cases of intermittent exotropia. In a review of the literature Coffey et al gave success rate of 28% for this mode of therapy in intermittent exotropia.[50] A good rule of thumb is to use 1D of over-minus correction for each 12Δ of exotropia and make adjustments as needed. Classically, this treatment is thought to stimulate accommodative convergence and in turn reduce the amount of exotropia. However, in cases of exotropia with normal AC/A ratio the amount of convergence induced by a typical 2 diopter overcorrection would be approximately 10Δ. This amount of convergence would only partially correct most cases of intermittent exotropia. An alternative explanation is that the minus lens overcorrection allows the exotropic patient to converge while not creating blur through the CA/C ratio.[51] That is, when an exotropic patient converges to compensate for the exo deviation they create active accommodation through the CA/C mechanism. For example a patient with a CA/C ratio of 1D to 12Δ will induce 2D of accommodation when converging 25 prism diopters. Regardless of the mechanism over minus correction can be used as an adjunct to vision therapy or as a passive therapy in a patient who cannot participate in a vision therapy program. It should be remembered when using an over-minus correction in school aged children, a near add is often required for optimal comfort with near tasks.

Occlusion

Some clinicians have advocated part time occlusion (3 to 6 hours per day) as a method to disrupt suppression and promote perception of pathological diplopia. In this approach, breaking down suppression can increase the frequency of diplopia which can act as a stimulus to fusional vergence and will in turn help promote alignment. If the child has a sufficient amount of fusional convergence to overcome the deviation, then alignment can be achieved with this approach. This approach can be quite effective in patients that are too young to undergo vision therapy. In addition, occlusion therapy can be used early in a vision therapy program to break down suppression. Coffey et al reported a success rate of 37% when pooling data from 7 studies in cases of intermittent exotropia.[50] However, most studies recommend that occlusion therapy be used in conjuction with other forms of treatment.

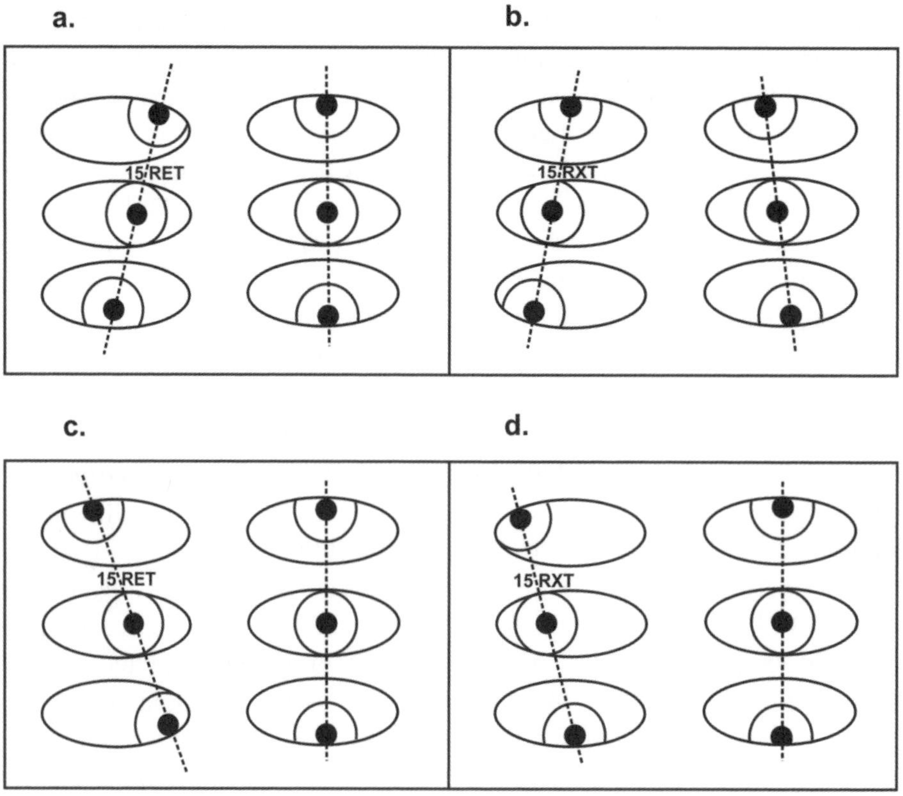

Figure 7-6. A and V patterns, a. A pattern in esotropia of the right eye. b. A pattern in exotropia of the right eye. c. V pattern in esotropia of the right eye. d. V pattern in exotropia of the right eye. (RET = right esotropia; RXT = right exotropia.)

Vision Therapy

In our experience, if the angle of deviation in PCX is less than 20-25Δ, our preferred treatment option is vision therapy, provided the patient is mature enough to participate actively in the program. The estimated success rate for vision therapy is estimated at 59%.[50] One critical issue in treatment is whether to disrupt suppression which may have to be done early in therapy. Breaking down suppression creates diplopia awareness which can act as a stimulus to fusion and help promote ocular alignment. Thus, occlusion therapy may be combined with vision therapy at the start of treatment. A more detailed description of vision therapy is given in Chapter 14.

Surgical

For deviations larger than 25Δ, we recommend beginning with a vision therapy approach but expect that surgery may be necessary to achieve comfortable alignment of the eyes at all distances and times of day. The surgical principles in PCX depend not only on the magnitude of the strabismus but also on whether the deviation is a basic exo deviation, divergence excess, or convergence insufficiency (see Chapter 14). The overall rate of success with surgical intervention has been estimated at 50 to 60 % and depends on the type and magnitude of the exotropia.[50,52,53] The surgery typically involves a recession of the lateral rectus and/or a resection of the medial rectus insertion. A recent study by Figueiria and Hing[53] found that surgery combined with orthoptic/occlusion therapy provided a significantly better result than surgery alone.[53] This study would support our general strategy of beginning with vision therapy in most cases of exotropia.

A AND V PATTERNS

The terms A and V patterns are used to describe significant changes in the horizontal deviation (eso or exo) as the eyes move from up-gaze to the primary position to down-gaze. A and V patterns are, therefore, a form of noncomitancy of the horizontal deviation. Specifically, an A pattern is present when there is an increased convergence (or less divergence) of the eyes in up-gaze and increased divergence in down-gaze. If a patient has an A-pattern esotropia, the eso deviation increases in up-gaze and decreases in down-gaze, whereas in A-pattern exotropia, there is decreasing exo deviation in up-gaze and increasing exo deviation when looking down (Figure 7-6). Conversely, a V pattern is indicated when the visual axes diverge in up-gaze and converge in down-gaze. The V-pattern esotropia increases in magnitude in down-gaze, whereas a V-pattern exotropia increases in up-gaze. These changes in the horizontal deviation with vertical gaze changes are clinically important because they significantly influence the diagnosis, prognosis, and management of strabismus.

Characteristics

An A or V pattern is diagnosed by comparing the alternate cover test results in the primary position to those found in the extreme up and down positions of gaze. By convention, an A pattern is indicated if the horizontal deviation changes 10Δ or more between up- and down-gaze. However, a V pattern is indicated when there is 15Δ or more change vertically. This larger measurement criterion for V patterns is attributable to a physiologic tendency for relative divergence in up-gaze.

In addition to A and V patterns, some patients may show an X pattern, in which divergence increases in up- and down-gazes (e.g., exotropia in both up- and down-gaze). This might be due to overaction of inferior and superior oblique muscles, causing a combination of a V and an A pattern.[54]

Estimates of the prevalence of A and V patterns vary widely, depending on the source and diagnostic criteria. Prevalence is probably close to half of all strabismic patients.[55] The relative frequency of these patterns, from most prevalent to least, is as follows: (1) V-pattern esotropia (by far the most prevalent), (2) A-pattern esotropia, (3) V-pattern exotropia, and (4) A-pattern exotropia.[56] The V patterns occur approximately twice as often as do A patterns, probably because esotropia is more prevalent than exotropia.

The etiology of A and V patterns is usually not paresis but mechanical in nature. The principal factors seem to be overactions and underactions of the oblique and vertical rectus muscles. For example, the most frequent cause of a V-pattern esotropia is the underaction of one or both superior oblique muscles. In down-gaze, the eso deviation is increased by the loss of abduction by the underacting superior obliques. In up-gaze, the eso deviation is decreased by the relatively increased abduction by the normally acting or overacting inferior obliques. Anatomic abnormalities of the bony structure of the orbit and abnormal insertions of muscle tendons have been cited also as etiologic factors in producing an A or V pattern.[13] A and V patterns are frequently associated with infantile strabismus, Duane retraction syndrome, Brown syndrome, acquired bilateral fourth nerve palsy, dysthyroid eye disease with inferior rectus muscle contracture, and orbital malformations found in Down syndrome. On the sensory side, ARC can occur in strabismic patients with A and V patterns; however, as the horizontal angle of deviation (H) changes in up- and down-gaze, the angle of anomaly may covary with it.

If a strabismic individual can achieve normal fusion in some field of gaze, that person usually adopts a head posture that allows fusion to occur. If a patient presents with a habitual chin elevation or depression, A and V patterns should be suspected. For example, a V-pattern esotrope who can achieve fusion in up-gaze may present with a chin depression and a "mischievous" appearance, whereas a V-pattern exotrope may display chin elevation and a "snobbish" appearance, because the deviation is reduced in down-gaze.

Management

We recommend moving the patient's head back (chin up) for measurement in down-gaze and the head down (chin down) for measurement of angle H in up-gaze. Clinicians can test for A and V patterns at either far or near distances, whichever they prefer.

Significant A and V patterns can often be treated surgically, usually by either operating on the oblique muscles or transposing the horizontal rectus muscles.[54] Surgical correction of an A or V pattern is indicated if the vertical noncomitancy contributes to excessive fusional demands or unacceptable cosmesis in cases of horizontal strabismus. An esotropia with an A pattern that has no oblique involvement may be treated by recession of the medial recti and transposed above the original insertion, approximately a muscle-width. The

Table 7-5. Characteristics of Microtropia

Mechanism	Unknown, often secondary to surgery or vision training for an infantile or primary comitant esotropia
Onset	From birth or the time of therapeutic intervention
Refractive error	Probably no relationship
Deviation	1-9Δ strabismic component; usually an additional phoric component; eso deviations much more common than exo or hyper deviations
Constancy	Usually constant in all fields of gaze and at all fixation distances
Comitancy	Usually comitant
Correspondence	Usually anomalous retinal correspondence relative to the strabismic component
Fusion	Peripheral fusion with some vergence ranges, some stereopsis, central suppression of the deviating eye
Amblyopia	Shallow amblyopia frequently present
Symptoms	Usually none
Prognosis	Poor for bifoveal fusion; usually a stable end-stage condition

specific surgical technique depends, of course, on the observed patterns of over- and underaction of the vertically acting muscles. For example, if there is also overaction of the superior oblique muscles in an eso A pattern, weakening procedures for these oblique muscles may be necessary. An underaction of the inferior obliques may also aggravate an A pattern and may require strengthening procedures. V-pattern esotropias may require recession of both medial recti and downward displacement of the original insertion. Because underaction of the superior oblique muscles will increase a V pattern, these muscles may require strengthening procedures. Similarly, overaction of the inferior obliques exacerbates a V pattern and may require weakening procedures.

A-pattern exotropia may require recession of both lateral recti, with downward displacement of the insertions. If the eyes are exotropic with an A pattern due to an overaction of the superior oblique muscles, weakening procedures for these may be required. V-pattern exotropias may be treated by recession of both lateral recti, with upward transposition of the insertions. If the inferior oblique muscles are overacting, the exo deviation tends to increase on up-gaze; these, therefore, may require weakening procedures.

Vision therapy is often helpful in cases in which the patient has some fusional vergence ranges, particularly in exotropic cases that are intermittent. When the exo deviation is small or moderate in the primary position, vision training has great value. However, in cases of large exo deviations with V patterns, surgery may be necessary. Otherwise, when the patient looks up to the sky or ceiling, where there are minimal environmental contours to stimulate fusion, the exo deviation will likely manifest.

MICROTROPIA

The definition of microtropia is disputed, and clinicians disagree as to its characteristics. The terms microstrabismus, monofixation pattern (or syndrome), and subnormal binocular vision have all been used to refer to the same or similar conditions. Microtropia is our term of choice for the condition having the characteristics described in the following section.

Characteristics

We believe that manifest deviation must be 1Δ or greater in magnitude to be classified as strabismus. A fixation disparity, however, is much lower in magnitude, usually not exceeding 20 minutes of arc. (See the discussion of fixation disparity in Chapter 3.) In our opinion, microtropia has been erroneously described by some clinicians as an "unusually large fixation disparity" We prefer to use the term microtropia to describe a frequently seen condition that has most of the characteristics listed in Table 7-5. There is a manifest deviation on the unilateral cover test from 1Δ to approximately 8Δ or 9Δ. This angle may show some variability in magnitude. Besides the manifest deviation, there is often a latent deviation (a phoric component) seen on the alternate cover test. On this test, one eye or the other is always being occluded, which reveals the fusion-free deviation. Clinically, the results of the unilateral cover test are compared with those from the alternate cover test. A larger magnitude is frequently seen on the alternate cover test, indicating a phoric component to the strabismus (Figure 7-7). These microtropic patients usually show foveal suppression of the deviated eye. Nevertheless, fusional vergence ranges can

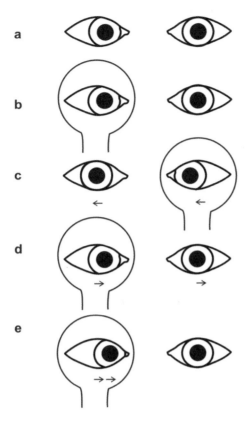

Figure 7-7. Microtropia of the right eye as shown on the alternate cover test. a. Cosmetically good in primary position, b. Occluder on right eye and no movement of the eyes. c. Occluder on left eye and movement of both eyes. d. Occluder switched to the right, esotropic eye and movement of both eyes, with left eye resuming fixation, e. Occluder remaining on right eye for approximately 1 minute, after which right eye slowly moved more inwardly, indicating a "phoric" component to the esotropia.

be measured and sometimes are almost normally sufficient. Usually there is ARC that is harmonious relative to the strabismic component of the deviation. Similarly, there may or may not be amblyopia. Peripheral stereopsis often is present, but central stereopsis is absent or greatly reduced, especially with random dot targets.

There are two major types of microtropia, primary and secondary. Primary microtropia is indicated if there is no history of a larger angle of strabismus. The etiology of this condition is unknown but, like PCE, there appears to be some genetic basis. Secondary microtropia is often the result of vision therapy or surgery for a larger angle of strabismus, particularly in cases of early onset. Other secondary causes may be aniseikonia, anisometropia, uncorrected vertical deviations, and foveal lesions.

Lang[57] reported that most patients with microtropia are microesotropes, but there are exceptional cases of microhypertropia that usually result from surgical intervention of a large-angle hypertropia.

Secondary microtropia is much more prevalent than primary microtropia.

There are specialized tests that help to identify microtropia. The unilateral neutralization test gives a direct measure of the manifest deviation seen on the unilateral cover test (Figure 7-8). When there is a phoric component, the alternate cover test is no longer useful in measuring magnitude of the strabismic component. To measure this horizontal angle of strabismus objectively, the examiner must simultaneously occlude the dominant eye and place the correct amount of base-out prism (in a case of esotropia) before the deviated eye to neutralize any movement of that eye. Consider, for example, a microesotropia of the right eye. The patient is instructed to look at a straight-ahead target while the clinician occludes the left eye. A small outward movement of the right eye is observed and estimated to be 5Δ. To measure this deviation, the doctor must simultaneously occlude the left eye and place the correct magnitude of base-out prism before the right eye to neutralize any movement of that eye (see Figure 7-8). If 5Δ base-out is placed before the right eye and there is no movement of that eye when the left is covered, then 5Δ is the measured magnitude. If there is eccentric fixation, that must be taken into consideration to calculate the true strabismic deviation (see Chapter 4). In microtropic patients who have a phoric component, the total angle of deviation should be measured with the alternate cover test in the standard manner.

In cases of microtropia where the patient has both ARC and eccentric fixation the diagnosis can be clinically challenging. When the angle of anomaly and the amount of eccentric fixation are both the same then there is no movement on unilateral cover test. This has been called microtropia with indentity.[57] These cases can be diagnosed using several procedures discussed in Chapter 5. The clinician can use visuoscopy to detect the presence of EF and can use the 4 base out test to detect a central scotoma in the amblyopic eye. These results combined with reduced stereoacuity would indicate the presence of a microtropia. The Bifoveal Test of Cüppers or the Brock Givner After Image test which both monitor ARC and fixation status can also detect microtropia with identity. (See Chapter 5.) When the angle of anomaly exceeds the amount of eccentric fixation then the microtropia is without identity. In these cases the clini-

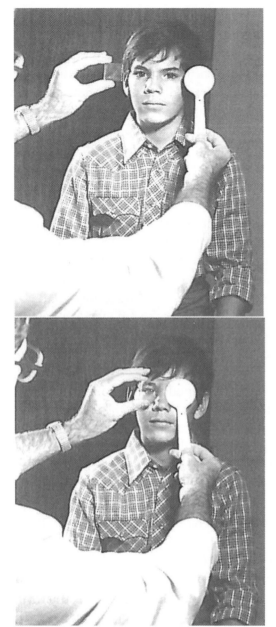

Figure 7-8. Unilateral neutralization test. Top. Preparing for the unilateral cover test for neutralization of an esotropia right eye with base-out prism, Bottom. Simultaneously covering the left eye with an occluder and the right eye with base-out prism. The prism power that equals the esotropic angle of the right eye neutralizes the angle of deviation so that eye movement does not occur.

cian will see movement on the unilateral cover test and the presence of eccentric fixation.

Another useful test for determining the clinical characteristics of a microtropia is the Bagolini striated lens test. A transluminator light (or a penlight) is the fixation target. The typical response of a microtropic patient on this test is a report of the two lines crossing at the light but a small gap observed in the line clued to the strabismic eye. The microtropic angle of deviation can be directly observed by using the unilateral cover test to verify the deviation. Perception of intersecting lines at the light

suggests harmonious ARC (i.e., an angle S of zero in the presence of a strabismus). A gap in the line seen by the deviating eye indicates central suppression. Harmonious ARC and deep central suppression are seen frequently in cases of microtropia. If there is any amblyopia, visuoscopy (also referred to as visuscopy) must be performed to check for the presence and magnitude of eccentric fixation, because this can influence interpretation of the cover test (as to magnitude of the strabismus).

Management

Microtropia in adults does not generally require vision therapy. These patients are usually symptom free, with no cosmetic problem. In addition, they usually have rudimentary binocular vision with fairly good fusional vergence ranges and peripheral (but not central) stereopsis. A small portion of adult microtropic patients, however, do have asthenopic symptoms related to the use of their eyes. Like the heterophoric patient whose fusional vergence is inadequate for visual comfort and efficiency, microtropic patients can have vergence and accommodative skills that are inadequate for their visual needs at school, work, and play. Prisms and added lenses do not seem to help in these symptomatic cases, possibly due to prism adaptation. We have trained the visual skills of many of these patients, often with good results. Vergence ranges increased to nearly normal levels, stereopsis increased slightly, and visual symptoms disappeared after a relatively short office and home training program, from 6 to 10 weeks in length. The microtropia still appeared on the unilateral cover test, but most patients were pleased with the outcome. However, we have also seen some symptomatic microtropia patients for whom no form of vision therapy relieved the symptoms. These patients had to avoid visual activities that exacerbated their symptoms which, in some cases, required a change in employment. In most symptomatic microtropia cases, we recommend vision training similar to that provided in cases of heterophoria.

Some clinicians report having cured microtropia in early childhood. von Noorden[18] discussed three patients younger than 5 years who had microtropia, anisometropia, and shallow amblyopia. These patients wore spectacle lenses for the anisometropia, and the dominant eye was patched. The results included elimination of the microtropia,

Table 7-6. Characteristics of Comitant Vertical Deviations

Mechanism	Innervational, anatomic
Onset	Birth to approximately 3 yrs
Refraction	Probably no relationship
Deviation	Usually small angles, 1-10Δ; often associated with moderate to large horizontal strabismus, eso or exo deviation
Constancy	Can be intermittent or constant, depending on magnitude and fusional status
Comitancy	Comitant, may be secondary to a spread of comitancy after a noncomitant deviation
Correspondence	Vertical ARC is rare but possible, more so, if the horizontal deviation is constant
Amblyopia	Less than in horizontal strabismus
Symptoms	More often than in horizontal strabismus
Prognosis	Poor if ARC; good if normal retinal correspondence
ARC = anomalous retinal correspondence	

20/20 (6/6) vision in each eye, and stereoacuity of 40 seconds of arc. It is possible that these patients were not actually microtropic but instead had anisometropic amblyopia with eccentric fixation (which von Noorden noted) in which the movement on the unilateral cover test reflected the eccentric fixation. Nevertheless, it seems prudent to treat any young patient with amblyopia, whether or not there is an associated microtropia, with patching and optical correction when required. Apparent spontaneous remission of microtropia in young children may occur.[58]

Early vision therapy in some primary microtropes with associated amblyopia has been effective and resulted in normal visual acuity and stereopsis in addition to elimination of the small strabismus. These microtropes, however, were known to have normal binocular development prior to the onset of the microtropic deviation.[59]

CYCLOVERTICAL DEVIATIONS

Cyclovertical deviations involve either the oblique muscles or the vertical rectus muscles. Vertically acting muscles have both vertical and cyclorotary actions in most positions of gaze. Therefore, innervational or mechanical abnormalities of these muscles usually result in both a vertical deviation and a cyclo deviation. Hyper deviations are also prevalent among patients with horizontal strabismus; nearly 40% of all esotropes have a small vertical component.[60] Although vertical deviations are found frequently in combination with horizontal strabismus, they can occur as isolated abnormalities. Because vertical fusional vergence is relatively weak as compared with fusional convergence or divergence, a small vertical deviation of even 1Δ or 2Δ may cause disturbing symp-

toms of diplopia, intermittent blur, eyestrain, and nausea. Moreover, a small vertical component can be the primary obstacle to fusion in some cases of horizontal strabismus. Most cyclovertical deviations are noncomitant (see Chapters 8 and 15). In the next section, however, we discuss comitant vertical deviations.

Comitant Vertical Deviations

Isolated comitant vertical deviations greater than 10Δ are rare. On the other hand, small comitant hyper deviations, as isolated conditions or associated with moderate or large-angle horizontal deviations, are common. Large angles of vertical deviation (greater than 10Δ) almost always show signs of noncomitancy, including those with paretic etiology and a subsequent "spread of comitancy." Amblyopia and ARC are less often associated with vertical deviations than with horizontal strabismus. The etiology of comitant vertical deviations presumably includes anatomic factors and abnormal innervation (Table 7-6).

The obvious conservative treatment for a comitant vertical deviation, either heterophoria or strabismus, is the prescription of vertical prism. Comitant vertical deviations of 10Δ or less can usually be managed successfully with spectacle prisms if the prism amount is split between the eyes and the frame does not have a large vertical dimension. Vertical prism corrections greater than 10Δ may result in cosmetic problems due to the optical displacement of the eyes. Vision training is a second-choice treatment option to increase vertical fusional ranges. However, vision training often is used in conjunction with prism therapy to help to relieve symptoms.

Cosmetic hypertropia or hypotropia greater than 10Δ often requires surgical management. In patients with a combined horizontal and vertical strabismus, in which the vertical component is less than 12Δ, surgical correction of the vertical deviation can often be accomplished by a vertical transposition (vertical offset) of the horizontal muscles. To correct a hyper deviation, for example, the insertions of the horizontal recti of the higher eye are lowered. This procedure is done in addition to the appropriate recession or resection procedure for the horizontal deviation. To correct for a hypotropia, the horizontal muscle insertions of the lower eye would be raised. Dale[4] reported that the correction ranges between 0.5Δ and 1.0Δ for each millimeter of offset surgery. For vertical deviations of 12Δ or greater, it is usually necessary to recess the appropriate vertical muscles. For example, if the patient has a comitant right hypertropia of 25Δ, the superior rectus in the right eye and the inferior rectus in the left eye should each be recessed to obtain the best possible comitant result.

Dissociated Vertical Deviations

DVDs, or so-called double hyper deviations, frequently are associated with infantile esotropia. (See the discussion of DVD earlier in this chapter.)

SENSORY STRABISMUS

A blind eye usually becomes a turned eye. When sensory fusion is lost, strabismus usually results. Severely reduced visual acuity in one or both eyes can be an insurmountable obstacle to sensory fusion. When the primary cause of a strabismus is a loss of vision due to visual or certain neurological diseases, then the term sensory strabismus has been used to describe the condition. Recently, some clinical researchers are advocating calling this condition strabismus with visual or neurological disease. The causes of sensory strabismus are therefore as varied as the causes of blindness or severe low vision. Some of the common causes in early childhood include ocular trauma, congenital cataracts, optic atrophy or hypoplasia, congenital ptosis, and high anisometropia. The second most common presenting sign of retinoblastoma in infancy is, in fact, esotropia.[61]

Sensory strabismus is usually comitant but, if the condition is of long standing, secondary contractures can occur, restricting the horizontal move-ment of the affected eye. When a patient presents with strabismus and reduced visual acuity in one eye, it is important clinically to establish which condition preceded the other. Is the strabismus secondary to the acuity loss, in which case a sensory strabismus is present? Or is the acuity loss due to strabismic amblyopia, which has a good prognosis for recovery if early patching and vigorous vision training are initiated?

The direction of eye turn in sensory strabismus appears to relate to patient age at onset. In a series of 121 sensory strabismus cases, Sidkaro and von Noorden[62] observed that esotropia and exotropia were about equally distributed if the onset was within the first 5 years of life. However, if the sensory obstacle occurred later than age 5 years, exotropia predominated by a large margin. This is consistent with our clinical observations that if vision is lost in adulthood, an exotropia rather than esotropia usually occurs. It is not clear why some patients become esotropic and others exotropic. Chavasse[63] speculated that there are various degrees of tonic convergence during early childhood, resulting in either esotropia or exotropia, but during adulthood there may be less forceful tonic convergence, in which case exotropia would predominate.

In many cases of sensory strabismus, the very nature of the condition precludes the restoration of binocular vision (e.g., optic atrophy). In some cases of congenital cataract or ptosis, early surgery and proper optical correction may offer some hope of recovering part or all of the vision loss. In most cases of sensory strabismus, however, therapy is directed toward improving the cosmetic aspects of the eye turn. If the deviation is relatively small, spectacle prisms may be used to correct the appearance of the strabismus (as described in Chapter 6). For larger deviations, cosmetic extraocular muscle surgery usually is advisable. The psychological consequences of a conspicuous, unsightly, turned eye are usually worth preventing, particularly for school-aged children. The standard operation is recession and resection of the appropriate horizontal eye muscles of the deviated eye.[18] Surgical results in sensory strabismus are often unpredictable, but adjustable sutures provide a means of making postoperative corrections. Long-term surgical results often are not as stable as in cases in which some form of binocular vision exists. The original deviation, or even a consecutive strabismus, can be the result over the years, requiring further operations to maintain acceptable cosmesis. The patient or parents must be informed of this possibility.

CONSECUTIVE STRABISMUS

Consecutive strabismus refers to an eye turn that changes from one direction to the opposite direction (e.g., when an exotropia becomes an esotropia postoperatively). There are very few spontaneous cases reported that are independent of a specific event, such as eye surgery or ocular trauma. Consecutive esotropia occurs almost exclusively after surgical overcorrection of an exotropia.

A common surgical goal in management of exotropia is to leave the deviation slightly on the eso side of alignment, approximately 10Δ eso, as there is a tendency for the eyes to diverge during the healing process. Occasionally, the overcorrection is excessive, and a cosmetic esotropia is evident. When this occurs, patients often report postsurgical diplopia. The reported prevalence of surgical overcorrections for exotropia varies, according to different authors, from 6% to 20%.[64,65] The immediate recommendation for small angles of consecutive esotropia is simply to wait and see whether the deviation resolves with the healing process. Many small overcorrections disappear with time, but larger deviations tend to increase. A large overcorrection with limitation of ocular motility on the day after surgery may require further immediate surgical management.[18] In most cases of overcorrection, another operation should not be performed until after 6 months, unless there is a significant degree of noncomitancy. Attempts to eliminate diplopia can be made with compensating Fresnel prisms or spectacle overcorrection using plus-fogging lenses over the deviating eye.

The prevalence of consecutive exotropia is lower than that of consecutive esotropia, ranging from only 2% to 8%, depending on the investigator. Consecutive exotropia can arise spontaneously, although most are surgically induced. As a rule, consecutive exotropia decreases over time. Therefore, a wait-and-see policy is appropriate unless the deviation is extreme or complicated by a marked reduction of ocular motility. Six months is a reasonable waiting period. Attempts to align the eyes and eliminate diplopia with base-in prisms or minus-lens overcorrection may prove beneficial.

In cases in which the AC/A ratio is moderate to high, we suggest prescribing between 2 and 4 D of minus-lens overcorrection for young patients as a temporary method for straightening the eyes. In cases in which lens overcorrection is indicated, we also recommend accommodative facility training to prevent asthenopia.

REFERENCES

1. CEMAS Working Group. A national eye institute sponsored workshop and publication on the classification of eye movement abnormalities and strabismus (CEMAS). In: Hertle R, ed.: The National Eye Institute Publications., 2001.
2. Pollard Z, Greenberg M. Unusual presentations of accommodative esotropia. Trans Am Ophthalmol Soc. 2000;98:119-24.
3. Parks M. Abnormal accommodative convergence in squint. Arch Ophthalmol. 1958;59:364-80.
4. Dale R. Fundamentals of Ocular Motility and Strabismus. New York: Grune & Stratton, 1982.
5. Calcutt C. Contact lenses in accommodative esotropia therapy. Br Orthop J 1989;46:59-65.
6. Grisham J, Gee C, Brott H, Burger D. Evaluation of Bifocal Contact Lenses in the Control of Accommodative Esotropia. OD thesis. Berkeley: University of California School of Optometry, Berkeley, 1992.
7. Rutstein R. Update on accommodative esotropia. Optometry 2008;79(8):422-31.
8. Watanabe-Numata K, Hayasaka S, Watanabe K, al e. Changes in deviation following correction of hyperopia in children with fully refractive accommodative esotropia. Ophthalmologica 2000;214:309-11.
9. Rutstein R. Spasm of the near reflex mimicking deteriorating accommodative esotropia. Optom Vis Sci. 2000;77:344-6.
10. Ludwig I, Parks M, Getson P, Kammerman L. Rate of deterioration in accommodative esotropia correlated to the AC/A relationship. J Pediatr Ophthalmol Strabismus 1988;25:8-12.
11. Bartlett J, Jaanus S, Piscella R, Sharir M. Ocular Hypotensive Drugs. In: Bartlett J, Jaanus S, eds. Clinical Ocular Pharmacology, 4th ed. Boston: Butter worth, 2001.
12. Raab E. Difficult Esotropia Entities: Principles of Management. In: Rosenbaum A, Santiago A, eds. Clinical Strabismus Management: Principles and Surgical Techniques. Philadelphia: Saunders, 1999.
13. Mein J, Trimble R. Diagnosis and Management of Ocular Motility Disorders, 2nd ed. London: Blackwell Scientific, 1991.
14. Semmlow J, Putteman A, Vercher J, et al. Surgical modification of the AC/A ratio and the binocular alignment ("phoria") at distance; its influence on accommodative esotropia: a study of 21 cases. Binocul Vis Strabismus Q. 2000;15:121-30.
15. Pratt-Johnson J, Tillson G. The management of esotropia with high AC/A ratio. J Pediatr Ophthalmol Strabismus 1985;22:238-42.
16. Nixon R, Helveston E, Miller K, et al. Incidence of strabismus in neonates. Am J Ophthalmol. 1985;100:798-801.
17. Friedrich D, deDecker W. Prospective Study of the Development of Strabismus During the First 6 Months of Life. In: Lenk-Schafer M, ed. Orthoptic Horizons: Transactions of the Sixth International Orthoptic Congress. Harrogate, U.K.: British Orthoptic Society, 1987.
18. von Noorden G. Binocular Vision and Ocular Motility: Theory and Management of Strabismus, 5th ed. St. Louis: Mosby, 1996.
19. Costenbader F. Infantile esotropia. Trans Am Ophthalmol Soc. 1961;59:397-429.
20. Ingram R, Barr A. Changes in refraction between the ages of 1 and 31/2 years. Br J Ophthalmol. 1979;63:339-42.

21. von Noorden G. *Infantile esotropia: a continuing riddle. Am Orthop J* 1984;34:52-62.

22. von Noorden G. *A reassessment of infantile esotropia. Am J Ophthalmol.* 1988;105:1-10.

23. Lang J. *Der kongenitale oder fruhkindliche strabismus. Ophthalmologica* 1967;154:201-8.

24. Wong A. *Timing of surgery for infantile esotropia: sensory and motor outcomes. Can J Ophthalmol.* 2008;43:43-51.

25. Pediatric Eye Disease Investigator Group. *Spontaneous resolution of early-onset esotropia: experience of the Congenital Esotropia Observational Study. Am J Ophthalmol.* 2002;133:109-18.

26. Taylor D. *Congenital Esotropia: Management and Prognosis.* New York: Intercontinental Medical Book, 1973.

27. Ing M. *The timing of surgical alignment for congenital (infantile) esotropia. J Pediatr Ophthalmol Strabismus* 1999;36:61-8.

28. Birch E, Stager S. *Long-term motor and sensory outcome after early surgery for infantile esotropia. J AAPOS* 2006;10:409-13.

29. London R, Griffin J, Mazer H. *Congenital esotropia: a documented case report. Am J Optom Physiol Opt* 1982;59:59.

30. Wilson ME, Saunders R, Trivedi R. *Pediatric Ophthalmology.* Berlin: Springer, 2009.

31. Prieto-Diaz J, Prieto-Diaz I. *Long term outcome of treated congenital/infantile esotropia: Does early surgical binocular alignment restoring (subnormal) binocular vision guarantee stability? Binocul Vis Strabismus Q.* 1998;13:249-54.

32. Havertape S, Whitfill C, Cruz O. *Early-onset accommodative esotropia. J Pediatr Ophthalmol Strabismus.* 1999;36:69-73.

33. Rowe F. *Long-term postoperative stability in infantile esotropia. Strabismus* 2000;8:3-13.

34. Shirabe H, Mori Y, Dogru M, Yamamoto M. *Early surgery for infantile esotropia. Br J Ophthalmol.* 2000;84:536-8.

35. Williams A, Hoyt C. *Acute comitant esotropia in children with brain tumors. Arch Ophthalmol.* 1989;107:376-8.

36. Lang J. *Normosensorial Late Convergent Strabismus. In: E C, ed. Transactions of the Fifth Meeting of the International Strabismological Association, Rome.* St. Louis: Mosby, 1986.

37. Marvo T, Kubota N, Sakaue T, Usui C. *Esotropia surgery in children: long term outcome regarding changes in binocular alignment; a study of 956 cases. Binocul Vis Strabismus Q.* 2001;15:212-20.

38. Prism Adaptation Prism Study Group. *The efficacy of prism adaptation in the surgical managment of acquired esotropia. Arch Ophthalmol.* 1990;108:1248-56.

39. Krzystkowa K, Pajakowa J. *The Sensorial State in Divergent Strabismus. In: Orthoptics: Proceedings of the Second International Orthoptics Congress.* Amsterdam, Neth.: Excerpta Medica, 1972.

40. Graham P. *Epidemiology of strabismus. Br J Ophthalmol.* 1974;58:224-31.

41. Jampolsky A. *Ocular deviations. Int Ophthalmol Clin* 1964;4:567-9.

42. Kraft S. *Selected Exotropia Entities and Principles of Management. In: Rosenbaum A, Santiago A, eds. Clinical Strabismus Management: Principles and Surgical Techniques.* Philadelphia: Saunders, 1999.

43. Hunter D, Ellis F. *Prevalence of systemic and ocular disease in infantile exotropia: comparison with infantile esotropia. Ophthalmology* 1999;106:1951-6.

44. Gregersen E. *The polymorphous exo patient. Analysis of 231 consecutive cases. Acta Ophthalmol.* 1969;47:579-90.

45. Burian H. *Pathophysiology of Exodeviations. In: Symposium on Horizontal Ocular Deviations. In: Manley D, ed.* St. Louis: Mosby, 1971.

46. Wirtschafter J, von Noorden G. *The effect of increasing luminance on exodeviations. Invest Ophthalmol.* 1964;3:549-52.

47. Burian H, Smith D. *Comparative measurement of exodeviations at twenty and one hundred feet. Trans Am Ophthalmol Soc.* 1971;69:188-92.

48. Scobee R. *The Oculorotary Muscles, 2nd ed. In.* St. Louis: Mosby, 1952.

49. Kushner B, Morton G. *Distance/near differences in intermittent exotropia. Arch Ophthalmol.* 1998;116:478-86.

50. Coffey B, Wick B, Cotter S, et al. *Treatment options in intermittent XT: a critical appraisal. Optom Vis Sci.* 1992;59:386-404.

51. Scheiman M, Wick B. *Clinical Management of Binocular Vision.* Philadelphia: Lippincott Williams & Wilkins, 2002.

52. Ekdawi N, Nusz K, Diehl N, Mohney B. *Postoperative outcomes in children with intermittent exotropia from a population-based cohort. J AAPOS* 2009;13:4-7.

53. Figueira E, Hing S. *Intermittent exotropia: comparison of treatments. Clin Exp Optom* 2006;34:245-51.

54. Pratt-Johnson J, Tillson G. *Management of Strabismus and Amblyopia: A Practical Guide.* New York: Thieme Medical, 1994.

55. Biglan A. *Pattern Strabismus. In: Rosenbaum A, Santiago A, eds. Clinical Strabismus Management.* Philadelphia: Saunders, 1999.

56. Breinin G. *The physiopathology of the A and V patterns. Trans Am Acad Ophthalmol Otolaryngol.* 1964;68:363.

57. Lang J. *Lessons Learned from Microtropia. In: Moore S, Mein J, Stockbridge L, eds. Orthoptics, Past, Present and Future.* Miami: Symposia Specialists, 1976.

58. Keiner E. *Spontaneous recovery in microstrabismus. Ophthalmologica* 1978;177:280-3.

59. Cleary M, Houston C, McFadzean R, Dutton G. *Recovery in microtropia: implications for aetiology and neurophysiology. Br J Ophthalmol.* 1998;82:591.

60. Scobee R. *Esotropia: incidence, etiology and results of therapy. Am J Ophthalmol.* 1951;34:817-33.

61. Ellsworth R. *The practical management of retinoblastoma. Trans Am Ophthalmol Soc.* 1969;78:462-534.

62. Sidikaro Y, von Noorden G. *Observation in sensory heterotopia. J Pediatr Ophthalmol Strabismus* 1982;19:12-9.

63. Chavasse F. *Worth's Squint or the Binocular Reflexes and the Treatment of Strabismus, 7th ed.* London: Bailliere, Tindall, and Cox, 1931.

64. Hardesty H, Boynton J, Keenan J. *Treatment of intermittent exotropia. Arch Ophthalmol.* 1978;96:268-74.

65. Dunlap E. *Overcorrections in horizontal strabismus surgery. In: Symposium on Strabismus, Transaction of the New Orleans Academy of Ophthalmology.* St. Louis: CV. Mosby, 1971.

Chapter 8 / Other Oculomotor Disorders

Neurogenic Palsies	213
General Considerations	213
Sixth Cranial Nerve (Abducens) Palsy	214
Möbius (Moebius) Syndrome	214
Fourth Cranial Nerve (Trochlear) Palsy	215
Third Cranial Nerve (Oculomotor) Palsy	215
Myogenic Palsies	217
Myasthenia Gravis	217
Dysthyroid Eye Disease	218
Chronic Progressive External Ophthalmoplegia	220
Mechanical Restrictions of Ocular Movement	220
Duane Retraction Syndrome	220
Brown (Superior Oblique Tendon Sheath) Syndrome	222
Fibrosis of the Extraocular Muscles	222
Adherence Syndromes	223
Orbital Anomalies	223
Internuclear and Supranuclear Disorders	224
Internuclear Ophthalmoplegia	224
Supranuclear Horizontal Gaze Palsy	225
Frontal Eye-Field Lesions	225
Occipital and Parietal Cortical Lesions	225
Brainstem Lesions	225
Supranuclear Vertical Gaze Palsy	225
Parinaud's Syndrome	226
Progressive Supranuclear Palsy	226
Parkinson's Disease	226
Nystagmus	227
Physiologic Nystagmus	228
Voluntary Nystagmus	228
Congenital Nystagmus	229
Nystagmus Blockage Syndrome	233
Latent Nystagmus	233
Rare Types of Nystagmus	233

Neurologic and muscular diseases affecting efficiency of binocular vision are discussed in terms of clinical diagnosis and management. A team approach often is required for proper management of these disorders.

NEUROGENIC PALSIES

General Considerations

Noncomitant strabismus is considered neurogenic palsy if it results from damage to one or more of the three cranial nerves subserving ocular motility. In the global sense, *palsy* refers to either a paresis or paralysis. If the nerve damage is complete and no innervation flows to the affected eye muscle, the strabismus is said to be *paralytic*. If disruption of innervation is partial, as is often the case, the term *paretic* is used. Paresis can be of any degree, from mild to severe, depending on the extent of the muscle's dysfunction. In cases of recent paresis or paralysis, the angle of deviation varies in magnitude in different fields of gaze. Also, the deviation varies depending on which eye is fixating. The *primary deviation* refers to the magnitude of strabismus when the unaffected eye is fixating; the *secondary deviation* is measured when the affected eye is fixating. In palsy of recent onset, the secondary deviation is larger than the primary deviation due to Hering's law of equal innervation (discussed in Chapter 4).

Some of many possible causes of neurogenic palsies that result in strabismus are direct trauma to the oculomotor nuclei or anywhere along the course of the nerves, inflammations, myasthenia gravis, multiple sclerosis, brainstem or neuronal tumors, and vascular disorders (e.g., aneurysms, hypertension, atherosclerosis, bleeding from diabetes). Table 8-1 lists the frequency of etiologic factors found by Rush and Younge.[1] The recent onset of diplopia associated with noncomitant strabismus at any age is a harbinger of active disease or injury. When this occurs, careful medical evaluation and management are indicated.

Patients with paretic strabismus often adopt an abnormal head posture, allowing them to maintain fusion in the least affected field of gaze. The head is usually turned in the direction of the action field of the affected muscle. (See the discussion in Chapter 4.) Some patients with noncomitant neurogenic strabismus turn their heads in the opposite direction to that expected, to increase the separation of the diplopic images so that one of the images may

Table 8-1. Etiologic Frequency of Oculomotor Palsy

Causes	Nerve VI (%)	Nerve IV (%)	Nerve III (%)
Vascular	18	19	21
Head trauma	17	32	15
Other known causes	18	8	15
Tumors	15	4	12
Aneurysm	4	2	14
Unknown causes	27	36	23

Source: Modified from JA Rush, BR Younge. Paralysis of cranial nerves 111, IV, and VI: causes and prognosis in 1,000 cases. Arch Ophthalmol. 1981;99;76-79.

Table 8-2. Differential Diagnosis of Paretic Strabismus and Developmental Strabismus

	Paretic Strabismus	Developmental Strabismus
Mode of onset	Usually sudden	Usually gradual or shortly after birth
Age of onset	Any age	Between birth and approximately age 6 yrs
Diplopia	Common	Uncommon
Comitancy	Noncomitant but can become comitant with time	Comitant; A or V pattern may be present
Head posture	Usually abnormal	Usually normal
Amblyopia	Rare, only if early onset	Common
Correspondence	Usually normal retinal correspondence	Anomalous retinal correspondence common
Trauma, neurologic or systemic disease	Common	Uncommon

be more easily suppressed or ignored. The same strategy may apply when some patients choose to fixate with the affected eye. The larger secondary deviation has increased separation of the double images.

Congenital torticollis of the head can arise from a structural deformity of the cervical vertebrae or the sternocleidomastoid muscle. This rare condition is easily differentiated from ocular torticollis (caused by extraocular muscle palsy) by direct questioning of the patient or parents or testing for a restricted range of head movement.

Recent diplopia, noncomitancy, and abnormal head posture are clinical features that distinguish acquired neurogenic palsy from developmental comitant strabismus. Table 8-2 lists differential diagnostic features.

In paretic strabismus, it is important to distinguish between a strabismus of recent origin, possibly due to active pathology, and a benign noncomitant deviation of long duration. Clinical features more commonly associated with deviations of recent origin are disturbing symptoms (e.g., diplopia, nausea, vertigo) and signs of abnormal head posture. These problems diminish or disappear when an eye is occluded. The later the onset of the deviation, the more likely is a report of diplopia.

In congenital or old cases of paretic strabismus, the clinician may find suppression, muscle contractures, and abnormal head posture. Old childhood photographs may reveal a head-tilt pattern of long standing. In congenital cases, the pathologic condition causing the deviation is usually inactive; however, if a patient reports a sudden onset of diplopia, even when the deviation appears to be comitant, it is advisable to suspect active pathology until proven otherwise.

Sixth Cranial Nerve (Abducens) Palsy

The most prevalent noncomitant deviation is acquired sixth nerve paresis. Congenital sixth nerve palsy is rare, and determining the cause is often difficult. Perinatal trauma is one possible etiology. The causes of acquired sixth nerve palsy are numerous. In older patients, the inciting event is often vascular in nature (e.g., ischemic infarction). In patients younger than 40 years, a frequent cause is multiple sclerosis. When a vascular lesion is in the brainstem, the damage usually involves other nuclear centers as well, with obvious clinical manifestations such as facial hemiplegia (damage to the fifth or seventh nucleus). Frequent causes are closed head trauma or a blow to the side of the head, where the sixth nerve is particularly vulnerable.

If a sixth nerve palsy occurs during visual immaturity, suppression, amblyopia, or even anomalous retinal correspondence can develop. In older patients, diplopia is usually reported. The deviation and diplopia increase in the field of gaze of the involved lateral rectus muscle. A compensatory head turn is made in the direction of the action field of the affected eye. If the paresis is severe, the duction (monocular) may be limited in the involved field of gaze and, generally, an abnormal version (binocular) movement is even more noticeable (because of increasing magnitude of the deviation) than is the abnormal monocular duction. Management of noncomitancy is discussed in Chapter 15.

Möbius (Moebius) Syndrome

One special condition involving bilateral sixth nerve palsy is Möbius syndrome. This congenital condition was once believed to be caused by a bilateral palsy of the abducens (sixth) and facial (seventh) nerves, because patients were found to have an esotropia, a bilateral inability to abduct the eyes, and a bilateral facial palsy (facial diplegia). Glasser,[2] however, pointed out that the etiology is usually much more complex and little understood, because of the many other associated conditions. Besides limited abduction and facial palsy, these children are found to have variable disorders in

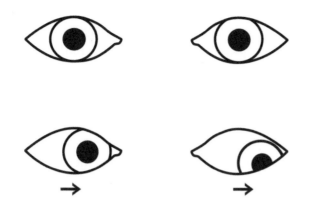

Figure 8-1. Falling eye syndrome on left gaze, with paresis of the superior oblique muscle of the fixating right eye.

several body systems, including an almost total lack of facial musculature; decreased bulk (atrophy) of one side of the tongue; mild to moderate mental retardation; congenital heart defects; limb and chest deformities; hearing, speech, and swallowing difficulties; and other manifestations.[3]

Ocular treatment usually involves correcting any significant refractive error and providing vision therapy for amblyopia if present. These patients should be encouraged to adopt a crossed fixation pattern, if they have not already done so, because abduction is limited. Surgical correction of the esotropia in the primary position might be attempted, but the results are frequently unsatisfactory.

Fourth Cranial Nerve (Trochlear) Palsy

The fourth cranial nerves emerge dorsally from the medullary velum and quickly decussate. This anatomic relationship places these nerves in a vulnerable position from a blow to the forehead. Traumatic closed head injury from a frontal blow is one of the main causes of superior oblique palsy, unilateral or bilateral. Even minor head injuries can result in nerve damage. The causes of fourth nerve palsies are numerous. Frequently, the etiology is vascular. The nutrient vessels to the nerve, the vasa nervorum, can be occluded, causing an ischemic infarction and the death of the nerve. Damage can also occur when blood leaks from vessels as a result of diabetes. In cases of unexplained nerve involvement, a glucose tolerance test is appropriate. Herpes zoster is another potential etiologic factor.

The most prominent sign of a recent superior oblique palsy is a hypertropia in the primary position that increases in down-gaze and with convergence.

Also in primary position, there is an excyclo deviation and often a small eso deviation. In the case of weakness of the left superior oblique muscle, for example, the compensatory head turn would be a right head tilt, a right head turn, and chin depression. (See the discussion of abnormal head posture in Chapter 4.) A positive Bielschowsky head-tilt test (left hypertropia increases on left head tilt) is an indication that the underlying disorder is an underactive left superior oblique muscle, possibly due to fourth nerve palsy. This is true even when there is spread of comitancy.

Patients with a fourth nerve palsy who choose to fixate with the paretic eye demonstrate the *falling eye syndrome* (more correctly, *falling eye sign*) (Figure 8-1). When the patient fixates with the affected eye, particularly in adduction, excessive innervation to the superior oblique muscle is necessary to maintain fixation. Because of Hering's law, the yoked contralateral inferior rectus muscle overacts, making the fixating eye appear to drop.

von Noorden et al.[4] reported that 21% of traumatic fourth nerve palsies in a large clinical series were bilateral. Other authors have reported even higher proportions of bilateral superior oblique involvement.[5] Severity of the paresis is often asymmetric (one eye higher than the other), which can mask the bilateral nature of the condition. One distinguishing feature of bilateral involvement is finding a right hypertropia on left gaze and left hypertropia on right gaze. Another differential observation is a positive Bielschowsky head-tilt test on either right or left tilt. For example, in a case of bilateral involvement in which the patient presents with a right hypertropia in the primary position, the right hypertropia increases on right tilt; on left tilt, a left hypertropia manifests and increases. Another particularly sensitive diagnostic indication of bilateral trochlear palsy is the patient's observation of a double excyclo tilt on a double Maddox rod test.

Third Cranial Nerve (Oculomotor) Palsy

Fortunately, congenital third nerve palsies are rare. The full syndrome includes (1) exotropia due to medial rectus involvement; (2) hypotropia due to weakness of the superior rectus and inferior oblique muscles; (3) limited depression in abduction due to inferior rectus weakness; (4) ptosis of the affected eye due to levator involvement; and (5) possible dilation of a fixed pupil that does not

Table 8-3. Features of Oculomotor (Third Nerve) Palsy

Exotropia due to involvement of the medial rectus

Hypotropia due to involvement of the superior rectus and inferior oblique

Ptosis due to involvement of levator palpebrae

Limited depression in abduction due to involvement of the inferior rectus

Chin elevation in bilateral cases due to limited elevation and bilateral ptosis

In some cases, labeled internal ophthalmoplegia, dilated fixed pupil of the affected eye(s). Other cases in which pupils are normal constitute external ophthalmoplegia

Potential for several unusual effects from aberrant regeneration of the third cranial nerve in congenital cases: jaw-wink reflex, widening of eyelids on depression, and retraction of eye on attempted elevation

react to direct or consensual light stimulation. If the fourth and sixth cranial nerves are uninvolved, the affected eye can be seen to abduct and intort with attempted depression (Table 8-3).

In cases of congenital third nerve palsy, there is often aberrant regeneration of the nerve (the so-called *misdirection syndrome*). Aberrant regeneration can consist of any of several features, all of which are not necessarily present in a given patient.[6]

1. Pseudo-Graefe's sign: elevation of the upper eyelid on attempted down-gaze.

2. Widening of the eyelids on adduction and narrowing on abduction.

3. A dilated, fixed pupil that does not react to direct or consensual light stimulation but that does react slightly on convergence or on adduction. This has been called the *pseudo-Argyll Robertson pupil*.

4. Retraction and adduction of the eye on attempted up-gaze.

Aberrant regeneration is believed to be due to axonal regrowth after a compression injury to the third nerve such as may occur during childbirth. New axons that are misdirected innervate inappropriate muscles, resulting in the paradoxical ocular movements and pupillary reactions characteristic of this syndrome.

Acquired third nerve palsy is a fairly common neurologic condition. Depending on the site of the lesion, the entire nerve can be affected (resulting in the characteristic signs described earlier for congenital third nerve palsy), or only a particular division or isolated root of the nerve can be damaged. Isolated palsies of various extraocular muscles supplied by the third cranial nerve occur less commonly than a more generalized condi-

tion. Any degree of paresis can be present. Deficiencies in elevation, depression, and adduction, along with ptosis, occur in various combinations with or without pupillary involvement. When there is extraocular muscle weakness along with pupillary involvement, the condition is called *internal ophthalmoplegia*. However, *external ophthalmoplegia* is indicated when extraocular muscle weakness exists without pupillary involvement.

Isolated superior rectus palsy is usually congenital. When the uninvolved eye fixates in the primary position, a hypotropia of the affected eye is seen. The hypotropic deviation increases maximally when the patient moves the affected eye into the field of action of the superior rectus muscle, the superior temporal field. Because most such palsies are congenital, the patients do not usually report any symptoms. The recommended surgical procedure for an isolated superior rectus palsy consists of an appropriate amount of inferior rectus recession and superior rectus resection in the involved eye. A 4-mm recession of the inferior rectus, by itself, may give up to 15Δ of vertical correction in the primary position.[7] A recession-resection operation of the same amount may provide as much as 40Δ of vertical correction.

Isolated medial rectus, inferior rectus, and inferior oblique muscle palsies are extremely rare. These three muscles all are innervated by the inferior division of the third nerve, so damage to that root tends to involve all three muscles. However, isolated palsies do occur occasionally for inexplicable reasons. In isolated medial rectus palsy, a noncomitant exotropia is seen along with limited adduction. The corrective surgical procedure is usually recession-resection of the horizontal muscles in the affected eye. The extremely rare isolated inferior rectus palsy can be congenital or acquired. When it is acquired, the cause is usually head trauma (e.g., a blowout fracture to the orbital floor). In the primary position, a hypertropia of the affected eye is found. An incyclo deviation of the involved eye is expected. If there is no restriction of the superior rectus as revealed by the forced duction test, a small hypertropia can usually be corrected surgically by resection of the affected inferior rectus. However, if a superior rectus restriction is found, it must be recessed as well. In large deviations, a combined recession of the superior rectus and a resection of the inferior rectus can correct up to 40Δ of vertical deviation in the primary position.

An isolated inferior oblique palsy is also extremely rare and can be either congenital or acquired. A hypotropia and incyclotropia are seen if the patient fixates with the nonparetic eye. The vertical deviation in the primary position, however, generally is not as large as in cases of isolated superior rectus or superior oblique palsy. If the patient chooses to fixate with the paretic eye (as in some acquired conditions in which the paretic eye has been the dominant sighting eye), a hypertropia of the noninvolved eye is found. As the patient moves the paretic eye into adduction, the contralateral hypertropia increases greatly. This observation is called the *rising eye syndrome* (more correctly, *rising eye sign*). A recommended surgical procedure for an isolated inferior oblique palsy is to recess the contralateral superior rectus and resect the contralateral inferior rectus muscle. This procedure gives greater comitancy when the paretic eye is adducted.

Double elevator palsy can be either congenital or acquired. All patients described as having double elevator palsy must demonstrate an inability to elevate the affected eye from any horizontal position—primary, adduction, or abduction. Some patients present with a chin elevation, indicating that they can fuse in down-gaze. Visual acuity is usually good in each eye. Patients often report diplopia with fixation in the primary position. Other congenital cases show a hypotropia of the affected eye, a pseudoptosis due to the hypotropia, and deep amblyopia.

At one time, double elevator palsy was believed to be caused by weakness of both the superior rectus and inferior oblique muscles of the affected eye, but the anatomy of the third nerve casts doubt on this explanation. Within the third nerve nucleus complex, innervation for these two muscles arises from disparate locations. Because the superior rectus is innervated by the superior division of the nerve and the inferior oblique by the inferior division, explaining the neurologic basis for double elevator palsy is difficult. One possible explanation is that the initial deviation is an isolated palsy of the superior rectus and, with time and another lesion, there is involvement of the inferior oblique. The features that distinguish the double elevator palsy then become evident. A second explanation

Table 8-4. Features of Myasthenia Gravis

Possibly unilateral, but usually bilateral, ptosis that is variable and subject to fatigue; often first sign

In 90% of cases, an oculomotor or strabismic deviation that can mimic any single or combined muscle palsy, including supra- and internuclear palsies; hence its label, the "great pretender"

More frequent in women than in men, particularly at ages 20-40 yrs

Frequently affects the muscles of mastication, swallowing, and facial expression

suggests that the condition is not a palsy at all but a restriction. In one study, three-fourths of the patients who were believed to have double elevator palsy were found to have restriction in up-gaze on the forced duction test.[8] Ziffer[9] stated that the causes of up-gaze limitations, either monocular or binocular, include restriction secondary to superior rectus paresis. It seems that an apparent congenital double elevator palsy can be caused by either a weakness or a restriction.

If there truly is a weakness of elevation, the *Knapp procedure* has proven to be effective in correcting the hypotropia in the primary position. The medial and lateral rectus muscles of the paretic eye are transposed to a position near the insertion of the superior rectus. If the elevation limitation is caused by a restriction, the surgical intervention is directed to releasing the restriction. The procedure in such cases often involves a recession of the inferior rectus muscle and the inferior conjunctiva.

MYOGENIC PALSIES

Myasthenia Gravis

Myasthenia gravis is a chronic, progressive disease characterized by skeletal muscle weakness and fatigue and has a predilection for the muscles of mastication, swallowing, facial expression and, particularly, eyelid and ocular motility (Table 8-4). Ptosis and diplopia often occur as the first signs of the condition, especially in adults. Ocular muscle involvement eventually occurs in 90% of all myasthenia patients and accounts for 75% of initial presentations.[10] The deviation can mimic any oculomotor palsy: In this sense, it is the great pretender. The onset can happen at any age, but the disease usually becomes manifest between the ages of 20 and 40, affecting women more often than men. Infantile forms are rarely encountered, but the course of the condition in infants and children differs from that in adults, as children exhibit a wider range of muscular involvement. The condition characteristically is variable, marked by periods of exacerbation and remission. Muscle function may change within minutes, hours, or weeks.[2]

Myasthenia gravis is a skeletal muscle autoimmune disorder distinguished by a reduction of the available postsynaptic acetylcholine receptor sites on the end plates at myoneural junctions. The anti-acetylcholine receptor antibody is present in approximately 80% of patients with the generalized disease and in approximately 50% of patients with myasthenia restricted to the ocular muscles.[11] Diagnosis of myasthenia gravis is based on demonstration of easy muscular fatigability and its rapid relief by systemic administration of an anticholinesterase agent such as edrophonium chloride (Tensilon). A period of 5-10 minutes of closing the eyes and resting also can temporarily restore functions; this can be helpful for differential diagnosis from causes other than myasthenia gravis.

Treatment of myasthenia gravis falls within the purview of a neurologist. Systemic anticholinesterase medications are given to treat the disease, but these are rarely successful in completely controlling ptosis and diplopia. In the purely ocular form of the disease, the administration of corticosteroids (e.g., prednisone) on an alternate-day schedule has yielded remarkably good results, approaching 90-100%.[12] Due to the variable nature of the condition, prism therapy is usually unsuccessful; the clinician often resorts to occluding one eye to relieve diplopia. Although myasthenia gravis may mimic any single or combined extraocular muscle palsy, including supranuclear and intranuclear ophthalmoplegia, eye muscle surgery is generally not indicated unless the deviation is stable over a long period of observation. A ptosis crutch fitted to a frame to eliminate the drooping lid or lids is occasionally beneficial. Frequent changes of Fresnel prism power can also be used to relieve diplopia. Thus, the ocular manifestations of the disease often are managed on a symptomatic basis.

Dysthyroid Eye Disease

The association of hyperthyroidism and eye disease has been known for two centuries. In 1835, Graves[13] described the eye signs of a hyperthyroid female patient in detail, particularly exophthalmos (proptosis). Hence, Graves' name became attached to the condition when exophthalmos is present. Graves' ophthalmopathy can appear at any time during the course of hyperthyroidism with its elevated levels of thyroid hormone. Systemic symptoms include nervousness, irritability, emotional lability, sweating, palpitations, difficulty breathing, fatigue, weight loss, increased appetite, leg swelling, and increased bowel movements. Commonly associated signs are goiter (enlarged thyroid), tachycardia, skin changes with abnormal pigmentation, and tremor.[14] Thyroid eye disease in children and adolescents is uncommon; the condition occurs most commonly in women 30-50 years old, and the prevalence peaks again in 60-year-olds. The overall female-male ratio for systemic hyperthyroidism is 4 to 1 but, in thyroid eye disease, the ratio is lower, approximately 2.5 to 1.0. [15] At the time of diagnosis, the eye symptoms and signs associated with hyperthyroidism occur in 20-40% of patients. Most patients present with the systemic symptoms. However, approximately 20% initially seek ophthalmologic or optometric care due to the ocular manifestations, without prior identification of systemic hyperthyroidism.[16] Graves' disease is an autoimmune disorder, although its etiology and pathology are not precisely understood. The goal of laboratory studies is to demonstrate either systemic hyperthyroidism or altered immune response to thyroid-related antigens, or both. Char[14] recommended the diagnostic laboratory test for thyrotoxicosis—determination of the serum thyroid-stimulating hormone level, which is abnormally low in this disease.

Proptosis of the eyes is a common sign associated with Graves' ophthalmopathy. Bilateral exophthalmometer readings in excess of 22 mm or a difference between the eyes of 2 mm or more is regarded by most clinicians as suspicious of orbital pathology. The average amount of proptosis in Graves' disease is not large (approximately 3 mm) as compared to controls.[17] There is usually some proptosis asymmetry. The eyelids usually are retracted in cases of Graves' disease, and the sclera shows superiorly and inferiorly (i.e., Dalrymple's sign). Eyelid retraction associated with proptosis is so specific to Graves' disease that it is used as the primary clinical indicator of the condition. Day[18] noted this finding in 94% of his series of 200 cases. In proptosis of nonthyroid origin, patients usually do not have eyelid retraction, although exceptions do occur. Because of the eyelid retraction, the patient may have the appearance of staring or being startled. Infrequent and incomplete blinking often occurs. On down-gaze, the upper eyelids usually lag, exposing sclera superiorly (i.e., von Graefe's sign). Exophthalmos is not always pathognomonic of thyroid eye disease. Many other conditions (e.g., high myopia, steroid use, Cushing's syndrome) result in proptosis or a pseudoproptosis. However, the combination of bilateral exophthalmos, eyelid retraction, stare, and an enlarged thyroid are virtually pathognomonic of Graves' disease.[14]

Proptosis in Graves' disease is caused by extraocular muscle enlargement. The muscles are usually enlarged two to five times their normal size due to fatty infiltrates, lymphocytes, macrophages, mast cells, and interstitial edema.[19,20] The increased muscle size is not due to the muscle fibers themselves, which histologically appear normal, but to inflammatory infiltrates, cells, and edema. Orbital connective tissue and extraocular muscle antibodies have been detected in the serum of patients with Graves' ophthalmopathy.[21] The immunologic mechanism of involvement is not well understood. Because of the enlarged muscles, there is a resistance to retropulsion (pressing the eye back into the orbit). The most commonly involved extraocular muscles in thyroid eye disease, in order of frequency, are the inferior recti (80% of patients), medial recti (44%), superior recti, and lateral recti.[22] Oblique muscles rarely are involved.

Inferior rectus involvement results in a tethering of the eye, restricting movement in up-gaze. In this case, the forced duction test is positive for a restrictive myopathy of elevation. Patients often report diplopia in up-gaze and, eventually, in the primary position; in fact, the most common cause of spontaneous diplopia in middle-aged or older patients is Graves' disease.[14]

Increased intraocular pressure (IOP) can occur due to the pressure of the muscle against the eye on attempted up-gaze. Some investigators believe that a 4-mm increase in IOP between inferior and superior gaze is highly suggestive of restrictive myopathy. Gamblin et al.[23] observed that all patients with long-standing thyroid exophthalmos had increased IOP, as did 68% of patients without measurable proptosis in the primary position. There is computed tomographic (CT) and ultrasound evidence of orbital involvement in almost all patients and clinical evidence of bilateral eye

Table 8-5. Classification of Ocular Changes in Graves' Disease

Class	Definition
0	No signs or symptoms
1	Only signs (upper eyelid retraction and stare with or without eyelid lag or proptosis); no symptoms
2	Soft-tissue involvement (symptoms and signs)
3	Proptosis
4	Extraocular muscle involvement
5	Corneal involvement
6	Sight loss (optic nerve involvement)

Source: Modified from DH Char. Thyroid Eye Disease, 3rd ed. Boston: Butterworth-Heinemann; 1997:46-56.

involvement in 80-90% of cases of hyperthyroidism.[24,25] Even in cases in which the condition appears unilateral, CT scans usually show enlarged extraocular muscles.[26]

Char[14] proposed an abbreviated classification system for the progressive eye changes found in Graves' disease (Table 8-5). The first two categories include minimal eye involvement, whereas the others represent more serious eye findings. Soft-tissue involvement, class 2, refers to symptoms of excessive lacrimation, sandy sensation, retrobulbar discomfort, and photophobia, but not diplopia. There can be injection of the conjunctiva and eyelid edema. Corneal involvement, class 5, refers to varying degrees of exposure keratitis due to the proptosis and lagophthalmos. Loss of sight, class 6, usually is caused by compression of the optic nerve at the apex of the orbit by the enlarged extraocular muscles.

Almost 90% of patients who develop the eye sign of Graves' disease undergo spontaneous remission of most signs and symptoms within 3 years of systemic treatment.[14] Eyelid retraction and lag on down-gaze usually resolve when hyperthyroidism is brought under control. Similarly, many patients with extraocular muscle involvement improve. Ophthalmic problems, such as exposure keratitis, should be monitored and conservatively treated during the course of systemic treatment. Systemic treatment of Graves' disease includes radiation of the thyroid, steroids, diuretics, and immunologic medication. If the patient's restrictive ocular motility does not respond sufficiently to systemic treatment, ocular muscle surgery usually is indicated. Similarly, if the proptosis does not diminish, the patient may benefit from orbital decompression surgery.

Several therapeutic approaches to the management of thyroid myopathy are available, but each has its limitations. The extraocular muscles are usually inflamed, enlarged, and fibrotic late in the disease. Most patients have either simple hypotropia or hypotropia combined with esotropia. Some patients assume an elevated chin posture because of the restriction of motility in up-gaze. Each of these factors must be considered in the choice of therapeutic options. Initially, the patient's response to medical treatment (antithyroid medication, corticosteroids, and immunosuppressive drugs) is evaluated. In cases of diplopia, prisms often are found to be helpful unless the deviation exceeds 10Δ. Because the deviation is usually noncomitant, prism spectacles need to be designed for specific uses at far and near. Presbyopic Graves' patients generally fare better with single-vision glasses than with bifocals. If the magnitude of the deviation is variable, Fresnel prisms are practical during this phase, as the prism power can be changed easily.

Muscle surgery should not be considered until the deviation is stable for 4-6 months. When muscle surgery is indicated, and it usually is after orbital decompression, it is advisable for the surgeon to use adjustable sutures along with a large recession of the restricted muscle. The adjustable sutures give the surgeon the opportunity to fine-tune the residual deviation the day after the operation. A single muscle operation is reportedly successful in correcting diplopia in 50-65% of patients.[27,28] Single binocular vision over a wide range of gaze is, however, an unrealistic expectation in most cases of Graves' ophthalmopathy, but the combination of surgery and prisms usually eliminates diplopia in the primary position and at the reading angle. Eyelid surgery for long-standing lid retraction or other lid abnormalities should be undertaken as the last step after orbital and muscle surgery.

Chronic Progressive External Ophthalmoplegia

Chronic progressive external ophthalmoplegia is a rare ocular myopathy that affects the extraocular muscles, levator palpebrae, orbicularis and, occasionally, other facial muscles, especially those used in mastication.[29] Chronic progressive external ophthalmoplegia is also known as *ocular myopathy of von Graefe*. The first presenting sign is often bilateral ptosis that does not improve with the administration of anticholinesterase agents, unlike the ptosis found in myasthenia gravis. There is usually a slowly progressive loss of ocular motility affecting elevation more than other fields of gaze. In extreme cases, motility is lost in all fields of gaze and the eyes appear frozen in place. The onset is usually before 30 years of age and may occur during early childhood. The condition appears to be genetic in origin, affecting men and women equally.

Treatment is based on the patient's symptoms. A ptosis crutch may be required to relieve the drooping eyelids. Prism therapy and surgical alignment of the eyes may be necessary to eliminate diplopia in some patients, often with satisfactory results.

MECHANICAL RESTRICTIONS OF OCULAR MOVEMENT

Noncomitancy may be caused by restriction of extraocular muscles. Several causes are discussed in this section.

Duane Retraction Syndrome

Although Duane was not the first to identify this retraction syndrome, in 1905 he rigorously analyzed a series of 54 cases and his name, subsequently, became attached to the condition. The syndrome is a congenital anomaly and accounts for approximately 1% of all strabismus.[30] The retraction syndrome has an unexplained predilection for the left eye (3 to 1) and seems to occur more often in females, although some evidence casts doubt on this last observation.[31] Approximately 20% of cases are bilateral.

The clinical characteristics in its classic form are as follows:

1. A marked limitation or absence of abduction, often associated with widening of the eyelids on attempted abduction

2. A mild to moderate limitation of adduction, often associated with an up-shoot or down-shoot of the eye on adduction

3. Retraction of the globe on adduction with narrowing of the eyelids

4. Esotropia of the affected eye in the primary position, frequently greater at far than at near. Exotropia and nonstrabismus are less often seen

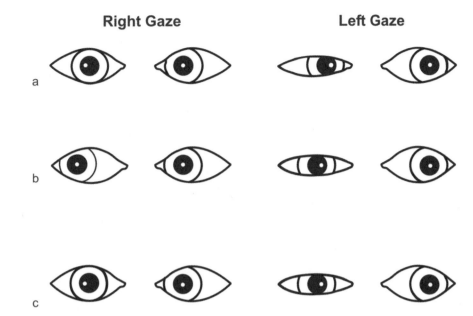

Right Gaze   **Left Gaze**

a

b

c

Figure 8-2. Duane retraction syndrome affecting right eye. Hirschberg testing (with corneal reflex) is shown, a. Type I. b. Type II. c. Type III.

5. Often, the necessity for a head turn in the direction of the affected eye to achieve limited range of binocular fusion

6. Poor gross convergence (remote nearpoint of convergence)

Duane retraction syndrome is thought to be caused by a miswiring of the eye muscles that causes some muscles to contract when they should not and other eye muscles not to contract when they should.[32] Evidence from several sources suggests that Duane retraction syndrome results from a lack of development of cranial nerve VI (abducens nerve). Instead of the lateral rectus being innervated by cranial nerve VI, the muscle is innervated by the inferior division of the third nerve. In most cases, on attempted abduction the lateral rectus does not contract. With adduction, innervation flows to both the medial and the lateral rectus simultaneously, although the medial rectus receives the greater proportion. This anomalous innervation pattern causes co-contraction of both horizontal muscles. Co-contraction results in retraction of the globe, partial limitation of adduction, and narrowing of the palpebral fissure. The anomaly of the abducens nerve is thought to be a disruption in embryonic development from either genetic or environmental factors.

In 70% of cases, Duane retraction syndrome is the only disorder that the individual has. In the remaining cases several conditions and syndromes have been associated with Duane retraction syndrome. These include malformation of the skeleton, ears, eyes, kidneys, and nervous system. The following syndromes have been associated with Duane retraction syndrome: Okihiro syndrome, Wildervanck syndrome, Holt-Oram syndrome, morning glory syndrome, and Goldenhar syndrome.

Significant variations from the classic form of Duane retraction syndrome have been reported by many authors. Huber[33] suggested the following classification, which describes three principal types (Figure 8-2):

1. Duane I: Marked reduction or absence of abduction, mildly defective adduction, retraction on adduction with eyelid narrowing. This is the classic and most prevalent form (70 to 80% of cases).

2. Duane II: Marked reduction or absence of adduction, normal to mildly defective abduction, retraction on adduction with eyelid narrowing. An exotropia of the effected eye is often seen in primary gaze. This is the least common form in most studies and occurs in about 7% of reported cases.

3. Duane III: Marked limitation of both abduction and adduction, retraction of the globe with narrowing of the eyelids on adduction.

The majority of patients with Duane retraction syndrome are asymptomatic. Many have a restricted range of binocular fusion and learn to turn the head habitually (rather than the eyes) to fixate. When strabismus is present, suppression is usually deep, preventing diplopia or other visual symptoms. In those few cases that do present with symptoms related to fusional control of the deviation, vision therapy can be attempted to build fusional reserves. (See Chapter 15 for a description of such a case.) Surgical intervention is usually considered only to reduce a cosmetically disfiguring strabismus or head turn and not necessarily to increase ocular motility or fusion ranges. When surgery is indicated, simple procedures generally are recommended, mainly medial or lateral rectus recessions.

Brown (Superior Oblique Tendon Sheath) Syndrome

The predominant feature of Brown syndrome is reduced or absent elevation on adduction. [34] The same degree of restriction is present on versions (binocular) and ductions (monocular). There also may be some limitation of elevation in the primary position and even on abduction in some cases. The condition usually affects only one eye, although we have seen several bilateral cases. Many patients maintain normal binocular vision in the primary position, but many have hypotropia, esotropia, or exotropia of the affected eye. Brown syndrome is a congenital anomaly with familial occurrence. Mirror reversal (i.e., opposite eye affected) has been reported in monozygotic twins. [35]

The clinical characteristics of Brown syndrome are as follows:

1. Absence or marked limitation of elevation on adduction

2. Normal or near-normal elevation in the primary position and on abduction

3. Possibly, depression of the affected eye (hypotropia) on versions (nasalward position of the eye)

4. Usually, widening of palpebral fissure on adduction

5. Divergence in up-gaze, usually a V pattern, with or without a strabismus in the primary position

6. Restriction to elevation on adduction with the forced duction test (see Chapter 4 for discussion of forced duction testing)

Several etiologies have been found in Brown syndrome. [34] The superior oblique tendon sheath may be fixed to and terminate at the pulley. If the sheath is short and is fixed at the pulley and the tendon insertion, it becomes a physical barrier to adduction of the eye. On adduction, the globe slips under the stretched sheath and, in some cases, there is an audible "click." The sheath prevents elevation on adduction. Other cases have been reported in which the tendon itself fails to slip through the pulley and restricts ocular motility in the same manner as just described.

Some individuals with Brown syndrome have experienced spontaneous recoveries. There is a sudden release of the restriction, the tendon moves normally through the pulley, and full motility is realized. It is interesting to note that more cases of Brown syndrome are found in children, suggesting that many cases do resolve spontaneously.

Other, less prevalent etiologies include an anomaly of the superior oblique muscle, paradoxical innervation analogous to the findings in Duane retraction syndrome, surgically induced restrictions, and restriction secondary to paralysis of the inferior oblique muscle.[36]

Many patients with Brown syndrome have normal binocular vision in the primary position, experience no visual symptoms, and have learned to move the head rather than the eyes to the affected field of gaze. Surgery is not recommended unless there is a significant strabismus, usually hypotropia, in the primary position or the patient has adopted a cosmetically unacceptable head turn. Brown[34] advocated dissecting and stripping the sheath while leaving the tendon intact. Although his cure rate was only 20%, some improvement was reported in 50% of the cases.[34] von Noorden[36] recommended performing a complete tenectomy of the superior oblique muscle, which dramatically improves the restriction. This, however, creates a weakness in inferonasal ductions, and further surgery often is required. Patients should be carefully selected for surgical treatment of Brown syndrome.

Fibrosis of the Extraocular Muscles

Generalized fibrosis syndrome is usually an autosomal dominant anomaly in which all the extraocular muscles, including the levator, are fibrotic. Both eyes are tethered downward, and the patient elevates the chin to fixate. A bilateral ptosis is usually evident. Surgical treatment is often unsatisfactory. One surgical approach is to recess both inferior rectus muscles and perform bilateral frontalis suspensions to correct the ptosis. There is a danger of causing exposure keratitis, which, if it occurs, would require further surgical intervention.

Strabismus fixus is a rare congenital condition in which one or both eyes are tethered in an extreme position of gaze, usually convergent and exceeding 100Δ. In most cases, this anomaly is cosmetically less acceptable than the generalized fibrosis syndrome. The eyes are firmly fixed in position, which is easily confirmed by the forced duction test. The patient must assume an extreme head turn to fixate with the preferred eye, as one eye is chosen over the other by habit. This anomaly is congenital and is believed to be due to fibrosis of the medial rectus muscles. The condition is treated surgically, preferably at an early age, by an extensive recession of the medial recti and the overlying conjunctiva. The eyes are anchored in a slightly abducted position, and maximum resection of the lateral recti may help to hold the eyes in a central position. Even though postoperative ocular motility will be very limited, cosmetic and functional improvement may be considerable.

Adherence Syndromes

Johnson[37] described two very rare restriction anomalies called *adherence syndromes*. These are usually acquired, often introduced by previous eye surgery; however, a few congenital cases have been reported. In the *lateral adherence syndrome*, the muscle sheaths of the lateral rectus and the inferior oblique muscles are joined by abnormal fascial tissue attachments. This union produces a limitation of movement in the field of action of the lateral rectus (i.e., abduction). The forced duction test reveals a lateral restriction to passive rotation of the eye.

In the *superior adherence syndrome*, there is abnormal adherence between the superior rectus muscle sheath and the superior oblique tendon that produces a limitation of movement in the field of action of the superior rectus. Diagnosis is often established during surgery using the forced duction test.

Treatment for these adherence syndromes requires loosening the adhesions by forcefully rotating the globe after detaching the lateral or superior rectus muscle.

Orbital Anomalies

A *blowout fracture* of the orbit may occur as a result of blunt trauma to the soft tissues of the eye, as when an eye is hit with a tennis ball or a fist or the face hits the dashboard in a car accident. A fracture usually occurs in the anterior and nasal orbital floor where the bone is thinnest and most vulnerable to impact forces. The maxillary and ethmoid sinuses may be involved. (A blowin fracture is also possible in this area, from trauma to the infraorbital rim; the maxillary sinus can buckle and rupture through to the floor of the orbit.[38]) Marked limitation of eye movements (elevation and depression), diplopia, and enophthalmos are common consequences. In many blowout fractures, internal eye damage may be absent because the fracture itself helps to cushion the blow. Of course, after an injury, the eyes must be thoroughly inspected for macular edema, retinal detachment, hemorrhage, oculomotor palsies, and other possible problems.

Depending on the size of the fracture, orbital contents can prolapse into the maxillary sinus. Orbital fat, fascia, the inferior rectus muscle, and the inferior oblique muscle can all become entrapped, thereby severely limiting eye movement (often elevation and sometimes depression). Hypotropia may be present in the primary position. A small crack in the orbital floor can incarcerate some orbital tissue, thus causing diplopia and other symptoms. After a recent blowout fracture, the most conspicuous clinical manifestations are swelling and ecchymosis of the eyelids and periorbital soft tissue. Initially, this swelling may cause a proptosis of the eye, but later, as the swelling subsides in 4-6 weeks, the loss of orbital fat may cause an enophthalmos. Radiologic investigation and CT scans of the orbit can provide evidence about whether an initial restriction of eye movement is due to local swelling or hemorrhage or to the entrapment of orbital contents.

In cases in which diplopia and oculomotor restriction persist past the initial healing phase, herniated orbital tissue must be extracted surgically from the bone fracture, and then the fracture must be repaired, von Noorden[36] does not recommend surgery for patients with orbital floor fractures who initially have no diplopia or in whom diplopia disappears within 2 weeks after injury. It is important to remember that diplopia after orbital fracture is not necessarily caused by entrapment of orbital

Table 8-6. Features of Internuclear Ophthalmoplegia

Adduction defect of one or both eyes on attempted horizontal versions

Abduction nystagmus on horizontal versions

Intact gross convergence in most cases of posterior lesions of medial longitudinal fasciculus (pons and medulla); absent gross convergence in anterior lesions of medial longitudinal fasciculus (midbrain)

Frequently, vertical nystagmus on up-gaze

Usually, absence of strabismus in the primary position although esotropia or exotropia seen in a few cases

tissue; associated extraocular muscle and cranial nerve palsy are common.[39] Surgical repair of the orbital floor is indicated when the forced duction test shows a mechanical restriction of elevation and a CT scan reveals entrapped tissue in the fracture.

INTERNUCLEAR AND SUPRANUCLEAR DISORDERS

Lesions between the nuclei of the third, fourth, and sixth cranial nerves, as well as lesions above these nuclei, are discussed.

Internuclear Ophthalmoplegia

A lesion in the medial longitudinal fasciculus (MLF) blocks information from the pontine gaze center and the sixth nerve nucleus to the contralateral third nerve nucleus. A lesion in this long internuclear pathway produces a characteristic set of clinical manifestations known as *internuclear ophthalmoplegia* (INO) (Table 8-6). The patient presents with deficient or absent adduction of the eye on the affected side on attempted version. In the subtle form, the adduction defect may be apparent only as a mild decrease in the velocity of adducting saccades. There is abduction nystagmus of the eye opposite the lesion on attempted version. The nystagmus may be present in the abducting eye only, or in both eyes, with the abducting eye having a larger amplitude of nystagmus. The dissociated or asymmetric horizontal nystagmus in these patients appears to be a secondary compensatory response to the weakness of adduction and appears not to be caused directly by the central defect.[36] INO is named for the side of the MLF lesion that is indicated by the eye with deficient adduction on conjugate gaze: For example, a left INO is indicated when the left eye lacks adduction and the right eye shows abduction nystagmus on attempted right gaze. In bilateral cases, there is usually abduction nystagmus of both eyes on lateral gaze, associated with little or no adduction of either eye (Figure

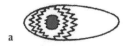
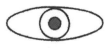
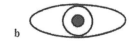
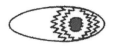

Figure 8-3. Bilateral internuclear ophthalmoplegia, a. Attempted right gaze showing adduction defect of left eye and nystagmus of right eye. b. Attempted left gaze showing adduction defect of right eye and nystagmus of left eye.

8-3). INO can be distinguished from an isolated medial rectus palsy, which also results in a loss of adduction, by the associated abduction nystagmus on lateral gaze.

The saccadic, pursuit, and vestibulo-ocular systems all are affected; however, *gross convergence* is *usually intact*. This presentation is seen in the most prevalent type, Cogan's posterior INO, due to a *pontine-level lesion* of the MLF.[40] A unique feature in pontine INO is that the medial rectus muscle contracts in response to a convergence stimulus but does not contract in response to a version stimulus. INO produced by a *midbrain lesion*, however, is usually bilateral with a *reduction or absence of gross convergence* (Cogan's anterior INO).[40]

There is often a coarse vertical nystagmus on up-gaze of both eyes in unilateral and bilateral cases. Most patients with INO have no strabismus in the primary position, unlike in medial rectus paresis. Occasionally, a horizontal strabismus is found superimposed on an INO, due to specific involvement of the respective nuclei (i.e., an exotropia associated with a lesion of the medial rectus component of the oculomotor nucleus [cranial nerve III] or an esotropia due to abducens nucleus [cranial nerve VI] or nerve damage).

There are two primary etiologies of INO. Bilateral INO in a young adult is most often caused by multiple sclerosis, a demyelinating disease, whereas INO in patients older than 50 years is frequently caused by a vascular lesion (e.g., an infarction). When multiple sclerosis is the cause, there are often other presenting symptoms such as decreased bladder control, limb weakness, unusual paresthetic sensations, or optic neuritis. Unilateral presentation almost always indicates an infarct (occlusion) of a small branch of the basilar artery and often is accompanied by vertigo and other brainstem symptoms.[40] Other rare causes of INO have been reported; these include brainstem and fourth ventricular tumors, hydrocephalus, infections (including those associated with the acquired immunodeficiency syndrome), pernicious anemia, head trauma, and drug intoxications (e.g., narcotics, tricyclic antidepressants, lithium, barbiturates, and other psychoactive drugs).[41]

Treatment options for INO are limited. Ocular manifestations are managed on a symptomatic basis. Patients usually do not present with a strabismus in the primary position and therefore do not report diplopia except on lateral gaze. They compensate by turning the head rather than the eyes for lateral fixation. Comfortable reading and safe driving, however, may require patching an eye—either total or partial occlusion. There may be some spontaneous or slow recovery of function with healing if the cause is of vascular origin. Patients with multiple sclerosis frequently experience periods of remission and recovery of some motor functions during the course of the disease. However, no treatment for multiple sclerosis is yet available that has proven effective in the long term.

Supranuclear Horizontal Gaze Palsy
Frontal Eye-Field Lesions

The two most common causes of lesions in the frontal cortex (Brodmann's area 8) are acute cerebrovascular accident (stroke) and head trauma. The frontal eye fields initiate voluntary saccadic eye movements, so a lesion on one side results in a conjugate turning of the eyes (and, usually, the head) toward the side of the lesion; the contralateral area 8 has unopposed action. If the lesion is isolated and the patient is sufficiently conscious, pursuit eye movements can be demonstrated on either side. Because the vestibular pathway is intact, the eyes can move into the field opposite the lesion by application of the doll's-head maneuver. Eventually, this gaze palsy may partially resolve, possibly as a result of other systems (e.g., the superior colliculus) generating saccades. [42]

Occipital and Parietal Cortical Lesions

An extensive lesion in the parieto-occipital lobe secondary to a vascular accident or tumor is the most likely cause of a gaze-dependent disorder of pursuit eye movements. The patient is unable to follow a moving target smoothly but uses a series of small saccadic steps for tracking. These saccadic steps are known as *cogwheel pursuits*. To a lesser degree, smooth pursuit tracking is reduced with age in many people, but the loss is usually symmetric in direction. The smooth pursuit phase of optokinetic nystagmus (OKN) is similarly affected when the stripes are rotated in the direction of the lesion, but it should be normal when the stripe rotation is reversed (i.e., toward the opposite side of the lesion). The associated and definitive clinical sign of this pathologic condition is homonymous hemianopsia.

Lesions located solely in the occipital region result in a visual field cut, often without pursuit abnormalities. Lesions in the right parietal region often produce visual neglect, where the patient does not attend to images in left visual space.

Patients having parieto-occipital lesions initially require management by a neuro-ophthalmologist, but they usually can be followed subsequently by the primary eye care doctor.

Brainstem Lesions

Brainstem lesions affect the descending fibers in the brainstem, from the cortical areas subserving pursuit and saccadic eye movements to the lateral gaze centers in the pons, specifically, the paramedial pontine reticular formation (PPRF). Stroke is the most likely cause of lesions in the rostral brainstem, whereas lesions at a lower level in the pons, involving the PPRF, can arise from several sources (e.g., vascular origin, demyelinating disease, and tumors).[42] If these descending fibers are interrupted, both pursuits and saccades are deficient or absent on the side of the "deprived" lateral gaze center. If a lateral gaze center itself is damaged, vestibulo-ocular responses can also be affected, as the PPRF is the beginning of the final common pathway to the horizontal oculomotor nuclei. Consequently, if a patient presents with a complete unilateral gaze palsy for all eye movements, the most likely cause is a lesion in the pons involving the lateral gaze center.

Supranuclear Vertical Gaze Palsy

Isolated lesions producing vertical gaze palsy are rare. Bilateral up-gaze deficits have been reported in the literature more often than have down-gaze

Table 8-7. Ocular Signs of Parinaud Syndrome(Dorsal Midbrain Syndrome)

Common
 Deficiency or loss of saccades in up-gaze
 Sluggish or tonic dilated pupils
 Light-near dissociation; good constriction at near
 Convergence-retraction nystagmus with oscillopsia (increased
   by rotating optokinetic nystagmus stripes downward)
 Papilledema
Less common
 Disturbances of down-gaze saccades
 Skew deviation
 Eyelid retraction (Collier's sign)
 Fourth nerve palsy (trochlear palsy)
 Loss of up-gaze pursuits

Table 8-8. Ocular Signs of Parkinson's Disease

Hypometric saccades in all fields of gaze, but initially in up-gaze
Saccadic "cogwheel" pursuits
Eyelid apraxia (difficulty in opening)
Decreased blinking
Sporadic oculogyric crisis

palsies. The reported cases usually involve vascular lesions or metastases in portions of the MLF connecting the fourth and third nerve complex or in connections with the superior colliculus.[12] Most cases of vertical gaze palsy involve generalized neurologic syndromes of which the gaze palsy is merely one, although possibly the first, of many expressions of the disease process.

Parinaud Syndrome

Often the first sign of Parinaud syndrome is up-gaze saccadic dysfunction. Initially, the patient finds that making up-gaze eye movements requires much effort; the eyes may swing back and forth in a serpentine movement when elevation is attempted. With elevation effort, the eyes often converge while simultaneously retracting into the orbits. Many patients later have convergence-retraction nystagmus with oscillopsia. The nystagmoid movements can be exaggerated by rotating OKN stripes downward, thus requiring upward saccades. Convergence-retraction nystagmus on vertical OKN testing is a common sign in Parinaud's syndrome. Other common signs include dilated pupils that are unresponsive to light, anisocoria, light-near dissociation (i.e., pupil constriction to a near stimulus but not to light), and papilledema (Table 8-7). The sluggish pupillary light response and nystagmus are indicators that the up-gaze restriction is not orbital in nature, as it is in Graves' disease. High-resolution CT scanning and magnetic resonance imaging are generally helpful in the differential diagnosis. Parinaud's syndrome usually indicates a neuro-ophthalmologic emergency.

Parinaud syndrome can be congenital or acquired. Its other names, *sylvian aqueduct syndrome* and *dorsal midbrain syndrome*, indicate its etiology. This syndrome frequently is caused by sylvian aqueductal stenosis (i.e., a restriction of cerebro-spinal fluid that flows between the third and fourth ventricles), resulting in hydrocephalus and papilledema. Some other causes are tumors of the pineal gland or in the region of the aqueduct or superior colliculus, neurosyphilis, multiple sclerosis, trauma, and stroke.[12] In cases of sylvian aqueductal stenosis, signs and symptoms usually are relieved by surgical insertion of a shunt to promote the flow of cerebrospinal fluid. Although tumors in this area often are inoperable, they frequently respond well to radiation therapy. The long-term survival rate for these patients is generally good.[43]

Progressive Supranuclear Palsy

Progressive supranuclear palsy is a generic label for a number of rare, degenerative diseases with similar features that affect pursuit and saccadic eye movements, the best known of which is Steele-Richardson-Olszewski syndrome. Affected patients typically are seen in the sixth or seventh decades of life with reports of being unable to move their eyes into down-gaze. The ophthalmoplegia progresses to loss of voluntary up-gaze saccades, loss of horizontal saccades and, finally, loss of pursuit eye movements. The oculomotor deficits are often compounded by a stiff neck. Vestibulo-ocular reflexes usually are intact, but severe neck rigidity may make their demonstration difficult. As the disease progresses, patients may develop strabismus and diplopia, loss of facial expression, and dementia. These patients usually have a progressive downhill course and die 8-10 years after the onset of signs. Ocular manifestations are treated symptomatically. Yoked base-down prisms may be helpful for tasks in down-gaze (e.g., reading and eating). Prisms or occlusion may be necessary to bring relief from diplopia.

Parkinson's Disease

Parkinson's disease is fairly common (0.1-1.0% of the population) and has conspicuous systemic and ocular manifestations. It usually occurs with old age. The condition stems from a depletion of the neurotransmitter dopamine secondary to the death of nerve cells in the substantia nigra, a basal ganglion nucleus of the upper brainstem.

The specific causes of nerve cell death are many, including carbon monoxide poisoning, viral infections, arteriosclerosis, syphilis, and tumors; it may even be part of the normal aging process in some people. Parkinsonian patients lose control of muscular activity. They tremble at rest and have trouble with fine motor coordination. There is often muscular rigidity, stiffness, and slowing of movements. In advanced cases, balance, posture, and walking are affected; patients often adopt a hurried, shuffling gait. Physical articulation of speech becomes difficult, and facial expression flattens. Early in the course of the disease, conjugate saccadic eye movements become hypometric in all fields of gaze, but up-gaze usually is affected initially (Table 8-8). Jerky, "cogwheel" pursuits are seen. Patients may also have difficulty opening their eyes (i.e., eyelid apraxia), and the rate of blinking decreases. Reports of diplopia often are associated with convergence weakness and a developing convergence insufficiency. Later in the course of this slowly degenerative condition, the eyes may periodically go into *oculogyric crisis*, in which they are locked in an extreme field of gaze for a few minutes up to a few hours.

There is no known cure for Parkinson's disease. Drug therapies have not proven successful as yet. Therefore, treatment addresses symptoms and is directed toward support and comfort. There often unpredictable periods of remission during which systemic and ocular signs diminish but, overall, the condition is progressive. Patients often are directed toward psychological support groups to help them adjust emotionally to the limitations of their condition.

NYSTAGMUS

The appearance of nystagmus in early childhood or later in life causes considerable distress for patients, family, and friends. Its presence usually is interpreted as a sign of serious visual dysfunction or, possibly, brain damage. Nystagmus (i.e., the involuntary rhythmic oscillations of one or both eyes) may indeed be the presenting sign of either a pathologic afferent visual pathway lesion or a disorder in oculomotor control. Thirteen percent of cerebral palsy patients have nystagmus, among many other visual disorders.[44] Approximately 10-15% of visually impaired school-aged children have nystagmus. Nystagmus can be conceptual-

Table 8-9. Clinically Relevant Characteristics of Nystagmus

Characteristic	Observations
Global observations	General posture, head position (turns or tilts), facial asymmetries
Type of nystagmus	Pendular, jerk, or mixed
Direction	Horizontal, vertical, torsional, or combination
Amplitude	Small (<2 degrees), moderate(2-10 degrees), large (>10 degrees)
Frequency	Slow (1/2 Hz), moderate (1/2-2 Hz), fast (>2 Hz)
Constancy	Constantly present, intermittent, periodic
Conjugacy	Conjugate (eyes move in same direction); disjunctive (eyes move independently)
Symmetry (oculus dexter and oculus sinister)	Symmetric (equal amplitudes); asymmetric (unequal amplitudes)
Latent component	Increase of nystagmus with occlusion of one eye
Field-of-gaze changes	Null point, dampening, or increase of nystagmus in any field of gaze or with convergence

ized as a disorder of the mechanisms that maintain stable fixation.[41]

Nystagmus, affecting approximately 0.4% of the general population,[45] is not a disease entity as such; rather, it is a sign of an underlying disorder. The clinician should attempt to describe the condition as either congenital or acquired and determine the general category of etiology (e.g., genetic, traumatic, toxic, metabolic error, developmental, visual deprivation). This discussion will focus on the most prevalent types of nystagmus: physiologic, voluntary, congenital, and latent. Rarer types, which may be harbingers of active neurologic disease, are presented later in Table 8-16 for the purpose of differential diagnosis.

Many clinical tests in the routine vision examination are complicated by the presence of nystagmus. The patient's inability to maintain steady fixation affects the accuracy of keratometry, retinoscopy, subjective refraction, the cover test, internal and external health inspection, and other measurements. For this reason, the clinician must exercise skill, patience, and persistence in clinical evaluation. The gross observation of nystagmus is necessary in all fields of gaze and at far and near distances, as many types of nystagmus show significant variation in these respects. Magnification (e.g., loop, binocular indirect ophthalmoscope, or slit lamp) is often useful for observing the characteristics of nystagmus. Table 8-9 presents characteristics of

Table 8-10. Characteristics of Physiologic Nystagmus

Type	Jerk; conjugate
Direction	Usually horizontal; fast phase of jerk toward side of gaze
Constancy	Occasional, usually when tired
Frequency	Rapid
Amplitude	Small, may be unequal in each eye
Field of gaze	Occurs in extreme horizontal fields of gaze beyond 30 degrees, occasionally in vertical gaze
Latent component	Can occur in extreme field of gaze when binocular vision is broken
Symptoms	None
Associated conditions	None
Etiology	Specific mechanism unknown but apparently caused by extreme general fatigue
Comments	Common condition relieved by rest or sleep; no other therapy recommended

Table 8-11. Characteristics of Voluntary Nystagmus

Type	Pendular saccades; conjugate
Direction	Horizontal
Constancy	Occasional, dependent on conscious effort, cannot be sustained for more than 30 seconds at a time
Frequency	Very rapid oscillations, 3-43 Hz
Amplitude	Usually small, 2 or 3 degrees
Field of gaze	Usually initiated by a convergence eye movement, probably accommodative convergence
Latent component	None
Symptoms	Oscillopsia, may be associated with malingering symptoms (e.g., blurred vision)
Associated conditions	None
Etiology	Not a true nystagmus; back and forth saccades without an intersaccadic interval; ability possibly hereditary
Comments	A trick of the eyes that is quite fatiguing, so the oscillation bursts are of short duration, prevalence is approximately 8%; may be associated with malingering behavior in school-aged children

nystagmus that are clinically relevant for differential diagnosis.

Physiologic Nystagmus

In a person who is very tired, it is not unusual for a jerk nystagmus to develop in extreme positions of gaze (Table 8-10). This is a normal type of nystagmus and of no particular consequence; it disappears after a good sleep. The oscillations are of small amplitude, conjugate, and rapid, and may be unequal in each eye. It is present only at the extremes of horizontal and, occasionally, vertical gaze. Because the condition is related to fatigue, it is usually intermittent but, if sustained, it must be distinguished from pathologic types of nystagmus. A reasonable clinical guideline is to regard as physiologic the fine conjugate jerk nystagmus detected beyond 30 degrees of gaze or beyond the range of binocular vision, unless there is a good reason to suspect otherwise. Alcohol intoxication causes physiologic nystagmus to decompensate, and the nystagmus becomes abnormal on moderate lateral shifts of gaze. This condition is used by law enforcement officials as an indication of whether a driver is operating a vehicle under the influence of alcohol.

Other common types of physiologic nystagmus that the clinician must recognize as normal are OKN and vestibulo-ocular nystagmus.[46]

Voluntary Nystagmus

Voluntary nystagmus might more properly be called *voluntary flutter*, because it is not a true nystagmus.

It is a series of rapidly alternating saccades, usually initiated willfully with a convergence movement, and represents nothing more than a trick with the eyes (Table 8-11).[47] This voluntary flutter is accompanied by oscillopsia and is quite fatiguing. It can be sustained for only a short period, 30 seconds or less. Approximately 5-8% of the population can demonstrate voluntary nystagmus, an ability that seems to run in families. [48] It is unlikely that preschool children would discover this ability but, occasionally, an older child has used this eye maneuver as part of malingering behavior, an emotional episode, or an hysteric reaction. Ciuffreda [49] has demonstrated that voluntary nystagmus can be part of a spasm of the near reflex if a patient voluntarily crosses the eyes.

The clinician can usually distinguish voluntary nystagmus by its distinctive features. The oscillations appear pendular ("saw-tooth"), conjugate, horizontal, and rapid (3-43 Hz) and are usually of small amplitude and short duration, due to their fatiguing nature. The rapid oscillations of spasmus nutans might be confused with voluntary nystagmus, except that spasmus nutans presents in infancy, not in school-aged children. Furthermore, spasmus nutans is much more sustained. Voluntary nystagmus, therefore, should be easily recognized.

Table 8-12. Characteristics of Congenital (Infantile) Nystagmus

Type	Pendular or jerk (or both); conjugate
Direction	Usually horizontal, rotary, rarely vertical; fast phase of jerk toward side of gaze
Constancy	Usually constant but can occasionally become quiet
Frequency	Variable, increases with peripheral gaze
Amplitude	Variable, increases with peripheral gaze and effort
Field of gaze	Often dampens with convergence and 10-15 degrees to one side (null point)
Latent component	Usually present; increased amplitude and frequency with occlusion of either eye
Symptoms	Generally, reduced acuity to varying degrees; in many patients, cosmetic concerns, head turns, rhythmic head movements
Associated conditions	Esotropia (common); amblyopia; moderate to high astigmatism; head shaking; 40% defective vestibulo-ocular and optokinetic nystagmus; occasional paradoxical response to optokinetic nystagmus
Etiology	Congenital; specific mechanism unknown; can be afferent or efferent pathway lesions; often hereditary pattern (X-linked, autosomal dominant, or others); efferent type possibly a defect in the pursuit system at the level of the brainstem
Comments	Improvement of condition with age; improvement of acuity and cosmesis possible at any age with spectacles, contact lenses, prisms, vision training, or auditory biofeedback

Congenital Nystagmus

The most common type of nystagmus is congenital nystagmus, apparently affecting men twice as frequently as women.[50] It is notoriously variable but, fortunately for the sake of differential diagnosis, certain clinical features are highly characteristic and distinguish it from other forms of nystagmus (Table 8-12). It is present at birth or shortly thereafter and, for this reason, is sometimes referred to as *infantile nystagmus*. The oscillations can be solely jerk (the most prevalent pattern), solely pendular, or a combination of the two. The oscillations can convert from one waveform to another spontaneously or may do so in different fields of gaze. If the waveform pattern is jerk, then the fast phase most often occurs in the direction of gaze.[51] Amplitude and frequency can vary from moment to moment and, on occasion, the eyes may become "quiet." The amplitude usually increases in some field of gaze and, for this reason, a patient may habitually assume a head turn or tilt to dampen the nystagmus as much as possible. The position of gaze in which the eyes are quiet is known as the *null region*. The nystagmus often is accentuated by active fixation, attention, or anxiety and may be diminished by convergence and purposeful eyelid closure.[52] It usually presents as conjugate and horizontal, but occasionally clinicians see vertical and torsional waveforms or some combination of these. When the nystagmus is horizontal, it usually remains horizontal even on up- and down-gaze. The condition rarely is associated with oscillopsia, even though the eye may be in constant motion, but one may find head nodding or shaking.

The specific neuropathology resulting in congenital nystagmus is not well understood in most cases, but the clinical conditions that cause it can be broadly classified as afferent and efferent. Afferent congenital nystagmus is associated with poor visual acuity. Congenital optic nerve atrophy or hypoplasia, congenital cataracts, ocular albinism, achromatopsia, and aniridia are all diseases of the eye or the *afferent* visual pathway that can result in congenital nystagmus. Visual acuity reduction usually is profound, and the prognosis for improvement poor. In these patients, who represent approximately 40% of all congenital nystagmus cases, the etiology is usually obvious on clinical examination.

The majority of congenital nystagmus cases, approximately 60%, are considered to be *efferent*, due to some disorder of the oculomotor systems. A disorder or lesion of the pursuit system at the level of the brainstem is suspected by some authorities.[41] Lo[53] reported CT scan abnormalities in 50% of congenital nystagmus patients. Magnetic resonance imaging scanning may identify an even higher percentage in the future. There is often a hereditary pattern of involvement, but some family members may have one waveform (e.g., jerk) and some another (e.g., pendular). In most efferent cases, the etiology is idiopathic. Patients with efferent congenital nystagmus usually have better visual acuity than do those with afferent types.

The prevalence of strabismus in congenital nystagmus is high, 40-50%.[54] The eye turn is usually esotropic; however, exotropias and hypertropias frequently are found. Identifying the strabismus may be difficult due to the pattern of nystagmoid

Table 8-13. Characteristics of Spasmus Nutans

Type	Pendular, eyes often asymmetric in amplitude
Direction	Usually horizontal, can be rotary or vertical
Constancy	Constant or intermittent
Frequency	Fast, 6-11 Hz
Amplitude	Small, approximately 2 degrees; eyes often asymmetric; appearance of monocularity in some because of asymmetry
Field of gaze	Present in all fields but variable with gaze
Latent component	None
Symptoms	Usually head nodding or wobbling; abnormal head position (tilt or chin expression) in 50% of cases
Associated conditions	Usually none; benign; occasionally, esotropia or amblyopia; a rare association with gliomas
Etiology	Mechanism unknown, may be hereditary
Comments	Onset not at birth but usually develops in first year of life; often lasts 1 or 2 years, then disappears with no permanent consequences; no treatment indicated; computed tomographic scan recommended to screen for gliomas

Table 8-14. Characteristics of Latent Nystagmus

Type	Jerk, conjugate
Direction	Horizontal
Constancy	Occasional, occurs on occlusion of either eye
Frequency	Variable
Amplitude	Variable
Field of gaze	Decreases in gaze toward covered eye; increases toward uncovered eye
Latent component	Manifest only under monocular conditions
Symptoms	Usually none as it is a latent condition
Associated conditions	Usually associated with one or more of the following conditions: congenital nystagmus, esotropia, amblyopia, disassociated vertical deviation, retrolental fibroplasia; occasionally occurs as an isolated condition
Etiology	Congenital condition; mechanism unknown; disturbed cortical binocularity, monocular optokinetic nystagmus asymmetry, abnormal localization, and proprioception; monocular reduction of illumination
Comments	Fairly common; complicates the assessment of strabismus and ocular motility; no treatment indicated

TABLE 8-15. Characteristics of Vestibular Nystagmus

	Central	Peripheral
Type	Jerk, conjugate	Jerk, conjugate
Direction	Often purely horizontal, vertical, or torsional	Usually mixed, never just vertical
Constancy	Constant	Intermittent, recurrent
Frequency	Increases with gaze toward fast phase, decreases or reverses to slow phase	Increases with gaze toward fast phase, decreases or reverses to slow phase
Amplitude	Increases with gaze toward fast phase; visual fixation tends not to reduce nystagmus	Increases with gaze toward fast phase; fixation tends to reduce nystagmus
Field of gaze	See Amplitude	See Amplitude
Latent component	Reduced by covering an eye if cerebellar disease; increased if vestibular disease	None
Symptoms	Mild vertigo, nausea, variable oscillopsia	Severe vertigo, nausea, persistent oscillopsia
Associated conditions	Rarely, deafness and tinnitus; usually other neurologic signs	Frequently, deafness and tinnitus
Etiology	Damage to vestibular nucleus or connections in brainstem or cerebellum (e.g., neuromas, demyelination)	Damage to labyrinth-vestibular nerve (e.g., vascular, demyelination, neoplastic)
Comments	Caloric testing useful; signs can mimic peripheral disease clinically	Caloric testing useful; signs do not mimic central disease; higher prevalence than central type

movements, so it is possible that the prevalence of strabismus in these cases is actually underestimated. The etiology of a strabismus can be completely independent of that causing the nystagmus, but most often the two conditions appear to be part of the underlying problem affecting the visual system. One controversial view is that most cases of esotropia associated with congenital nystagmus are secondary to the nystagmus and originate as an attempt to stabilize the eyes. This condition is known as *nystagmus blockage syndrome*.

Congenital (infantile) nystagmus must be differentiated from other types of nystagmus that occur very early in life, such as *spasmus nutans*. The diagnosis

Table 8-16. Rare Types of Nystagmus

	PAN	Seesaw Nystagmus	Gaze Paretic Nystagmus	Muscle Paretic Nystagmus	Upbeat Nystagmus	Downbeat Nystagmus
Type	Jerk usually acquired, can be congenital	Pendular, eyes move in opposite vertical directions	Jerk conjugate and equal between eyes	Jerk; fast phase toward the affected field more in affected eye	Jerk	Jerk
Direction	Beats to left, then to right in 3-min cycles	Conjugate torsional oscillations with disjunctive vertical movements	Horizontal but sometimes with torsional component	Horizontal or vertical in direction of affected muscle	Vertical, slow phase downward	Vertical, slow phase upward
Constancy	Constant with pauses as it changes direction	Intermittent, transient	Constant	Constant or intermittent depending on lesion	Periodic, usually in primary gaze and up-gaze	Intermittent, periodic, depends on head and body posture
Frequency	Fast, variable	Slow, ≤1 Hz	Variable	Varies with gaze, increasing in affected field	Variable, fast	Variable, fast, increases with head hanging and convergence
Amplitude	Variable	Variable, usually small	Usually small, sometimes large	Variable	Types: large increases in up-gaze; small increases in down-gaze	Small, maximum when eyes turned laterally and slightly downward
Field of gaze	Increases in extreme horizontal gaze	Torsional movement in all fields but seesaw in up-, down-, and primary gaze	Increased amplitude in affected field of gaze	Increased amplitude in affected field of gaze	Not present in all fields of gaze (see Amplitude)	Most prominent when looking down and laterally, not present in all fields
Latent component	None	None	None	None	None	None
Symptoms	Oscillopsia, impaired visual acuity, possible alternating head turn	Decreased visual acuity, occasional bitemporal hemianoptic field defect	Inability to hold eye in affected field of gaze	Often associated with diplopia if of recent onset	Infrequent oscillopsia	Oscillopsia

Table 8-16. Rare Types of Nystagmus--continued

Associated neurologic signs or conditions	Smooth pursuit usually impaired; gaze-evoked and down-beat nystagmus possibly accompanying multiple sclerosis, syphilis, head trauma	Bitemporal hemianopsia, septo-optic dysplasia; seen in some comatose patients after severe brainstem injury	Cerebellar disease, especially flocculus lesions, one type related to vestibular disease	Associated with paretic strabismus, sometimes ophthalmoplegia	Posterior fossa disease	Multiple sclerosis, hydrocephalus
Etiology	Vestibulocerebellum or craniocervical disorder, multiplesclerosis, trauma, intoxication, encephalitis, vascular disease	Sellar or parasellar tumor disease of the mesodiencephalic junction, trauma, vascular disease	Lesion in frontal gaze center or brainstem projections or pontine gaze centers	Single-muscle weakness, paresis, myasthenia gravis	Types: (1) lesion in anterior vermis of cerebellum or medulla; (2) intrinsic medullary disease or structural deformity	Compressions at foramen magnum level (Arnold-Chiari malformation), encephalitis, alcohol, spinocerebellar lesions, magnesium deficiency
Comments	Acquired PAN treated successfully with baclofen (anti-spastic agent); may continue during sleep; can occur as a side effect of some anticonvulsive drugs	Rare; usually acquired, although congenital type seen; rise of intorting eye and fall of extorting eye in acquired cases, opposite in congenital cases	Same in the two eyes; fairly prevalent form of nystagmus	Asymmetry between the two eyes, which distinguishes it from gaze paretic type; little or no nystagmus in unaffected eye	Nystagmus possibly increased by barbiturates, phenothiazides, phenytoin sodium (Dilantin)	May be congenital or acquired; reports of improvement using base-out prisms in spectacles and drug therapy (clonazepam)

PAN = periodic alternating nystagmus.

is apparent if the nystagmus is associated with an obvious afferent lesion (e.g., albinism, congenital cataracts, optic atrophy), but efferent etiologies can present the clinician with a diagnostic challenge. In summary, the most distinctive feature of congenital nystagmus, besides its early onset, is its variability. Congenital nystagmus, although often constantly present, can vary in frequency, amplitude, and type and alternate between pendular and jerk waveforms. There is usually a latent component. A family history may reveal a genetic condition. Spasmus nutans is an altogether different type of nystagmus and has a later onset than congenital nystagmus. It is characterized by high-frequency, small-amplitude oscillations that often are intermittent and asymmetric when comparing each eye (Table 8-13). For further information on differential diagnosis, the reader is referred to an extensive review by Grisham.[55]

Nystagmus Blockage Syndrome

A less well-known form of congenital jerk nystagmus is associated with esotropia. The amplitude of nystagmus is reduced or absent with convergence when the fixating eye is adducted. The medial rectus muscle, which holds the fixating eye in adduction to "block" the nystagmus, becomes hypertonic, which eventually results in esotropia. The mechanism is not fully understood, but this association of congenital nystagmus and esotropia is known as *nystagmus blockage syndrome*. Often there is an accommodative element to the strabismus as well.

The syndrome has these main features: First, the onset is in infancy. Jerk nystagmus precedes the onset of a variable esotropia that may be alternating or unilateral. Amblyopia is common, although some infants appear to cross-fixate so that amblyopia is prevented. Second, there is an abnormal head posture, whereby the head is turned toward the adducted, fixating eye (i.e., a left head turn if the left eye is the fixating eye). Third, the fixating eye remains adducted with occlusion of the fellow eye. The condition can, therefore, initially simulate a paralysis of the lateral rectus muscle. With further testing, abduction can usually be demonstrated, indicating a pseudoparalysis of abduction. Fourth, on adduction of the fixating eye, the nystagmus is reduced or absent, but nystagmus intensity increases as the fixating eye moves toward the primary position and into abduction. Generally speaking, the treatment of nystagmus and esotropia in nystagmus blockage syndrome is more difficult than management of either condition independently. Surgery often is necessary to compensate for both the head turn and the strabismus.

Nystagmus "blockage" compensation can also occur with induced fusional convergence by using base-out prisms. Binocular visual acuity may improve significantly. (See the section Optical Management in Chapter 15.)

Latent Nystagmus

A conjugate jerk nystagmus evoked by occlusion of one eye is a latent nystagmus (Table 8-14). It often is associated with strabismus, particularly congenital (infantile) esotropia, double hypertropia (dissociated vertical deviation), and amblyopia.[56] This congenital condition might occur independently of other visual conditions; however, a latent component to congenital nystagmus often is seen, and a jerk pattern can be superimposed on a pendular waveform. The jerk pattern of latent nystagmus is characterized by a fast phase in the direction toward the fixating eye and by the increase of nystagmus amplitude on temporal gaze. Visual acuity is better with both eyes open than with either eye occluded. No specific therapy is indicated, as the condition is only manifest with monocular occlusion.

Rare Types of Nystagmus

There are many types of nystagmus that can present at any age due to acquired pathologic factors (e.g., developmental anomalies, trauma, drug toxicity, vascular accidents, and endocrine imbalances). Fortunately, most of these conditions are extremely rare, but the prevalence increases in old age. Table 8-15 lists characteristics of vestibular nystagmus, and Table 8-16 lists the clinical characteristics of several other rare types of nystagmus. As a rule, the clinician should be very familiar with the previously described common types of nystagmus. If a nystagmus case does not fall naturally into one of the common diagnostic categories, refer to Tables 8-15 and 8-16 in an attempt to establish the probable diagnosis. It seems prudent that all patients having nystagmus, except for physiologic and voluntary nystagmus, should be examined by a neurologist or neuro-ophthalmologist.

REFERENCES

1. Rush J, Younge B. Paralysis of cranial nerves III, IV, and VI: causes and prognosis in 1,000 cases. Arch Ophthalmol. 1981;99:76-9.

2. Glasser J. Neuro-Ophthalmology, 3rd ed. Philadelphia: Lippincott Williams & Wilkins, 1999.

3. Wishnick M, Nelson L, Huppert L, Reich E. Mobius syndrome and limb abnormalities with dominant inheritance. Ophthalmic Paediatr Genet. 1983;2:77-81.

4. von Noorden G, Murray E, Wong S. Superior oblique paralysis. A review of 270 cases. Arch Ophthalmol. 1986;104:1771-6.

5. Neetens A, Janssens M. The superior oblique: a challenging extraocular muscle. Doc Ophthalmol. 1979;46:295-303.

6. Dale R. Fundamentals of Ocular Motility and Strabismus. In. New York: Grune & Stratton, 1982.

7. Jampolsky A. Vertical Strabismus Surgery. In: Symptoms on Strabismus, Transaction of the New Orleans Academy of Ophthalmology. St. Louis: C.V Mosby, 1971.

8. Metz H. Double levator palsy. Arch Ophthalmol. 1979;97:901-3.

9. Ziffer A. Monocular Elevation Deficiency (Double Elevator Palsy). In: Rosenbaum A, Santiago A, eds. Clinical Strabismus Management: Principles and Surgical Techniques. Philadelphia: Saunders, 1999.

10. Osserman K. Ocular myasthenia gravis. Invest Ophthalmol. 1967;6:277-87.

11. Soliven B, Lange D, Penn A. Seronegative myasthenia gravis. Neurology 1988;38:514.

12. Burde R, Savino P, Trobe J. Clinical Decisions in Neuro-Ophthalmology 2nd ed. In. St. Louis: Mosby, 1992.

13. Graves R. Newly observed affection of the thyroid gland in females. Lond Med Surg J. 1835;7:516-20.

14. Char D. Thyroid Eye Disease, 3rd ed. In. New York: Churchill Livingstone, 1997.

15. Jacobson D, Gorman C. Endocrine ophthalmopathy: current ideas concerning etiology, pathogenesis and treatment. Endocr Rev. 1984;5:200-20.

16. Gorman C. Temporal relationship between onset of Graves' ophthalmopathy and diagnosis of thyrotoxicosis. Mayo Clin Proc. 1983;58:515-9.

17. Jamamoto K, Itoh K, Yoshida S, al e. A quantitative analysis of orbital soft tissue in Graves' disease based on B-mode ultrasonography. Endocrinol Jpn. 1979;26:255-61.

18. Day R. Ocular manifestations of thyroid disease: current concepts. Trans Am Ophthalmol Soc. 1959;57:572-601.

19. Kroll H, Kuwabara T. Dysthyroid ocular myopathy. Arch Ophthalmol. 1966;76:244-57.

20. Daicker B. The histological substrate of the extraocular muscle thickening seen in dysthyroid orbitopathy. Klin Monatsbl Augenheilkd 1979;174:843-7.

21. Kendall-Taylor P, Perros P. Circulating retrobulbar antibodies in Graves' ophthalmopathy. Acta Endocrinol. 1989;121(suppl 2):31-7.

22. Scott W, Thalacker J. Diagnosis and treatment of thyroid myopathy. Ophthalmology 1981;88:493-8.

23. Gamblin G, Harper D, Galentine P, al e. Prevalence of increased intraocular pressure in Graves' disease. Evidence of frequent subclinical ophthalmopathy. N Engl J Med. 1983;308:420-4.

24. Grove AJ. Evaluation of exophthalmos. N Engl J Med. 1975;292:1005-13.

25. Dallow R. Evaluation of unilateral exophthalmos with ultrasonography: analysis of 258 consecutive cases. Laryngoscope 1975;85:1905-18.

26. Enzmann D, Donaldson S, Kriss J. Appearance of Graves' disease on orbital computer tomography. J Comput Assist Tomogr. 1979;3:815-9.

27. Dyer J. Ocular muscle surgery in Graves' disease. Trans Am Ophthalmol Soc. 1978;76:125-39.

28. Evans D, Kennerdell J. Extraocular muscle surgery for dysthyroid myopathy. Am J Ophthalmol. 1983;95:767-71.

29. Kiloh L, Nevin S. Progressive dystrophy of the external ocular muscles (ocular myopathy). Brain Res. 1951;74:115.

30. Archer S, Sondhi N, Helveston E. Strabismus in infancy. Ophthalmology 1989;96:133-7.

31. Tredici T, von Noorden G. Are anisometropia and amblyopia common in Duane's syndrome? J Pediatr Ophthalmol Strabismus 1985;22:23-5.

32. Gurwood A, Terrigno C. Duane's retraction syndrome: literature review. Optometry 2000;71:722-6.

33. Huber A. Electrophysiology of the retraction syndrome. Br J Ophthalmol. 1974;58:293-300.

34. Brown H. Congenital Structural Muscle Anomalies. In: Allen J, ed. Strabismus Ophthalmic Symposium I. St. Louis: Mosby, 1950.

35. Katz N, Whitmore P, Beauchamp G. Brown's syndrome in twins. J Pediatr Ophthalmol Strabismus 1981;18:32-4.

36. von Noorden G. Binocular Vision and Ocular Motility 4th ed. St. Louis: Mosby, 1990.

37. Johnson L. Adherence syndrome: pseudoparalysis of the lateral or superior rectus muscles. Arch Ophthalmol. 1950;44:870-8.

38. Raflo G. Blowin and blowout fractures of the orbit: clinical correlations and proposed mechanisms. Ophthalmic Surg. 1984;15:114-9.

39. Wojno T. The incidence of extraocular muscle and cranial nerve palsy in orbital floor blow-out fractures. Ophthalmology 1987;94:682-5.

40. Cogan D. Neurology of the Ocular Muscles, 2nd ed. Springfield, Ill: Charles C Thomas, 1956.

41. Leigh R, Zee D. The Neurology of Eye Movements, 2nd ed. Philadelphia: Davis, 1991.

42. Mein J, Trimble R. Diagnosis and Management of Ocular Motility Disorders, 2nd ed. Oxford: Blackwell Scientific, 1991.

43. Beck R, Smith C. Neuro-Ophthalmology: A Problem-Oriented Approach. Boston: Little, Brown, 1988; 179-782.

44. Scheiman M. Optometric finding in children with cerebral palsy. Am J Optom Physiol Optics 1984;61:321-3.

45. Anderson J. Latent nystagmus and alternating hyperphoria. Br J Ophthalmol. 1954;38:217-31.

46. Leigh R, Averbuch-Heller L. Nystagmus and Related Ocular Motility Disorders. In: Miller N, Newman N, eds. Walsh and Hoyt's Clinical Neuro-Ophthalmology, 5th ed, vol. 1. Philadelphia: Lippincott Williams & Wilkins, 1998.

47. Stark L, Shults W, Ciuffreda K, et al. Voluntary Nystagmus Is Saccadic: Evidence from Motor and Sensory Mechanisms. In: Proceedings of the Joint Automatic Control Conference. Pittsburgh: Instrument Society of America, 1977.

48. Zahn J. Incidence and characteristics of voluntary nystagmus. J Neurol Neurosurg Psychiatr. 1978;41:617-23.

49. Ciuffreda K. Voluntary nystagmus: new findings and clinical implications. Am J Optom Physiol Optics 1980;57:795-800.

50. Anderson J. Cases and treatment of congenital eccentric nystagmus. Br J Ophthalmol. 1953;37:267-81.

51. Nelson L, Wagner R, Harley R. Congenital nystagmus surgery. Int Ophthalmol Clin. 1985;25:133-8.

52. Shibasaki H, Yamashita Y, Motomura S. Suppression of congenital nystagmus. J Neurol Neurosurg Psychiatry 1978;41:1078.

53. Lo C. Brain Computed Tomographic Evaluation of Non-comitant Strabismus and Congenital Nystagmus. In: Henkind P, ed. ACTA, Twenty-Fourth International Congress of Ophthalmology vol 2. Philadelphia: Lippincott, 1982.

54. Mallett R. The treatment of congenital idiopathic nystagmus by intermittent photic stimulation. Ophthalmol Physiol Optics 1983;3:341-56.

55. Grisham D. Management of Nystagmus in Young Children. In: Scheiman M, ed. Problems in Optometry: Pediatric Optometry vol 2. Philadelphia: Lippincott, 1990.

56. Harley R. Pediatric Neuro-Ophthalmology. In: Pediatric Ophthalmology 2nd ed. In. Philadelphia: Saunders, 1983.